A Secret Never to be Told

Unravelling the mystery of my missing mother

Alison Cobb

First published in Great Britain in 2022

This first edition published in 2022 by
Lapwing Publishing Services
2 Siren Cottages, Horsgate Lane, Cuckfield RH17 5AZ

http://www.lapwingpublishing.com

British Library Cataloguing-in-Publication Data
A catalogue record for this book is available from the British Library

ISBN 978-1-9993226-3-2

Printed and bound by TJ Books, UK

Cover design: Jana Lenzova
Magpie illustrations: © Honor Ash

This book is dedicated to Steve,
who taught me what fun life can be, and how to make the most of it.

One for sorrow,

Two for joy,

Three for a letter,

Four for a boy,

Five for silver,

Six for gold,

Seven for a secret never to be told.

(Traditional English magpie superstitions)

Contents

Contents (continued)

Preface

I was brought up as a very special child. Given pets and toys and treats and taught tricks and jokes and songs by my father, by his friends and colleagues and by all the grown-ups that I knew, I was always aware of having a lot of attention paid to me, always carefully included, and being much loved. I was very lucky. I was an only child with a hugely extrovert father, an Irish orthopaedic surgeon, and we were almost part of each other, bonded together, until he went away as an army surgeon in World War II. His beloved fiancé then took over, and later still I was looked after by aunts and uncles in Dublin.

All these kind people, and especially my father, were compensating for a disaster in my background that they did not want to tell me about. Their kindness greatly supported me and gave me a childhood many children would envy. Such love and care bulwarked me against the fact that I did not have a mother.

Why not? All my friends had them. Where was mine? She, and all her half of the family, were missing. All my father's family and closest friends said nothing. My father, my nannies, my nursery governess, my father's fiancé, my aunts and uncles, my cousins, even the headmistress of my boarding school all knew the secret, and did not tell me. When, at 13, I did discover the truth, I was terrified. I did not dare tell anyone what I now knew. Finally forced to say, my headmistress said I was 'wicked' for finding out.

I have taken nearly a lifetime to piece together what really happened. Still some pieces remain unknown, and I am 87. I greatly hope that anyone reading this book will understand how horrific it is to have such an important secret hanging over your life, and how that secret crawls about among all the people who know, doing harm and hurting wherever it goes. By telling here how unhelpful it was for everyone to say nothing, maybe in future people will find the courage to take a big gulp, and say what they know as soon as they do. Resolution and even cure could come that way.

Much of this is a description of my childhood and written through the eyes of a child. Then, I did not know the words 'homosexual', or 'paedophile'. We girls at Pony Club dances knew over-active fathers who might try to feel us up behind a curtain, and warned each other to avoid these 'dirty old men'. I have used the words that we children spoke. I knew no special word to describe our shy and anxious manservant, and would never have thought of him as 'gay'. I do not wish for the use of yesterday's inappropriate words to cause distress today and have mostly tried to avoid them.

So here is some truth. Quite hard to take, but far better to tell than keep quiet. This kind of secret should always be told.

Chapter 1
The Icy Lie

My friend Nick and I are in bed together for warmth, our bodies touching, the eiderdown drawn up tight around us. It is black night both indoors and out. There is ice on the inside of the window panes, and our face flannels are freezing stiff on the edge of the basin. We are in bed up in one of the attics at Somerleyton Hall, where Nick lives. Our fingers are painful with cold, and sore from tussling with sprigs of holly.

We are talking in whispers so as not to wake Nanny next door. This is Nick's night nursery on Christmas Day 1939, and it is about five in the morning. We are undoing our Christmas stockings. We are both six years old.

Nick says, in a hoarse whisper, as he tears off the paper from a little parcel: "Soldiers," and he jabs me with one.

Feeling them carefully in the dark, I reply "On horses?"

"Cavalry", Nick says. "Lancers. Feel this," and he prods me with the lance.

Nick's 11-year-old brother Bill has a huge army of lead soldiers, passed on by his father, which he can deploy all over the nursery floor. Nick knows what they all are, but is only allowed to play with them if Bill lets him. So he is very proud of the four mounted figures Father Christmas has brought him, lancers riding two horses rearing up, and two cantering, so that only one hind leg is in touch with its square plinth.

Then he says, "I think I've got a torch here."

He hands it to me and it does feel just like a torch.

"You're right, it must be", I whisper back. "But I can't make it work. You do it."

He finds the switch, and turns it on, so now we are making progress. After total blackness, what a wonderful difference a little light makes. The lit torch lies on the eiderdown. We unwrap in the dark and then hold our present in front of it to see what we have.

Nick hands me some jelly babies, "Bite the heads off first."

We are getting very excited, and tearing the paper off faster and faster.

"I've got a pencil sharpener with two holes", I say.

"Why does it have two holes? Is it rude?"

"One for the wooden part, and one for the lead, see?"

"Two holes for two different things. I'd like one of those", he says. "You are lucky."

"Not lucky. Father Christmas tries to think of things you want."

Then Nick discovers a very small penknife, not very sharp, but I envy him, and say, "I hope I get one of those". Maybe later on I can tempt him to swap it with my pencil sharpener.

We were getting near the end. I undo the next thing very slowly to make it last. It is irresistible.

"Toffees," I excitedly exclaim to Nick.

We guzzle them. They taste of black treacle and are very hard to chew. We need to keep swallowing a lot of saliva with loud sucky noises that we hope Nanny will not hear.

Then Nick has a pen that writes with three colours.

"There you are," I say. "It's not luck. Father Christmas knew you wanted that pen, didn't he?"

Down by the heel of the stocking I find a little wooden dog, with black leather ears, on a round stand. Elastic runs through the dog's joints and tail, and when I push the button under the stand, it collapses. When I let go, it stands up.

"This dog dies, and comes to life again," I say, showing Nick.

"Like Jesus" he replies.

And then I ask: "When do we get our other presents, the big ones?"

Nick's mother is going to be my Godmother, and I told her I wanted a pony, so I hope she has told my father. He knows already, really, because I never stop asking for one. But if she asks him too, that will help.

Nick whispers, "We get them after church."

Nick's family owns the church, I think. At least, it is in their park not far from the house. They go every Sunday, and Nick's father reads the lesson. I am going to wear my new yellow tweed coat to church this Christmas Day. It has a proper waist, a flared skirt, six brown buttons and a brown velveteen collar. And I shall wear my new lace-up shoes, and I am going to show Nanny that I can do them up myself. I hope.

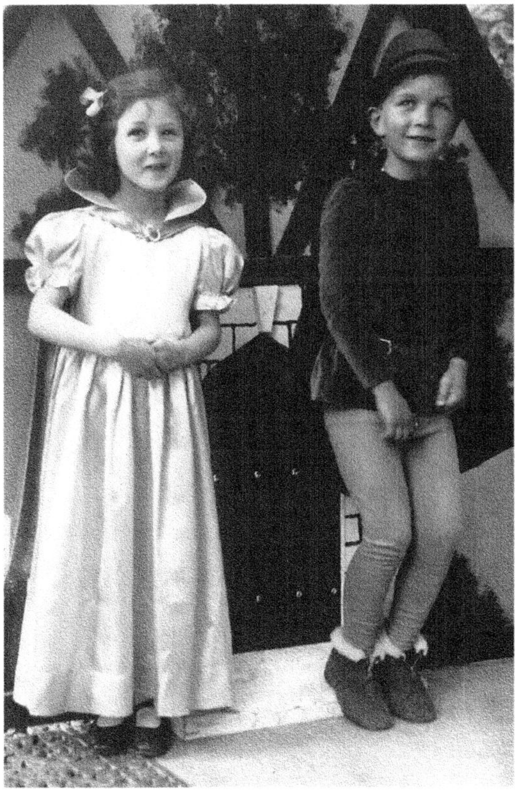

Fancy Dress party at Somerleyton Hall, Suffolk. Alison and Nick Crossley as Snow White and a Dwarf. Both aged six.

Suddenly, in his ordinary voice, a voice that could easily wake Nanny, Nick announces, to my astonishment: "I don't believe in Father Christmas. Father Christmas is a lie."

He sounds very angry.

"Shhh. He can't be. You're mad. Look what he's given us."

"He is, I know."

"Don't talk so loud. How do you know?"

"Smell this dog."

He has just taken the paper off a small stuffed dog, fawn and white, with a cheerful snub nose. I smell it.

"What does it smell of?" I ask, "Father Christmas?"

"No, of course not. *Who* does it smell of?"

I give it another sniff.

"Your Aunt Noonie?"

"Yes it does. That's definitely the smell of her cigarettes. She must have given it to me."

"So how did Father Christmas put it in your stocking?"

"Well he didn't, did he? *She* put it in."

It has to be true. That dog's smell is unmistakable. Nick's Aunt Noonie smokes oval Turkish cigarettes, with a distinctive rich dark smell, and the dog smells strongly of them.

I try to imagine the grown-ups, at night, creeping up to the nurseries where they are never normally seen, with stockings full of things they have just wrapped, and putting them on our beds. It seems impossible: actually unimaginable. But this must be true. There can be no other explanation. They did it.

Most of our presents are lying all over the eiderdown, with paper everywhere. I cannot bear to undo any more while I think about this.

I would not have minded if they did it and said it was them. But pretending it is Father Christmas leaves a horrid cold feeling in the pit of my stomach. I am deeply shocked. If there is no Father Christmas, what are they thinking of, Nick's mother and father, and his Aunt Noonie; and Nanny too, because she would not have allowed visitors to her nurseries without a challenge? Come to think of it, Nanny is definitely in it too. We had knelt at our beds the evening before, in front of Nanny, and prayed that Father Christmas would bring us, "and every good child" (a bit that Nanny put in), something nice. She made us do that and she knew perfectly well that it was not true. I do find it frightening.

Almost at the end Nick says, "No lumps of coal. They wouldn't dare."

So we are just peeling the tangerines from the bottom of the stockings, when Nick looks at me with his nice brown eyes, nearly black in the torchlight, and says: "You know what this means, don't you?"

"What?" I ask.

"If Father Christmas is a lie, then what about God?"

"But if they know that, why don't they tell us?" I wailed.

"Shut up!", Nick hissed.

But it was too late. My shriek of despair had woken Nanny. She came in, and was cross with us for waking her, for opening our presents so early, and being in bed together.

There are so many things grown ups do not tell you. They know these things perfectly well, but they would rather not say. Sex is one thing, of course, and I can see how they are embarrassed to tell about that. But there are other more important truths that it really would be a help to know. They leave you stranded up there on a cloud, fog everywhere, and there is a fearful distance to be falling, falling down to the real world.

This book is about finding out.

Chapter 2
Singing in the Bath

When I was three, my own Nanny (not Nick's) got sacked for teaching me to say 'Pardon'. She and my father had a furious argument over which was ruder, 'What?' or 'Pardon?' My father won, and she had to go. Her crime was one of my earliest memories. I was not sad she went, because she was quite a bully about saying 'Pardon'. I had a lot of earache then, and I suppose she said something I did not hear properly, so I asked "What?"

She said, "*What* did you say?"

"What?" I asked again.

"Did you say, '*What*'?"

"Yes, 'what'."

"Well, what *do* you say?"

"I don't know."

"*Don't* say 'What', say 'Pardon'."

"Why?"

"'What' is rude. 'Pardon' is polite."

"Why?"

"Don't keep saying 'Why'. That's rude, too."

Any time I said 'What' to her, she went pink with anger and her eyes bulged, and she said, very loudly, "Don't say '*What*'. What *do* you say?"

And I replied, sulkily, "Pardon".

My father thought he won, and did not know that she still believed she was right. For a while I managed to say 'Pardon' to her and 'What' to him, but one day I made a mistake, said 'Pardon' to him, and that was it. He came into the nursery and told her to go, while she was doing the ironing, and she cried, her tears sprinkling down all over the clothes and hissing on the iron. She left the next day. Although I did not like her much, I felt guilty and ashamed because it was my mistake that had been her undoing. I have never said 'Pardon' again.

My childhood was full of contradictions of this kind, but I knew whose side I was on. I always danced to my father's tune. I sang his songs, said what he said, did whatever he asked me to do. It was fine like that: it was the way to get the best out of him, and we hugely enjoyed each other's company. He was a big, brave, boisterous Irishman who loved the world to go his way and was unusually good at making it do so. He lit up life wherever he went. I loved him.

I was brought up the only child of a single parent. Many people think being an only one is sad, but there are great compensations: the best of these for me was being the close friend of my father. I had no mother, so he brought me up. He had a job to go to, of course (he was an orthopaedic surgeon), so I had a series of Nannies.

Most of their time, I remember, the Nannies washed and ironed my clothes, and sat me on my pot (for what seemed an agonisingly long boring time, and left a red ring round my bottom), gave me spoonfuls of horrible Milk of Magnesia, took me for walks in my pram, and tried to make me eat food I hated, like meat. I always had to leave a little on the side of my plate 'for Mr. Manners', whoever he was. He was not a real person, I knew. Mr. Manners did not lurk in the kitchen waiting for our plates to come down from the nursery so that he could gobble up the gristle and bacon rind we had left for him. He was just someone who existed in the imaginations of all Nannies, but not those of anyone else. I used to compress the food I did not like into a tight lump on the edge of the plate for him, but usually Nanny prodded it with a fork to see how much was there, and if she judged it excessive (nearly always) she tried again to make me eat it.

When I would not eat, every Nanny always exhorted me to 'think of the starving children of Europe' and I knew that these poor children were real. I could not imagine them, or what starving felt like, or where Europe was, so I used to say "Why not do it up in a parcel and send it to them, then?" and that could make any Nanny very cross.

Although they told me what to do, I do not remember that they ever read to me, played with me, or talked with me. Those things may not have been part of their training. The Nannies came and went, and apart from the 'Pardoner', I cannot remember any special one. What I do remember is the creak of the wooden ironing board, and their grey uniforms, with hats like stiff headscarves tied at the back. They twiddled my hair up in strips of rag at night, which was terribly painful in bed because in whatever direction I lay little hairs pulled at my scalp and made it hard to sleep. Nannies did it to make me have ringlets, which my grandmother wanted, though she only came once from Dublin to see them. They washed my face, and scrubbed my knees, which then felt raw and cold, before putting me in my smocked organdie dress to go to the photographer and be told to watch the dickie bird.

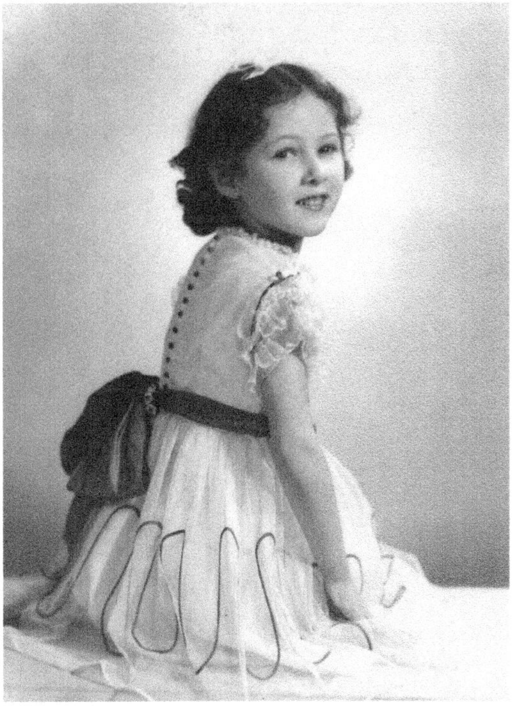

Alison aged 5 in an organdie dress at the photographer. She has had her neck washed and knees scrubbed and they are cold and sore. She is told to 'Watch the dickie bird'.

The Nannies never stayed long, so I suppose they must have met with other forms of disapproval, though whether they disapproved of us, or my father of them, I do not know. The very worst Nanny was Nanny Took, who used to come whenever one of my Nannies left. She was a temporary Nanny who went round Norfolk from home to home, stepping in to replace holidaying or sacked Nannies of children who later became my friends. We all discussed her, later, when Nanny days were over, and said how much we had hated her. She was not just strict, she was tough. She walloped us all with the back of a Mason Pearson hairbrush on places that really hurt, like knuckles, or on our upper thighs, where the red wheals would not be seen by parents. She did it for the smallest of crimes, like not holding our spoons and pushers in the correct hands. Mercifully, she never stayed long. I later heard grown-ups saying to each other how wonderful she was, and I was shocked that they thought that. Imagine, Nanny has walked out, how are you going to cope with these small children? Just telephone Nanny Took and she'll be round the same day, simpering away, secretly armed with her horrible hairbrush.

I had a bath with my father every morning. That is to say, he had the bath, and I sat on the edge and watched him. We used to sing, in the white foggy steam, about what we would do with the drunken sailor, and early one morning we heard a maiden singing, and "Alas my love you do me wrong", and "Danny Boy", and "I might as well be, where the Mountains of Mourne sweep down to the sea" and many, many more: some not altogether polite, though never with rude words in them. There was the young man with a stutter, who had been advised to sing his proposal in order to get all the words out:

> Oh Hell, oh Hell, oh Helen I love you,
> Your feet, your feet, your features are divine,
> I swear, I swear, I swear that I'll be true,
> Oh Hell, oh Hell, oh Helen do be mine.

And sometimes we sang of the natural world:

> The higher up the mountain, the greener grows the grass,
> And there goes a billy-goat a-sliding on his
> If you don't believe me, if you think I'm telling a lie,
> Just ask the girls of Derbyshire, and they'll tell you the same as I.

I was probably only five years old when we sang this, and quite unaware of the missing word there: I just thought the song went like that. I was much older and singing it in the bath myself, when I suddenly realised it did not rhyme or scan. We also sang a very nice song about a bad bullfighter, who was a dirty dog, and stole away the girlfriend, and so we planned, with mighty effort, to kill him.

The bathroom was all white, except for the big black and white linoleum squares of the floor. It faced east, and the early morning sun, dappled through the moving leaves of the lime tree outside, poured in. Singing sounded good there, it was bold and clear, and we sang at the tops of our voices. My father had rather a good baritone voice, and sing as I would, mine was not nearly as loud as his.

He sat in a bath that seemed as big as a single bed, with huge taps that he could turn on and off with his toes. On the white tiles on the wall an extending arm was fixed with a round enlarging mirror on it, which was pulled out for shaving. He used Ingrams Shaving Cream, which you can still get, and the smell of it still reminds me of all the nicest things I know about men. Apart from shaving, he had no use for soap and never washed in his bath. He just lay there, with the biggest natural sponge I have ever seen, resting on his groin.

From the bath he sorted out his life, on the telephone. The telephone came in from the bedroom on a long twisted flex, and the earpiece was covered with shaving soap. When I was four and a half or five he often made me use it, and when I put it to my ear it crackled and squeaked and left my ear and hair uncomfortably sticky.

"Get the hospital and tell my stooge [he jokingly called his greatly liked and trusted Registrar, Richard Howard, his "stooge": I had no idea then that this was a pejorative term] to start operating: I'm going to be late", he would say, and I, knowing the number of the hospital would ask for the orthopaedic block and then for Richard, and tell him to start operating. They always put the easy cases, the ones Richard would be able to do, at the start of the list.

He also used me to arrange his social life. "Did I take Pinkie or Ione out last time?" he would ask. "Pinkie I think," I said. "OK then, try Ione: see if she'll come out with me tonight or tomorrow night." And I tried her, and she always said yes.

My father was a hairy man. He was thickly covered with hair, and he even had hairs on the last joints of his fingers and toes. He needed me to sit on the edge of the bath, he said, because if I were not there to frighten them, birds would fly in through the window and make nests in the hairs on his chest. When I believed him, I thought it was a lovely idea, and wished he would let them try. Later on, when I did not believe him, I knew better than to tell him. He was not the sort of man you could challenge.

Just before he finished he put his head under water and bubbled noisily. I knew then to get his huge towel and hold it above my head with my arms spread wide. Then he rose, half the bath water pouring from his wet curly coat, stepped backwards out of the bath, and backwards into his towel on to the cork bath mat. I never saw anything he did not want me to, because if I lowered the towel below my eyes he flung the monster sponge at me, full of water, shouting "Hands up!" I got soaked, and learned the lesson. These days of course, young ladies know more about anatomy. I could have too, I suppose, if I had had brothers.

I remember now proving how little I had ever seen of adult male anatomy, in my late teens. Visiting Florence with a group of girls from my finishing school, we history of art students were climbing a fig tree full of ripe fruit just above the old Roman amphitheatre at Fiesole, the little hill town outside Florence. Screwing up our eyes in the blinding sunlight, we were relieved to be in the green shade of the tree. Having eaten as many of those honeyed fruits as we could manage (we did regret it later, of course), we started to climb down, and there sitting in the lowest fork of the tree was an unknown young man showing off an erection which he evidently wanted us to examine. I looked, then climbed quickly over him and told our teacher. I said he seemed to have been badly injured in an awful place, the wound was swollen and purple, and I thought we ought to try to help him get to hospital. Fortunately, other girls knew better.

After his bath, my father, dry and dressed, brushed his black hair with two oval brushes on which he poured Bay Rum. The spicy smell of it prickled my nostrils. Tucked into a corner of the looking glass where he did this was a list of orthopaedic operations which were either unsatisfactory, or could not be done at all. The list came from Professor Girdlestone at Oxford, who taught him orthopaedics, and who had said: "If any of you want to be rich and famous, you need to think of a way of making a better job of one of these."

As he brushed his hair, every morning, he read them through. One day he did think of a better way of doing a more satisfactory operation, but the war intervened; he needed many examples before he could publish, and was not able to until after he came back.

He went down to the dining room for breakfast. He lifted me onto the high shelf of the fireplace, so I faced him, and asked me to tell him where he was going today. "The Norfolk & Norwich," I guessed, "Grove House Nursing Home, The Jelly Lind (the children's hospital was named after a famous Scandinavian soprano, Jenny Lind, but when I was five her name was unknown to me), or King's Lynn, or Lowestoft, or Yarmouth?" These were the hospitals for which he was the orthopaedic surgeon, and on many of his visits I went with him. However, while I was on the shelf, I was not allowed to wriggle or fidget, and I promised I would not try to get down until he said I could and came to lift me off. The shelf seemed very high, and below were hard shiny red and yellow tiles.

One day he realised he was late, and went off in a rush forgetting to take me down. My new nursery governess found me up there about half an hour later, was too small to reach me, but got Roper the butler to come and try to lift me off.

I made a frightful scene. I screamed and yelled and kicked at Roper as hard as I could, and tearfully said that I had been told to stay there and not fidget and certainly not get down until my father lifted me off. In the end they had to telephone the hospital and Richard had to continue operating while my father returned and got me. He said I was quite right, but Dickie, the nursery governess, was very angry with him. She was always on my side, which I liked. We slept in the same bedroom, and I can remember watching her put little dots of Pond's Vanishing Cream on her face, and rubbing it in every morning. It is extraordinary how certain smells can arouse my oldest memories.

"What are you doing, Dickie?"

"Putting on Pond's Vanishing Cream."

"Will you vanish?"

"No, but after a bit, the cream will."

Although Dickie was very good at teaching, I had a poor view of her intellect. It seemed to me awfully stupid to bother with the cream, if it was going to disappear.

Sometimes my father said: "Let's go and eat grapes." Grapes were very special then, but private patients always had them. Sometimes they felt too ill to eat them, and sometimes it appeared they thought my father was so wonderful they would have given him everything they had in the world, so a few grapes were nothing.

At the private block of the Norfolk & Norwich or in the nursing home we went into each of his patient's private rooms in turn, and stood by their beds that had wheels on, like my pram, for him to talk to them at length. As he did so, he helped himself to large bunches of their grapes, giving me some of them too.

"Of course you'll walk again," I heard him say. "I know you will. Your operation went perfectly. We'll start you practicing very soon; tomorrow or the next day. I'll be there to help you." And then, grinning, he said: "I'll make you. As a matter of fact I can make anyone do anything. You will walk. Watch this. Alison looks perfectly happy, doesn't she, eating your grapes? Well, I can make her cry by just looking at her."

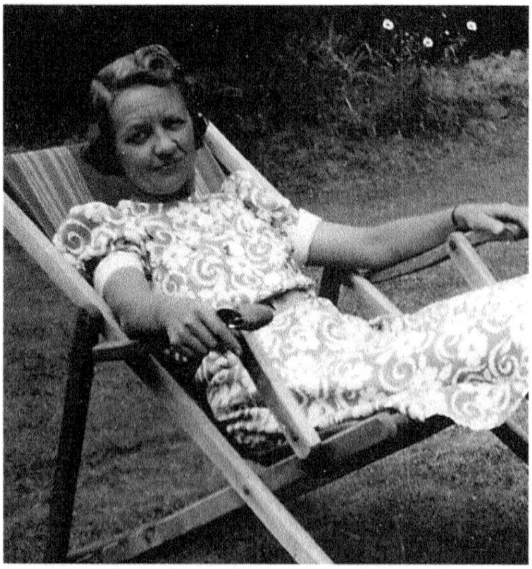

Dickie (Marie Hansen), Alison's Danish nursery governess. Dickie was a natural teacher and Alison's best friend.

"Oh, for God's sake, Tommy," the patient said, "Don't, for heaven's sake, don't."

In complete silence, my father then glared at me across the bed. His awful face struck me with terror. His look full of such hatred really upset me. It was impossible not to stop myself crying, and I wept.

"There you are," he said, coming round the bed to comfort me, "She is crying. You'll walk."

On other days I went with him in the car when he was holding a clinic at Lowestoft, Yarmouth or King's Lynn; quite a long journey in those days, and we talked all the way. My father drove with considerable verve. He did not shoot, but he loved chasing pheasants, and when I see one walking in the road today I still feel a rush of anxiety because once we would have dashed up first one bank and then the other, trying to squash it, and often nearly overturning the car in the process. If he did succeed in running it over, it was always too damaged to be eaten. It wasn't shooting, but I think he thought it was sport.

Sometimes he said: "You can drive if you like, to stop you feeling sick". I was too young to drive, of course, but I could sit on his knee and steer.

"I'm making the engine go, but you are watching and steering. I haven't got my hands on the steering wheel, see? So it's entirely up to you."

Looking out of the front window, not seeing the trees and hedges flashing by the side window, and concentrating so hard, I really did not feel sick at all.

"Exciting bit coming in a minute. Roundabout. You are not strong enough to steer her round a roundabout. This Phantom Three is the first Rolls Royce with an aeroplane engine. Let's see if she'll fly."

I could not think how, but I hoped and supposed and trusted that she would.

"Hold her very steady. It's all up to you. We've got to get her up to sixty. I'll hold you. You hold the wheel. Set her at it, straight ahead, straight over."

The silver lady on the bonnet wobbled and shook. With a bump, a leap and a roar of excitement, we flew straight over the top.

"There you are, see? She flew."

If he wanted it to fly, it flew. It did not occur to either of us that it would not. Perhaps that was not the way to deal with a roundabout. He could make things happen. He was magic.

From the age of about five or six he insisted that I use the map to tell him where we were going. He was quite savage about getting it right. I think often he knew the way, and just wanted me to learn to map-read. When I made a mistake, he gave me one more chance to try again, and if I got it wrong a second time, he put me out by the side of the road, often on one of those little grass triangles with a signpost on it, and drove off. He did not say whether he was going for ever, and I did worry terribly about that, though I knew better than to cry, but actually, in about five minutes, he reappeared and let me back into the car. Then he pointed out how I had made the mistake, and said "Don't do that again". We used the Ordnance Survey map, and he wanted to be told about rivers, railway lines and churches with towers or steeples that we passed. It was very frightening, but a wonderful training. I soon learned to read a map, and never to make mistakes: I would think that I am at least as good as a SatNav today.

When we got to the hospital, sometimes I could go in and sit in Sister's office drawing with the crayons I had brought, but I was often left in the car and told not to fidget with anything, or get out, no matter who told me to, until he came back. I am one of the few people who does like the smell of hospitals: they remind me of my father. They seem not to have quite the same smell today: I suppose because there is less ether about.

Dickie, my governess, had to fit lessons around these spur-of-the-moment arrangements, and yet I believe she taught me all I know. She was a huge improvement on Nannies. She taught me to write and read and draw and paint and she taught me arithmetic and my times tables. We learned to plant seeds in the garden together, and we used to go for walks taking a paper bag of bread for the goats in Cringleford: first they ate the bread, and then, with equal enthusiasm, the paper bag. I tried on my own, and was disappointed to find that I could not eat even a tiny torn off piece of a paper bag.

Dickie read to me endlessly, until I could read to her. She taught me to sew and knit and sing, and talk in Danish, because she was Danish (her real name was Marie Hansen). Unfortunately, without practice, regrettably, I have completely lost my ability to speak Danish, and now can only just distinguish its sing-song notes on the radio from other Nordic languages. She taught me long division and, for me, mathematics has never progressed much beyond this milestone. But the best thing about her was that we really liked each other: she was my defender and my friend, and I was hers.

Once my father took me with him to see a private patient in his own home. He did not want me to catch the polio his young patient might be having, so he said I could not come in.

"But I tell you what," he said. "You get in the back on the floor, and make yourself as small as possible, and I'll cover you up with the rug. Now when I've finished I'll say to his mother and father: 'Alison's in the car. Do come out and say hello to her'. And then I'll open the door and we won't be able to see you. And I will say, 'Oh no, where's Alison? She's gone.' And we will all be terribly worried, and then after a bit, I'll pull the rug off you, and there you will be. And then we will all be so relieved, we'll be laughing. But of course you absolutely mustn't move. Not a sign, quite still, OK?"

I was squashed into the square hole in the floor beside the big transmission in the back of the car, absolutely boiling hot under the fur rug, but I did not move. It was already dark when he came out. He later explained that he was upset because the little boy was extremely ill with polio, and if he survived, was going to be badly paralysed. So he just got in the car and drove off. When we got home he got out and slammed the door and went into the house.

A moment later Dickie came out shouting "Where is she, where is she? It is hours after her bedtime, what have you done with her?"

And then my father guiltily remembered, opened the door and lifted the rug. I was very stiff and red with the heat, and Dickie came and gathered me up and shouted: "What on earth did you do that for? Look at her, the poor thing is absolutely bright red. How could you do that?"

I was glad Dickie was so angry, but I did feel a bit sorry for my father all the same. He was not used to anyone shouting at him.

I had far more possessions than most children. Despite my indifference to much of them, I was overrun with dolls, stuffed toys, tricycles, a fairy bike, dolls' house, gramophone, records, jigsaws, Plasticine, Minibricks, Meccano, a magic lantern, crayons and paints. Grateful patients often gave things to me instead of to my father. Once a nun, a Little Sister of the Poor, broke her leg. She came to his consulting rooms as a private patient, with the Mother Superior, who explained that it would not be possible for her to undress in front of a man. My father gently explained that before he could help her he did need to know what was wrong and that he was used, professionally, to seeing women undressed. So he was allowed to see, and arrange for her treatment, and recovery in a private room at the hospital. She was charged nothing. "If you park outside my consulting rooms in a Bentley, you pay a Bentley price. But for a Little Sister of the Poor, hopping on one leg, in agony, there is no charge," he often said, of his sliding scale of fees. By way of thanks, the whole convent sat down and made me a hamper full of dolls' clothes, every stitch sewn by hand, embroidered, smocked, with French knots, and handmade lace inserts, and pretty, tiny ribbons. They had the smallest mother of pearl buttons, and exquisite buttonholes. I felt bad about this, because I really had no interest in dolls.

Instead, I was always asking for a pony, and no one gave me that. I was not going to be allowed one until I was six years old because my orthopaedic surgeon father believed that riding too young might be one of the causes of the bandy legs to be seen on so many jockeys.

When I pleaded, I was given a long-haired black and white kitten. His head was black but he had a white nose and mouth. London Zoo had just acquired its first black and white cuddly bear from China: a panda. Pandas were fashionable. Even in Norfolk we were subjected to story-book pandas, colouring-in pandas and stuffed pandas from tiny to huge. I was given all of them, but I ignored them in favour of what seemed to me much more like the real thing: my handsome cat, called Panda.

I learned, after a few battles, that you do not fight cats. It is impossible to make them do what you want, but you can tempt and cajole them into doing many things they might ordinarily not want to do. I used to dress him up in my exquisite dolls' clothes and walk him about the garden in my dolls' pram, and he lay there quietly purring.

I asked again, about a year later, but still no pony. Instead, we got an affectionate, slithery, black and tan dachshund puppy. Roper said she was a German dog, and when the war came, everyone would stone her. I was terrified of that: I thought we hated Germans, not German dogs. My father named her Gretchen.

"Heil Hitler, Gretchen," he said, and she would come across the room to him and jump into his lap. She was too long to sit up and beg by herself, but he held her up, her back leaning against his stomach. Then he took her right elbow in his hand, and squeezed it, saying "Heil Hitler!" In a reflex action, her paw shot up in a perfect Nazi salute, much to my father's satisfaction.

I made a set of show jumps for Gretchen on the lawn. No jump was more than nine inches high. We had a brush fence, a triple bar, a brick wall and a high jump. I made a ditch too, but Rose the gardener hated it because he could not mow the lawn properly, and he kept filling it in. Gretchen would do anything for cheese, so I begged a piece from Chef, and, armed with a pointing stick and the cheese, I urged Gretchen round the circle of jumps. At dinner parties in summer time, I was woken up and got out of bed in my nightdress to demonstrate Gretchen's prowess. Children make good animal trainers, my father explained to his guests, because they cannot imagine what an animal is unable to do. A child may have completely unrealistic expectations, but sometimes, surprisingly, they succeed.

While the guests were having drinks before dinner, sometimes we made a bit of money out of them. We would bet them that I could not carry my father across the room. He was six foot and weighed 13 stone. I was four and a half years old and probably weighed about three stone. If we were going to do this one, we always practised it before the guests arrived. Everyone would say that this was a completely impossible task and the only way we could do it was by cheating.

"But suppose," my father said, "Suppose we succeed without cheating? You can be the judges of that. You can watch as closely as you like. It's impossible, isn't it? Surely that's a very safe bet? Yes, well it might hurt Alison a little bit, but bet enough to make it worth her while. Now, what are we bet?"

And he went round the room collecting offers.

Set up, I then took off my shoes, tucked my skirt into my knickers and knelt on all fours. The tops of my feet were flat on the floor, my heels turned outwards. Very gently and carefully, my father, in his socks, placed his heels on the balls of my feet, and the rest of his feet were supported on my out-turned heels.

"Ready?" he asked. "Move when I say."

He leaned over and put his hands lightly on my shoulders.

"Left", he ordered.

And I moved my right hand and left leg forward a short pace.

"Now right", he said, and we took another step. At that age, one's feet and ankles are so soft they can take a great weight without hurting. It just felt like a big squeeze, that is all. So we crossed the room, and won the bets.

Sometimes we did the bottle on the five-pound note trick. You persuade a guest to lend a five-pound note (a lot of money in those days), put it on a sturdy flat table and upend an empty wine bottle on it. Then you say "I bet you, you cannot get the note out without touching the bottle." Neither pulling gently, nor snatching suddenly releases it, and after a bit the guest gives up. My father would then suggest: "If Alison can get it out, maybe she can keep it?"

To this day I can hardly bear to tell how to do this trick; it is such a useful one.

But what I did when the guest had given the go ahead was gingerly take hold of a corner of the note, keep it just taut, clench my other fist and gently thump it on the table. The vibrations of the thumping release the note a tiny bit at a time, and in about a minute, I had it in my hand and the bottle was still upright. And everybody laughed. My father, of course, kept all our winnings, but he said they would go towards a pony one day.

I had no idea how other children came by their ponies. Did they do tricks for them, or for something else they badly wanted? Did they even do tricks at all? I didn't really care. I loved doing tricks myself. It made my father very proud of me, and I knew we were a tough team: my father and I.

Chapter 3

Swastika Rose

I have an old sepia photograph of my father as a young child. My Aunt Mabel, my father's older sister, who gave it to me, told me the story attached to it. Here is a little boy of three (it says on the back of the photograph, though I think he looks more like four) with golden, shoulder-length curls. The year is about 1907 and it is a photograph taken before his hair was cut for the first time. My grandmother loved her son's long curly locks. My grandfather thought he looked like a 'girly boy' and wanted something done about it. So without telling his wife he decided to take his son to the barber, but to placate her had the boy photographed before the deed was done.

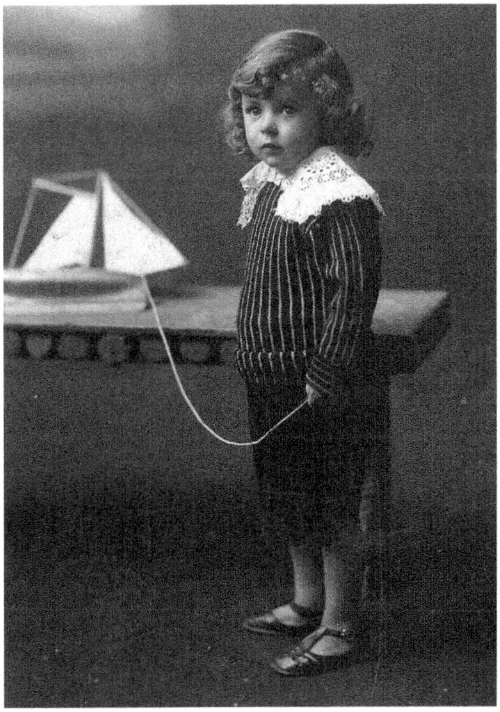

Alison's father Herbert Alfred Brittain aged 4: just before he had his hair cut for the first time. His father called him 'a girly boy'.

Very unusually for my father, who, by all accounts, even at the age of three, was never frightened, in this photograph he looks more than apprehensive: he looks terrified. What is frightening him? He may not have been told what is going to happen. He has been tethered to a table by a string attached to a toy yacht. He wears a stripy top and dark shorts to below the knee, and has on a lace collar, too big for him, but which gives a slightly nautical impression. I guess that it is, like the yacht, a photographer's prop. His legs are bare, and he wears sandals too small for him. He looks very uncomfortable: either the collar was scratchy, or his sandals were pinching his toes. Or he just feels silly holding the string.

He may be confused by the large, dazzling lights on him, while the rest of the studio disappears into darkness. The room probably smells musty and dusty. He wants to suck his thumb. His father warns him not to, and to stand absolutely still. He has to stand all alone in this pool of hot lights, and suddenly the photographer's head disappears under a black hood. To be told to stay still when every instinct is for fright and flight is no recipe for happy smiles.

Then there was probably a flash and a bang when the picture was taken, a funny smell, and the photographer, now the enemy, pops up from behind the camera, grinning.

But his troubles for that day have only just begun: worse is to come. He is marched off to the barber, sat in a high chair in front of a mirror, has a robe tied around his neck, and has to watch as all his hair is cut off, and falls to the floor around him. Samson cannot have been more shocked when he saw what Delilah had done. He cannot recognise himself: he is transformed.

Then, at last, his father takes him by the hand and they go home. He feels relief as they walk up to the door, and secure in the sight of his mother coming to greet them. But she looks at him with horror, and bursts into tears. My heart goes out to him: poor little boy. What a cruel way to become a man.

When he was about five years old his mother used to ask him, "Herbert, we have been invited out to tea: now, are you going to be a good little boy, or a bad little boy?" If he said he was going to be good, his mother took him with her, with his brother and sisters. If he said he was going to be bad, she left him behind, because she knew he meant it. Even as a very small child he had rules outside the nursery that applied only to him. Rarely for such a little one, he always knew his own mind, and was completely uncowed.

Once, when the family was going to go on holiday and he did not want to go, he managed to get all the suitcases down from the attic and take them off to the pawnbroker without anyone noticing. He was in bad trouble when he finally confessed under duress, the day the family was trying to pack up to go, and they had to be redeemed. I have not been told what he did with the money, or whether he had to go on the holiday after all.

After my grandmother died, when my father was 41, he inherited an enormous silver cup. It was a family heirloom, and its story tells quite a bit of my family's story. I remember the cup standing on our sideboard in my childhood. It was engraved with the names of all the winners of the Wall Jump, the most difficult high jump, at the Dublin Horse Show. The name recorded for the last three times, and therefore the outright winner of the cup, was Swastika Rose. My father was both proud and ashamed of this inheritance. The cup must have been quite valuable: it really was a mighty trophy, but I have no idea what happened to it or where it is now.

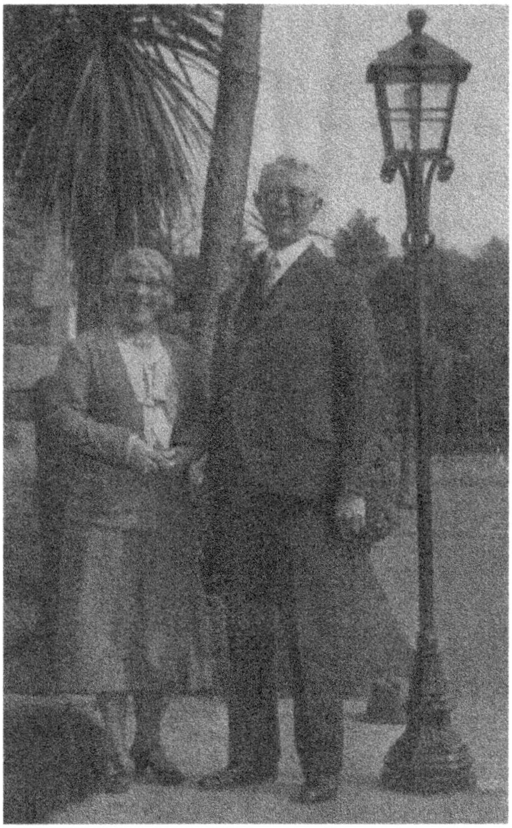

Alison's grandparents in 1932 at The Great Southern Hotel, Parknasilla, County Kerry: a grand hotel built for a railway that never reached it. Elizabeth McLamon and John Wesley Brittain.

I never knew my grandfather at all. I was only four when he died: too young to remember meeting him, though I believe he must have seen me. I expect I looked like any other baby to him. All I can remember is the photograph of him sitting very upright, a tall (6 foot 2 inches) good-looking man with white hair, wearing Lenin spectacles, a separate stiff collar and a three piece suit. He lived in Dublin, and I in Norwich, so I suppose we would not have seen much of each other anyway.

My grandfather was Irish. His Christian names were John Wesley, which my father would never have told me. Grandpa was therefore, obviously, a Methodist, and he was said to be a God-fearing, honourable, hard-working and kind man, who is reported to have taken a great interest in all the many members of his workforce, and to know them all, and their spouses and children, by name, and to be extremely solicitous for them if they were ever sick or in debt.

He had originally trained in a draper's shop, and, orderly and hard working as he was, he could yet be led astray, it seems, by his fascination with hats. Until he made money he was said to be very cautious about spending, but he was 'as far as presents went, generous to a fault'. Aunt Mabel writes in her memoirs: 'One day he would say to Mother, 'Come into town, and I'll buy you a hat'. I have seen him buy two hats for her at 25 or 30 guineas each, an alarming price at that time, when models from Paris could be got for as little as 5 guineas'.

As a young man, my grandfather ran a laundry in Belfast, and later went over to England to learn more of the laundry business (laundry was always pronounced '*larn*dry' by my Dublin relatives). There was great unemployment in Dublin, and he wanted to start a business there, which would give work to many people in need. The other reason he chose Dublin, recorded by Mabel, is that he said he thought that unlike Belfast, Dublin people were inclined to be lazy, and would therefore be more likely to send out their laundry. Once he was familiar with the latest laundry methods, he came back and started his new laundry. Mabel writes of the time they were in London, 'All the hot summer of 1911 the names for the new laundry were discussed, discarded and discussed again. Daddy's parents came from Belfast on a visit and were taken to the 'White City Exhibition' which was in full swing that Coronation Year (George V). Very large picture hats were the fashion, held on the head by highly ornamented, and very long hat pins. Grandma bought some of these at a stall at the Exhibition, and Daddy's attention was drawn to one of an extraordinary shape. He enquired of the salesgirl, and she gave him a leaflet explaining that it was one of the oldest good luck signs in the world – a swastika. It was also explained that it must be straight and not tilted, as the latter brought ill luck. (It may be remembered that Hitler's was tilted.) Daddy came into the house that evening calling 'Mother, where are you? I've got the name of the new laundry' – so the Swastika Laundry Ltd was registered in 1912, and certainly brought us good luck'. Imagine that hat. Did he buy one for Granny? How on earth did you wear a great picture hat shaped like a swastika, pinned to your head with a long ornamented pin, and keep it upright, not tilted?

Grandpa always said the swastika was lucky, a Buddhist sign of peace, and you could see it on the fly-leaves of Rudyard Kipling's Jungle Books. There, he was right. Like Kipling's swastika, Grandpa's was upright and not tilted, so the rise of Hitler throughout the 1930s did nothing to shake his faith in the name, and it persisted until well after the Second World War. Dubliners always referred to it as the 'Swasteeka', to rhyme with beaker.

My father's younger brother, Uncle Eric, told me that laundrymen agreed that The Swastika was the biggest laundry in the world. Not that the premises were the biggest, nor that they covered a huge amount of territory, but that the Swastika took in the largest number of bundles. A bundle is a unit of laundry: the dirty clothes sent from one person, or one family. The reason there were so many bundles was that many people in Dublin then were poor, and most owned only two sets of clothes. Irish complexions are so beautiful, and the light there is so exquisite, because so much gentle rain falls. Dublin is damp. The problem was not so much the washing of clothes, but the drying. Even with a week to do it, clothes might not get dry. So customers wore a clean shirt and pair of underpants one week, and sent the other shirt and pants to the laundry, and so could always go to work looking respectable. Hence the huge number of bundles (or of course, Grandpa might have been right, and Dubliners might have been inclined to be lazy: 'laid back' might be a better description).

Uncle Eric told me they once actually had a clever mystery thief, who had worked out this laundry system. He was probably an employee, who presumably had put his own two shirts on a horse: at least it seemed he owned no washable clothes himself. One bundle of clean laundry was missing every Friday, and it reappeared dirty the next Friday, and the Laundry had to send a letter of apology every week to whoever was the real owner.

When I was 10 and evacuated to Dublin during the latter part of the war, Uncle Eric, who had inherited the laundry, took me round it. It was an enormous dark shed with lights hanging down over the work surfaces, smelling strongly of soap, and full of men and women working. Loudspeakers played 'Music While You Work', which could be heard all over the factory, but not in Uncle Eric's office. A wash of steam constantly curled up to the ventilators in the roof from the great vats of clothes churning round. Women pushed the edges of a sheet between the huge rollers that ironed it, and afterwards folded it so skilfully and rapidly you could hardly believe they had done it. Only men operated the dyeworks. There were circular vats as big as ponds full of the different colours, one man in charge of each. They tested the strength of the dye by tasting it, and so the green dye man had green fingers and mouth, and the blue vat man had blue, and so on. They must have lost the sensitivity in their fingers: the dye water into which they dipped them to 'taste' was boiling. They looked fantastic, the stains on their skin must have been permanent, and I now wonder what their friends said to them if they went for a pint or two of Guinness after work.

Dirty laundry was collected, and delivered clean in several very pretty yellow vans drawn by two black horses harnessed side-by-side. Irish draught horses were, and still are, very fine looking animals. They are not heavy horses with feathered feet like Shires, but a bit lighter, like very heavy hunters, or the police horses of today. They say the English brought a lot of good stock over to Ireland so that they could breed useful horses for the military there. The Swastika horses lived in a field and were stabled beside the laundry, and the site at Ballsbridge was right next to the Dublin Horse Show grounds. Once, a delivery man suggested to my grandfather that he should enter one of the horses in a jumping class at the Show. "Rose is a wonderful jumper, Sir, I know, I've seen her. She jumps like a great big bird."

An experienced horsewoman, a friend of the family, was asked if she would like to try her, and so she and Rose entered the lists to jump one single object in the Dublin Horse Show: the Wall. This contest was called the 'Puissance'. This terrifying obstacle was set at five feet high, and a new course of stones was put on after every jump. Contestants went to and fro, and as soon as one of them hit it, they were out. There was a long run up to the wall, diagonally across the show ring, and I like to think of Rose gathering speed across the grass and thrusting her great black form up into the air with her powerful hindquarters, tucking her huge hind feet tightly against her belly to clear the stones, and landing with a tremendous thump. If she was an Irish draught horse, she was a great big galumphing mare, with a very brave heart. She was no bird.

Rose won that year, and she won the next, and the next, and thus she won the cup outright. My father liked the idea of Rose winning a cup, but he hated the thought of the Laundry. He had been to public school in England, and I am

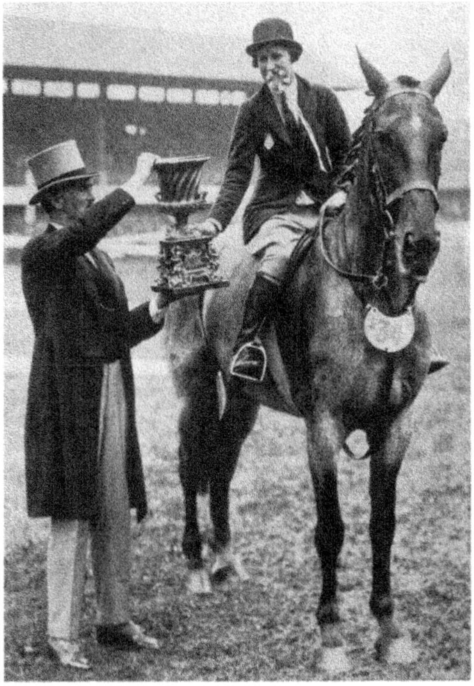

Swastika Rose winning the Challenge Cup for the wall jump (reproduced from The Illustrated Sporting and Dramatic News, August, 1935). © Illustrated London News/Mary Evans Picture Library.

sorry to say that he did not want to own up to three things he disliked: having an Irish father, who was a Methodist, and "took in other people's dirty washing for a living", as he said.

My very first memory of going over to Dublin was in 1938 and flying in a cold and noisy open bi-plane. The pilot sat in front, and I sat on my father's knee in the back seat. I snuggled under my father's coat, but even then the icy wind tore past, and I was silenced by the roar of the engine. I remember the plane was bright red, and shook violently as it took off. Granny was cross when we got there about me being so cold and deaf. I do not remember Grandpa being there. He must have died before that visit.

Sometime earlier, perhaps a year before, I remember my father going over to Dublin on his own. I had never seen him cry, and I was shocked and horrified to see him do so. On this occasion he came into the nursery to say goodbye to me because he was going to Dublin. His eyes were red and streaming tears, his nose was running, and his voice was hoarse and blurred. He said that Grandpa had gone to feather (I was sure he said 'feather', but he must have meant heaven). He picked me up, hugged me and kissed me, leaving wet on my face, and quickly went. I was upset and crying myself because I knew something was terribly wrong, but I did not know what it was. I asked Dickie if he was really crying, and if so, why?

"Your grandfather," I heard Dickie repeat, "has gone to feather, and your father has gone to Dublin to be with your grandmother, and help her. He will come back in a few days."

"Will grandpa come back from feather?" I asked.

"No, I'm afraid not, Darling", Dickie said.

'Feather' sounded to me like an awful place to go to, since it made people cry who never had before. I felt very sorry for my grandfather, and hoped my father would never go there.

I slept badly and had nightmares while my father was away. When he came back he said to Dickie: "I can't ever sleep. I stay up all night reading. She can come and lie in my bed and I'll read to her if you're tired."

So I went to his room and got into his bed. It was uncomfortable. There were lots of little yellow capsules in it, and they rolled into the dip where I lay, like stones in your shoes. So my father read to me. He found a story in the Bible that he thought I would like. It was about a king who wanted to get rid of three men. He thought he would cast them into a burning fiery furnace. He was so full of fury that his face changed: I imagined it like my father glaring at me across a hospital bed to make me cry. And he ordered, "Heat the furnace seven times higher" until it was absolutely huge. But Shadrach, Meshach and Abed-nego believed in God, who would not let them burn, and you could see them in flames, walking about inside the fire. I found this an awful, absolutely terrifying scene, and cried loudly in fear. So my father had to take me back again to Dickie. In the morning I told Dickie about the story, and she went to my father and said that the Bible was full of good stories, why had he had to choose such a bad one? I was only a little girl and he should try to think what he was doing to me. After that I would not let him read to me for a long time.

If you had asked me I would never have said that running a laundry was a good way to make a lot of money, but it seems my grandfather had a protestant work ethic and, surprisingly, The Swastika did make my grandparents rich. They had six living children. They had a big late Victorian stone house in Anglesea Road, a desirable residential part of Dublin. It had a 16 acre garden (a sort of miniature Buckingham Palace) with a tennis court, and there were magnificent greenhouses, and many gardeners (one of whom looked after a beehive), and surely there were many indoor servants too. Indeed, after my grandfather died, Granny on her own needed seven members of staff to look after her. The final house sale lists hundreds and hundreds of pelargoniums in the greenhouses. Perhaps geraniums red and delphiniums blue were fashionable plants in those days.

When I was about 20 I asked my well-loved Aunt Mabel, my oldest Aunt, the oldest child in the family, how it could be that we were both Irish, and protestants, when everyone else in Ireland was catholic. She gave me a deeply unfashionable answer. Astonished at my ignorance (I was brought up in England, after all), she claimed "Oh Darling, *we* are the Protestant Ascendancy". Even if she had been right in this grand and confident assertion, I am sure it is absolutely not something one would say today.

Many English protestants were brought over to Ireland by Oliver Cromwell in the 17th century to control the catholic Irish. The old catholic Norman and Irish aristocracy were dispossessed of their lands, which were given to English gentlemen who fought for Cromwell. These became the 'Protestant Ascendancy', who for the 17th, 18th and 19th centuries held sway in Ireland, helped by new laws passed to support them. The ordinary foot soldiers were called Planters, because they were planted on the Irish to keep them in order. They lived in small semi-fortified towns with a barracks to house the necessary soldiers, and hated and feared the Irish. When I lived in Dublin in 1944, and one of us children committed some minor crime, our Nanny would exclaim, "You're a bold bad girl, and Oliver Cromwell is coming to get you". In the 1970s, when the British were locking up the IRA men in Long Kesh prison in the North, the most popular song in Southern Ireland for 16 weeks had a line in it that went 'Cromwell's men are here again'. If, more than three centuries later, the Irish still cannot forget Cromwell's men they must have been terrible, and I really hope that I am not descended from them.

I have never heard of any lands, castles, or that lovely Irish word, 'demesnes', belonging to our family, and if we were the Ascendancy there should be memories of those, at least, even if we no longer held them. We might have been foot soldiers, Planters, I suppose, but there is an alternative possibility, which I prefer.

I did ask Aunt Mabel if she was sure we were the Protestant Ascendancy, and how she knew it, and challenged like that she said, "Well, maybe Darling, we were yeomen farmers."

Henry II brought Normans and Bretons over to Ireland in the 12th century to help subdue the Irish, and we may have been descended from them. Our surname, Brittain, is said to be the ethnic name for a Celtic-speaking Breton. But why were our family protestant? Henry II, the Normans and the people of Brittany (Bretons) were all Christians, like the Irish. There were no protestants until Henry VIII wanted to get divorced and fell out with the Pope. Then when the English became protestants, the people of the old religion were called 'Roman' catholics. However, during the Irish potato famine in the late 1840s, protestant Church of Ireland pastors offered soup to the starving, if they would relinquish catholicism and become protestants. The poor souls who gave in were called, derisively, 'soupers'. It is possible that our ancestors were Bretons who arrived in Ireland with Henry II in the 12th century, and, coming from Brittany, they were Bretons and so named simply 'Brittain'. The Normans and Bretons sent by Henry II to rule over the Irish are famous for having happily integrated with their neighbours: they married the Irish, lived like the Irish, and in particular they spoke the Irish language. They were, in the famous saying, 'More Irish than the Irish'. That makes them Celtic-speaking Bretons, then. Having been dispossessed by Cromwell, over the next 300 years they may have become less and less successful, until, in the famine, they were starving. One explanation for the surname Brittain, and the protestant religion, could be that we 'took the soup'. I could forgive our family for this much more easily than for being Cromwell's men.

One more little fact supports the Breton suggestion. Blood group B is common in the Far East, but rare in Western Europe, except down the Atlantic coast of the continent. Here, Basques, Bretons, Cornishmen, the Irish, the Welsh and the Scots commonly have blood group B. I used to give blood, and I remember one day an old, smelly, sit-up ambulance coming for me at work, to collect some of my blood that was urgently needed at the hospital. Eight of us were sitting there, minding our own business, when I leaned to my neighbour and asked him, "What is your blood group?"

"B Rhesus Positive" he replied.

"Me too," I said, and we then asked all the other donors. All of us turned out to be B Rhesus Positive, which we agreed is so rare that we might have been our area's only supply. We hoped our victim recovered, with the help of our eight pints of blood. He or she might well have been Irish, too.

So, with my rare blood group B, I think that makes it a little more likely that we might be descended from 'soupers'. If only I could choose, I would much prefer that.

My father had no truck with the Protestant Ascendancy, or anything else Irish. He felt sure he could get further if he moved to work in England: that there would be better opportunities for doctors there. His mother had christened him, her eldest son, Herbert Alfred. He changed his name to Tommy after he went to live in England, and when his mother came to visit him he refused to speak to her if she called him by the names she had bestowed.

He told me once, of the 'Paragon', a hated cousin of his with whom he was always being compared unfavourably by his aunt, his mother's sister. The Paragon, Arthur, was a little older than my father, and was sent to Sedbergh School in the Lake District a few years before my father. He was expelled, but that news did not get out until much later. Then he became a medical student at King's College Hospital, London, but he never qualified. And all those years, to their chagrin, my grandmother and father were regaled by Arthur's smug mother with stories of Arthur's successes, and my poor father was forever being told of the conquests he had to live up to. Finally, the young man emigrated to Australia, and my father hoped that was the last he would hear of him. Many years later, when Uncle Eric was visiting us in Norfolk, they started remembering the Paragon, and my father wondered how he ended up.

"He wrote me a begging letter from Australia," said my father, "saying he was married and 'the little woman' had had a baby daughter, and was lonely, and longed for a wireless to keep her company. Would I by any chance have six pounds to spare for that kindness? I was so bloody pleased the Paragon was reduced to begging from me that I sent it to him. Straight away."

"You didn't?" said Eric. "But didn't you hear about our father, and me?"

"What about you?"

"Well he wrote begging letters to both of us."

"Oho! How much?"

"We didn't know he'd written to each of us until we had paid up, I'm sorry to say. He asked me for a tenner, and our father for 100 pounds, and he got both."

"Oh no", my father said, his hand over his eyes, "Oh *no*!"

"Still, never mind, it got worse for him. He ended up committing suicide in Sydney Harbour, wanted for murder."

"Oh jolly good," my father said.

My grandmother had one of the first motor cars, and a chauffeur, who was never allowed to exceed 12 miles an hour. The reason for the car (of which my grandmother was truly afraid) was probably to do with Grandpa's brother, George Armstrong Brittain, who also went to England to learn a trade. He worked in a bicycle shop in Oxford in partnership with a Mr William Morris. A family story goes that one day Mr Morris said he thought they should give up bicycles, and try making cars, and my great uncle replied, "Ah no, they'll never catch on", and went back to Dublin. He did, in fact, become interested in cars, and even aeroplanes, and Mr Morris (who became Lord Nuffield) remembered his erstwhile partner, and very decently gave him the sole right to sell Morris cars in all Ireland, which made him a good living; but it must have been salt in the wound, even so.

Some of my aunts and uncles by marriage remember my grandparents from the time when they first met them. One said he was astonished, when taken to visit his future in-laws, to discover no books in their house. This was pretty mean of him, because, in the final sale, shelves and shelves of books are catalogued. And of course there must have been a Bible, though that may have been kept by the bed. He cannot have looked properly. Another aunt-by-marriage said naughtily that the daughters were absurdly overdressed, and that it was very embarrassing to have to greet them drinking morning coffee in Switzers department store in Dublin, because then everyone knew you knew them. My Aunt Mabel writes that their father 'took a great interest in our clothes, and liked us to wear real silk stockings, for which he would willingly pay. We each got six pairs every Xmas as an extra present – he bought 30 pairs every year in Brown Thomas!' She continues that, when she was 17, her parents bought a holiday house in Greystones, Co. Wicklow, 'a small seaside village much favoured by retired people in those days. We were very happy in Greystones, although the aforesaid retired people were not at all friendly, it then being a crime to be in business! We managed alright without them.' Sadly, it seems that my happy nouveau riche and overdressed aunts were made mock of because their father was 'in trade'.

The only thing I ever heard my father say about his father was that he would not allow swearing, so the boys had to say "DAMson jam" when they were cross. My grandmother apparently said, with emphasis, "PUDC!" which sounded explosive and angry, like a swear word, but actually stood for 'Pembroke Urban District Council' (why? I have no idea), and so was harmless. Maybe "Oh Hell, oh Hell, oh Helen I love you" came from his childhood too.

Not only did Grandpa not allow any members of his family to swear, but they also were never to drink alcohol, or play cards on Sundays. He held firmly to these rules himself, until comic chance intervened. He took his two youngest daughters on a cruise to South Africa in 1933, when they had just grown up. The first night out from Southampton, the wine waiter approached them at dinner and asked what would they like to drink?

"Something with fruit juice?" my grandfather suggested, not very wise in the ways of the world.

"How about a Gimlet, sir?" replied the wine waiter. "That has lime juice in it."

"Let's try a Gimlet each," my grandfather ordered.

So they tried them, liked them, and had three doubles each and every evening of the voyage, there and back.

The sons, my father and Eric, much older and wiser than their sisters, met the threesome after their cruise, off the boat at Southampton.

"Was it fun? Come on, let's celebrate," said my father. "We're going to a hotel for the night, and first we'll all have dinner."

While dinner was being ordered, a waiter asked what they would like to drink. My father ordered gins and tonic for himself and Eric, and lemonade for the others. Grandpa intervened.

"You know" he said, "On this cruise, one of the nicest things was a delicious drink we discovered, with lime juice in it. I wonder if they have it here?"

"Probably", my father said. "What was it called?"

"It was called a Gimlet."

"Was it now? A Gimlet. And how many of these delicious drinks did you happen to have?"

"Well, we had three each every evening."

"Ha!" shouted the brothers. "Ha, Ha. Yes I bet they have them here. But before we order, let's just check that you know what's in them."

"Lime juice," said Grandpa, "I said. And could we order doubles please, to save the waiter coming and going?"

"Indeed we could. What fun. Well done. We never thought you'd be up to it. You must have had a great holiday. Three double Gimlets a night." The brothers eyed each other, nodded, and one of them said: "You do know, don't you, that the other ingredient of a Gimlet is gin?"

At which my grandfather, greatly humbled, settled for lemonade, and, sadly, never allowed alcohol to pass his lips again.

He died seven years before my grandmother, and I heard my father say that after his death she really came into her own, and kicked up her heels. I could not imagine this, because to me she was a little old lady with white hair and a black dress who walked with a stick. How could she kick up her heels? But she did.

She made friends with many widows like herself, who needed ways to fill their days. They used to go off on holiday together to a hotel in Greystones, where once the family had had the holiday house, and had felt they were ostracised for being 'in business'. Unattractively named Greystones has been described to me as a very 'English' town outside Dublin. There, in her widowhood, my grandmother learned to play bridge, and to have a glass of sherry every now and then. Grandpa, in heaven, would not have approved, but somehow she seemed able to ignore that. She became completely passionate about cards: obsessed, she lived for them – an absolute bridge fiend. One night she telephoned my Aunt Ann, her youngest daughter, and said with great excitement: "Oh Ann, Ann, I have just done something I've wanted to do all my life."

She must have meant ever since she learned to play bridge.

"I'm so excited," she said. "So triumphant. Do you know, this evening I actually bid, and made, a grand slam."

That night she died in her sleep, which was a wonderful way to go. Except, of course, that shortly afterwards she should have gone up to heaven and rejoined her entirely good, blameless and temperate husband, and she may have had some explaining to do.

Chapter 4
The Moonbeam Babes

Sometimes my father had breakfast in bed. I had already had mine before I went to see him, and the smell of his was nauseating to me, especially the fried eggs and the coffee. His tray was crammed with the usual stuff: a plate of sausages, bacon, eggs, tomatoes, mushrooms and fried bread. The blue and white coffee pot, milk jug, sugar bowl and gigantic cup and saucer had Norfolk windmills on them. Somehow there was also squeezed onto the tray a toast rack, butter, marmalade, mustard, salt and pepper and table napkin in a silver ring. When I was four I used to sit on his bed and talk to him while he ate it, before he had his bath.

One morning Roper brought the tray in and my father asked him to switch on the electric fire. It had two long bars, and a big shiny curved reflector. Roper, balancing the whole tray on one hand, bent down to the switch, and the tray tipped and everything fell off and spilt all over the green carpet. The fried eggs lay close together, like the eyes of a huge flatfish, swimming in a sea of black coffee with waves of bacon and islands of fried bread. I thought I might be sick.

"Roper, you're a twerp!", my father shouted from his bed, as Roper rushed downstairs to order, from an irate Chef, another complete breakfast.

Very interested in this nice sounding new word, I asked "What is a twerp?"

"Someone very silly." My father said.

Roper came back, still flustered, with a dustpan and brush with which he tried, rather hopelessly, to clear up the mess.

I had just been staying with my friend Judy at her house in Hethersett. I often stayed with her, and Judy was part of my life. Judy was thin like me, and quite a lot smaller than me. I was three months older than she was. I could nearly always win physical battles with her. I used to shout "I'm bigger and older and stronger than you are: give that to me." And I wrenched whatever it was from her. It sent her mad with rage, and she used her strong powerful nails to scratch me. As an only child, learning to get on with other children came late to me, but before I decided to grab something I took into consideration the punishment I would get from those nails.

I really loved Judy's Mummy. That is what I always called her, 'Judy's Mummy', not Mrs Holmes, or Aunt Noel, until after I was nearly grown up myself. She was a sweet, gentle woman with kind eyes and a pretty face in a halo of naturally wavy light brown hair. She paid children a lot of attention, which was nice for us. She fussed over Judy all the time as if she were a fragile doll. When I was there she fussed over me too. We could not go out without wearing the right clothes and shoes. We had to be warm enough and not too hot. We had to wash our hands and dry them properly when we came in. We must try to eat up all the food we were given. We often ignored her. We were supposed to come in when they rang the bell above the stables, but we often pretended we had not heard it. Judy's Mummy was never very cross. We made houses in the woods. We stole an egg from the hen house and tried to fry it in butter in a tin lid over a candle (not a success: we burned our fingers). We put holly branches in her older brothers' beds to annoy them. This was most satisfactory: they roared with rage. It was a very different life from what I was used to at home, and I loved it.

When I got home, I said to my nursery governess, Dickie: "Judy's got a mummy, hasn't she? And Sara's got a mummy, and Bridget's got a mummy. Where is my mummy?"

Dickie said I should ask my father.

"Do you think she has gone away?" I asked.

"Yes, I think so," said Dickie.

"Do you think she's gone to feather, and is not coming back?" I wondered.

"Yes, maybe," Dickie said. "Don't worry about it, Darling."

That afternoon my father's girlfriend, Ione Barclay, came to take me to tea at Colney with her mother and father. Colney Hall, home of the Barclays (of the bank), was a vast house, a huge Victorian red brick pile with horns and antlers on the wall up the wide uncarpeted stairs and lion skins hanging down over the lavatory doors; so frightening that however much I needed to I couldn't bear to go into one, and had to hang on until I got home.

There was the biggest gun-dog kennel I had ever seen, in the middle of the lawn in front of the ha-ha. It was a proper gun-dog kennel, only three times the size of a normal one, built of bricks, the pitched roof was slated and the concrete run was surrounded by tall iron bars. It was empty. I once asked Ione's youngest sister Sonia (who many years later became my father's second wife, my stepmother) what sort of an enormous dog they kept in it.

"It wasn't a dog, Darling, it was a couple of lions," she said.

"Why did you keep lions?"

"My uncle went big game hunting in German East Africa, and he shot a lioness and then discovered she had two little cubs. He felt sorry for them so he brought them home. He called them Mitzi and Fritz and they were great pets. When they were small they were allowed to run loose in the grounds, and we often watched them enjoying themselves chasing the postman on his bicycle as he rode across the park to the Hall."

How glad I am that I was not that postman. A zoo owner once introduced me to a playful tiger cub that grabbed me by the thigh and bit my knee: the pressure behind those teeth and claws, even in a cub, is terrifying, and they dig in like Stanley knives. The postman cannot have been at all amused. He must have been tough and courageous, and even when the cubs were small, he would have had to pedal extremely fast, covering about half a mile of gravel drive in each direction.

"And in the evenings," Sonia continued, "they came into the room where we sat after dinner, and shared it with all the family, lying down in front of the warm fire like two big dogs."

"They sound nice", I said.

"Well yes they do, don't they? But it ended up very sadly".

"What happened?"

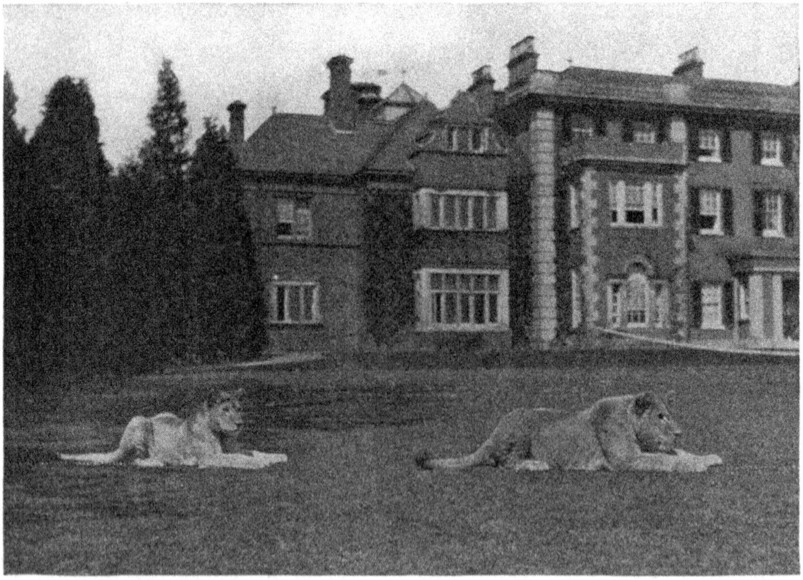

A photograph in 1911 of Mitzi and Fritz relaxing on the lawn at Colney Hall (reproduced from The Tatler, August 1911) © Illustrated London News/Mary Evans Picture Library.

"When they were about two years' old a man from the RSPCA came to the front door. My father already had his pack of chow-chow dogs then and they made a hell of a racket when they saw someone they didn't know. They bit anyone they could get at so they had to be dragged away and shut in his room before the door could be safely opened. The RSPCA man said, above the din, that he had heard we had pet lions. 'So what?' we shouted back. He felt it was his duty to warn us that as lions get older they get fiercer and rather untrustworthy. 'Not Mitzi and Fritz,' we said, 'they're very friendly'. The RSPCA man still thought he should advise us to find a safe home for them: a zoo or something. 'What?' we said, 'Send little Mitzi and Fritz away to a zoo? Poor things! Oh no, we wouldn't do that.' So he went away."

"I'm so glad you didn't send them away," I said.

"Ah, but not long after that, my Uncle Terence was killed by them."

Apparently, the RSPCA man told them that if they were going to keep these dangerous animals, they should be more careful. They should be kept in their cage at all times, and no one should ever go in with them while they were being fed. After that there was no more lying by the fire after dinner. They were no longer let out of their gun-dog kennel and had to be fed, watered and hosed out through the bars. The family felt very sorry for them.

The Barclays' oldest son and heir, Terence, the one who had shot the lioness, was in the army. When one day he came home on leave, he said he could not believe his pet lions were really dangerous. He had known them since he had rescued them as tiny cubs, and they had always liked him. So he opened the door, and went in to talk to them and rub their foreheads. One of the lions rushed at him and attacked, and savaged him terribly. His courageous sister managed to pull him out, and he might have survived today with antibiotics. But his wounds went septic, and he got blood poisoning and died of it.

Countless years later I was staying with Judy, and she said "You must go and talk to Mr Bell, our gardener. He used to work at Colney, you know".

Mr Bell said he first started working there when he was 14, raking the gravel and sweeping up the leaves. And that if any of the gardeners spotted Captain Barclay coming out of the house to walk round, they all had to go and hide, at once, in the potting shed, so that he could have the place to himself. I asked Mr Bell if he remembered the lions, because somehow I was not quite sure that I believed Sonia.

"The lions," he said. "No. They were no longer there when I started. But they had been there, and there had been a tragedy, because they had killed young Lieutenant Barclay, the oldest son, and the family was very upset. Almost the first work I had to do was climb up on the marble fireplace in the hall. I was chosen because I was so agile then. I had to cut a great big picture out of its frame there, and roll it up. It was a picture of Daniel in the Lions' Den, and after the trouble the family couldn't abide having it in the house."

So it was true. And I do wonder where that picture is now. When the Barclays left Colney, did they find it, with the removal men, rolled up in the attic? Or was it still there for the next person to find? As the Barclays owned the famous bank, it may have been quite a good picture.

I recently went to Colney Church and found Terence's gravestone. On it is written 'In Loving Memory of Terence Henry Ford Barclay, Lieutenant

Scots Guards, eldest son of Hugh and Louisa Barclay who died at Colney on 27.12.11 from the result of an accident, aged 29 years'. On the simple chancel screen inside the church, it states 'He died from injuries received from a captive lion at Colney'. His younger brother Evelyn (who later became my step-grand-father), eventually inherited Colney.

Evelyn could be a rough and very forthright person. I heard recently that some years after the tragedy a relative died in Ireland and Evelyn went over with his brother-in-law to sort things out. They had a bit of time on their hands before catching the night boat back, and Evelyn suggested: "While we're here let's go up to the Zoo and see those two lions that ate up old Terence." The brother-in-law was very shocked, and would not go.

At tea that day, Ione sat next to me near her mother at one end of the table, and her father Evelyn sat at the head of the table, a long way down at the far end. He still kept a pack of chow-chows: ugly, bristly, stiff-legged dogs with sinister black insides to their mouths. They had ginger hair and fierce tempers; not so very different, I suppose, from their erstwhile contemporaries the lions. Evelyn had a cup and saucer four times the size of my father's big one, and filled the saucer with tea again and again for each of his chows. He was so extremely fond of his chows that he had bought a little cottage for them, at Mundesley, on the North Norfolk coast, so that they could enjoy seaside holidays.

At that time I did not know that Captain and Mrs Barclay lived at either end of the house and had not spoken to each other for years. When the gong went, they met for meals in the dining room, which was once the ballroom, with leather-covered screens around the ends of the long table to keep draughts out. He always sat at one end of this refectory table with his chows, she at the other end with her dachshund. She drank China tea, he and his chows drank Indian.

The Hon. Mrs Barclay (Noons or Noonie) was my friend Nick's aunt (the giver of the cigarette-smoke-smelling stuffed dog). She was amusing, entirely good, reasonable and responsible. She wore tailored tweed skirts, soft jerseys, pearls and good flat shoes. My father obviously had a very soft spot for her, and had she been unmarried, I guess he might have wanted her even more than he did her beautiful daughter Ione. She lived with her dachshund in an elegant pale green drawing room, with a sweet-smelling wood fire burning. There were many silver-framed photographs on the grand piano of her daughters and other members of her family wearing trains with a trio of ostrich plumes, like the Prince of Wales' Feathers, on their heads, being presented at Court, and there were signed ones of Queen Mary, and the King and Queen. Noons was a magistrate, and a girl-guide leader for her area. She and my father used to telephone each other with answers to crossword clues, and have naughty bets on how long Queen Mary, or George Bernard Shaw would live after having broken their hips in old age. It was an easy bet: Noons always lost, because she was admiring and loyal, and wanted the victims to live as long as possible. My orthopaedic father knew perfectly well that you did not survive long with a broken hip when you were old, so of course he won. When I was about 15, Sonia told me of a tremendous breach between her mother and father, which she had witnessed out of her nursery window in the attic.

One day the guides were in the Colney woods learning woodcraft with Noons instructing them. Sonia could see from her nursery window that an excellent tea had been prepared for them for when they had finished, with cucumber sandwiches, scones and jam, and fruit cake, all laid out on trestle tables with white table cloths on the terrace above the lawn outside the house.

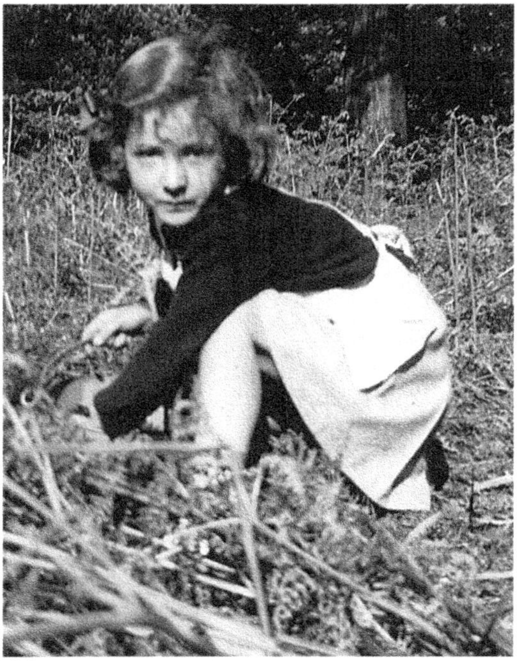

Exploring the garden. Alison aged about five.

Evelyn Barclay lived in a large cold room with coconut matting on the floor. It smelt strongly of dogs. His straight grey hair would not lie down smoothly, and stuck out in tufts. He smelled of Vicks Vapour Rub, a eucalyptus ointment to be rubbed on your chest to help you breathe when you had a cold. It is still available today. But he never seemed to have a cold: I think he must just have liked the smell. He always wore fawn corduroy trousers, and we were told when he died that he had 32 pairs of tailor-made corduroys, as yet unworn, in his wardrobe. He also had garages full of very fine motor cars: Lagondas and Rileys with open tops. He had many cages of canaries, and seven dog beds with chows in them around the floor. The chows were famous for their tempers, likely to attack everyone who came to the front door, and especially they bit poor Noons, again and again, giving her wounds that sometimes needed the doctor to come. When the bell rang the butler had to take a footman with him to drag the dogs away before he could open the door. The footman usually got well bitten himself in the process. I heard that in later years, Colney was sold and a former footman bought it. Was he the one that kept getting bitten, finally acquiring a just reward for his pains? The chows had taken most of the stuffing out of the only piece of furniture in the room, a sofa on which Evelyn sat, listening to the radio at full blast all day.

Evelyn always went to The Theatre Royal in Norwich for the Thursday matinee. This particular day was a Thursday, and in the matinee all the dances were performed by Miss Vera's Moonbeam Babes, the eight- to ten-year-old girls of a local dancing class. Evelyn was very partial to the Moonbeam Babes, and as they had delighted him with their performance, he went backstage and said: "Guess what, my Darlings, there's a lovely tea for you at home. I'll get some taxis, and you jump in and come and have it with your old uncle Evelyn." They jumped in, arrived at the Hall, went round the back to avoid the chows, reached the terrace, fell on the tea and ate it all up. Sonia saw that Evelyn had a Moonbeam Babe sitting on either knee when a long crocodile of blue-uniformed girl guides snaked up from the woods, Noons at the rear, to find that their tea had been eaten. Surely this, or something very like it, must have been the cause of the trouble.

Anyway, the day I went to tea, there they were, not speaking, and Evelyn was putting down saucers of tea (with milk and sugar) and shouting: "Come on my old Coppa, drink it up, drink it all up."

Dogs having tea was a new idea for me, and I asked Ione's mother "Why is he doing that?"

"Because he is very silly", she replied, quietly.

"Aha", I thought, and I pointed at him and said: "You're a twerp".

"I'm a what?" he bellowed.

"You're a twerp," I said again, louder. "You're very silly, giving your dogs tea, so you're a twerp."

This caused great guffaws of laughter. Evelyn was red in the face with excitement.

"Come here my Darling," he shouted. "Come here at once and sit on my knee and tell me that again. I don't think I heard it right."

So I walked the full length of the table and got on his knee and looked him in the eye. The veins on his cheeks and nose were all broken and his purple skin was covered in little red squiggly lines. He looked at me in a very hard way I did not like, but I said again to him "You're a twerp", and he was obviously delighted. The women at the other end were giggling too.

"They're really silly", he said, "They are. You tell them what they are, too. Go on, I'm waiting."

So I pointed at each of them in turn, and shouted "You're a twerp and you're a twerp too". Everyone seemed really pleased.

My father came to have a drink and pick me up, and on the way home he said: "Noons says you called her a twerp. Did you?"

I could tell I was in trouble, so I did not answer.

"Did you?" he asked.

"Yes," I confessed.

"Why", he said, "for God's sake why on earth did you do that?"

"Ione's father said her mother was silly," I replied. "You said Roper was a twerp when he spilt your breakfast. You said it meant he was very silly."

"Oh God," my father said. "Well, you're going to have to write her a letter saying you're sorry." On pink paper, with hand-ruled pencil lines, and a great deal of Dickie's help, I wrote the first letter of my life. I found it deeply humiliating: 'Dear Mrs Barclay', I wrote, 'I am sorry for calling you a twerp. Love from Alison'.

Chapter 5
Mickey Mouse

My father felt very cold at night. Norfolk houses were not centrally heated in those days. He slept in a double bed, with two hot water bottles, six or seven blankets and, on top of them, two stuffed quilts with lead in the corners. If he did not have that much weight on him, he could not sleep. Much later, when Gretchen had puppies, we kept two of them, and Anna and Ferdie became his living hot water bottles, and slept right down the bed with him, one for each foot.

We often went to stay at Somerleyton with Nick's mother and father. My father complained to me that there were never enough blankets on any bed there, though he had his own ways of dealing with it.

The Somerleytons had fragile bones and loved hunting and skiing: an ill wind, he said, which blew no one any good except an orthopaedic surgeon. My father had mended the bones of several members of the family. The first time, he told me, he was on a modest skiing holiday on his own in Kitzbuhel, Austria. He got a message in his boarding house that there was a call for an English doctor at the hospital. When he got there, Lady Somerleyton was still saying, with some emphasis: "Get me an English doctor."

She was in great pain. Doctors in the hospital were trying to set her broken femur without any anaesthetic. There was no anaesthetic in the hospital. So my father went out and bought a bottle of brandy, and said: "You're going to have to drink an awful lot of this, I'm afraid."

"I can't," she said, in anguish. "I'll be sick."

"You're not going to be sick," he said. "You can have it with water or soda or something, but you have got to get it down. We're going to have to set this bone for you. Alcohol is a great pain killer, and it is the only one we've got."

So she obediently drank it, was not sick, and they set the femur. When I asked how, he said that they set it by pulling hard at her leg to get the two overlapping parts of her broken thigh bone apart so that they could be properly re-aligned, touching, ready to grow together again, and mend. This manoeuvre, he said, can cause death from shock unless the patient is deeply anaesthetised, so it says much for the power of the brandy. Not surprisingly, united against the common enemy of Austrian doctors, she and my father became good friends.

He had also told various Somerleyton family members, as he circled round them on his horse while they lay injured on the plough in the hunting field, that he would first catch their horse and then call an ambulance at the next telephone box, and see them in the Norfolk and Norwich Hospital that evening. Then he galloped off to catch the horse, telephone, and follow hounds. When he was hunting, nothing stopped him. He loved it. He said, "Once your blood is up, you cannot stop. No one would expect you to". He hunted throughout the season on Thursdays and Saturdays. My father did not operate on those days, but he always turned up in the hospital after hunting to see his patients. Staff and patients were quite used to seeing him in his riding clothes: his boots, his jodhpurs, his scarlet coat, his stock and even his face all covered in mud. He liked speed in all its forms, and so he hunted with the Norwich Staghounds, which could gallop for ten or more miles non-stop at a stretch, in pursuit of a red deer that until then had lived in a deer park. The object was to capture the deer and return it to its park at the end of the chase, not to kill it. Its ear was notched to mark it before it was released, so that it was only hunted once in its life.

Once, he mended the broken leg of a Somerleyton horse. He put a massive plaster-of-Paris cast on its whole foreleg, and the horse was kept in a sling, hooves only just touching the stable floor, so that at first it could put no weight on the damaged leg. In those days, horses with broken legs were shot. Maybe they still are. The sling was gradually lowered so that the leg took more weight, and it mended perfectly, and the horse was able to be ridden out hunting again. People said my father was a miracle worker, which embarrassed him.

Shortly after the horse recovered, my beloved cat Panda broke his leg. He came in one morning with a dangling front leg. He was taken to the vet, and kept there. Then suddenly I had to go and stay at Somerleyton, and my father took me in the car.

"What is going to happen to Panda?" I asked.

"The vet says it is very doubtful if he can mend his leg."

"So what is going to happen to him?"

No answer.

I realised, with horror, that he was cheating. They were going to kill Panda because he was unmendable. And I was to be kept out of the way until, hopefully, I had forgotten him. But there was not a chance of that. I still haven't forgotten him, a lifetime later.

"You're going to kill him, aren't you?" I said. "You mustn't, please don't, I couldn't bear it. You mustn't, you mustn't," I was crying now. "You can't, he's mine, and I haven't even said goodbye to him."

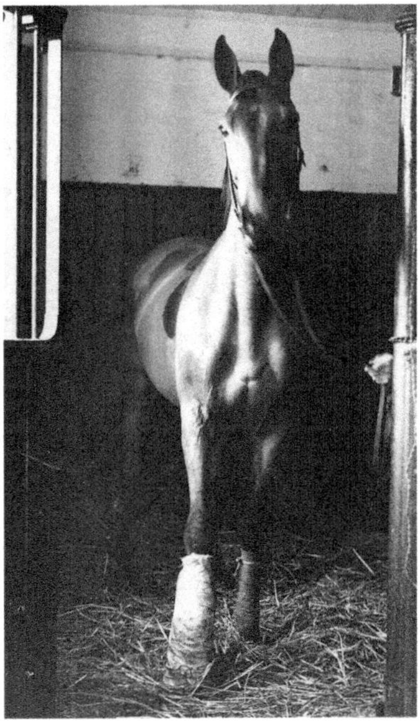

A horse at Somerleyton treated by Tommy with foreleg in plaster-of-Paris.

Silence.

"Tell me the truth" I cried, "Tell me the truth, please. You always make me tell you the truth, now you've got to tell me. You're going to kill him, aren't you?"

"Well, if he cannot be mended he will be in great pain, and it might be kinder to kill him."

"What do you mean, he can't be mended? Of course he can. You mend him. You can mend anything. You can mend people, and mend a horse, so how can you possibly think you can't mend a cat? Will you try? You haven't given him a chance yet. Promise me, promise me, you'll try."

I was now weeping uncontrollably, which my father could never stand.

"Stop snivelling", he said.

"No I won't," I sobbed. "Not till you promise to try and mend Panda's leg."

He gave a big sigh, and said "All right, I'll try".

"Promise?" I insisted, "Promise?"

"Promise", he replied.

He took Panda to the childrens' hospital, the Jenny Lind, and there set his shoulder and put him in a cast that went right round his body, as well as down his front leg, which stuck out in front of him. He put him in a wicker bassinet in the middle of the oldest childrens' ward, with a net over him. The sick children managed to persuade Panda to lie there quietly, and eat and drink again. There, to my father's horror, the Daily Mirror got to hear about it, and printed a double page with photographs of Panda, headed 'Miracle Surgeon Mends Cat's Leg in Hospital'. He came out to Somerleyton to fetch me, showing me the pictures of Panda in the Jenny Lind.

"Look what you've made me do," he said. "Cats are not supposed to be in hospitals, and surgeons who try it could get struck off. I was hoping to sneak him in and that no one would notice."

"But you have mended him?"

"I've set his shoulder bone. It might still go wrong. We're not out of the woods yet, and it will be some time before he can come home. But I did try."

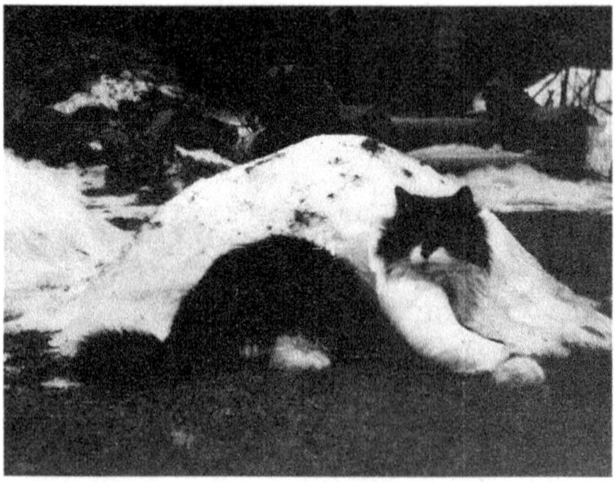

Panda, Alison's pet cat, treated by Tommy with foreleg and shoulder in plaster. Tommy said an orthopaedic surgeon could be struck off for treating an animal.

I cried with relief, and hugged and kissed him.

In the end, and after some months of recovery, my spirited black and white Panda was completely normal again.

I would be six years old just before Christmas of 1939, and so old enough not to get bandy legs if I learned to ride. So I rode every day at Somerleyton, with Nick. I always liked sharing a bedroom with Nick

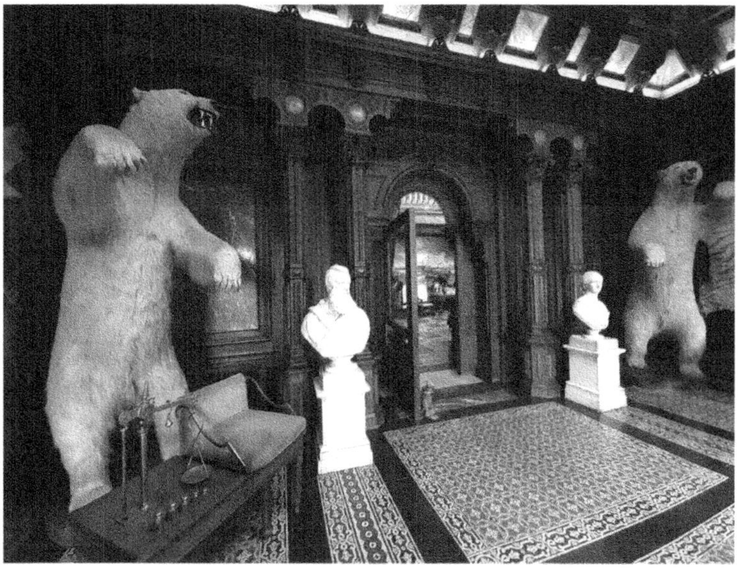

Stuffed Polar bears nine feet tall, guarding the front door of Somerleyton Hall. Shot by Savile Crossley (later 1st Lord Somerleyton) in 1897.

on the top floor in the nurseries, with his Nanny next door, but I used to feel terrified walking into the house, because the entrance hall was a huge dome of stained glass beneath which, guarding either side of the door, two enormous stuffed polar bears stood on their hind legs snarling. The polar bears were more than twice as tall as me. They had been shot by a previous Lord Somerleyton. The kind butler Coley knew how frightened I was, and always came to the hall smiling, to take my luggage and lead me in by the hand.

When we went riding the groom towed me along on a leading rein, on Nick's old pony, saying: "Sit up straight, Miss Alison. Look out between his ears. Heels down a bit, feet straight forward. Keep your hands down."

But Nick could ride by himself on his new pony, and he could trot and canter. I envied him.

And then, when we next went to stay at Somerleyton, it was just before Christmas. Down in the drawing room, just after church on Christmas day, my father asked me, "You still want a pony for Christmas?"

"Yes, yes, of course" I eagerly replied.

"What's wrong with Panda and Gretchen?"

"I love them, but they are not ponies."

He kept me in suspense for what felt like minutes, and then told me that my Christmas present was to be what I had been so longing for, and had never quite dared hope I would get.

"I've got you a pony," he said. "Mickey Mouse."

Mickey Mouse was mine! My very own pony. I had a hot electric feeling between my ears and eyes, and I was jumping up and down with excitement. I leapt at my father to hug him, and he beamed with pleasure at my joy.

I had sometimes ridden Mickey Mouse in a riding school in Norwich. He was a very small black gelding, not grossly fat, like a Shetland pony, but about the same height. He stood at eleven hands, or three feet eight inches high. He had white rings round his eyes. He may have had some Exmoor pony in his ancestry, because that is the natural colour of the skin round their eyes: it looks like makeup, and it made him look alert. So he was called Mickey Mouse. He had been trained to obey voice commands, so that if you said "Trot" he trotted, and if you said "Stand" he stood. He was the easiest pony to handle and ride I have ever known, the dream first pony.

I loved every bit of him. I loved putting my nose near his nostrils and smelling his sweet breath. I loved running my fingers through his long winter fur. I loved cleaning out his hooves, and brushing him, and hissing as the groom did, to drive away the dust. I loved him so much that to this day, when the dentist warns, "This might hurt a little. Think of something nice," a picture of Mickey Mouse springs into my mind, with his warm body, gentle nature and lovely smell. I can stand any pain if I think of him. His image even helped with the pains of giving birth to my babies at home (they are grown up now, with children of their own, but I still haven't told them that: they might not like it).

I wanted him to live in our garden, but he had to go and live in a livery stable with my father's huge hunter, Caravan. But we went there together to ride, most afternoons. My father strongly believed that hacking daily, jogging down the roads for an hour or two, got both your horse and yourself fit for hunting. He called it, as I expect the French (some of whom seem so concerned with their innards) might call it: 'shaking up your liver'. Mercifully he would have nothing to do with a leading rein, and I learned to trot and canter the first day. He never gave me any instructions about how to ride.

Then my father said we would go and spend the weekend with Bridget's mother and father at Mulbarton, and it was going to be really exciting, because we were going to ride there, across country. It was a lot further than I had ever ridden, but he was sure I could do it.

We set out on Friday afternoon when he had seen his last patient. Little Mickey did not exactly jump fences, he squeezed through. He climbed down into the bottom of ditches, and scrambled up the other side, while Caravan and my father flew over the obstacles, waiting impatiently for us to appear. We had to go across a flooded field. Mickey started to paw the water, showering it up all round him. I pulled his reins up really short, and he suddenly put his head down to drink, pulling me off, over his head. I fell into the water, and he galloped off. My father galloped off too, and I was left there, sitting in about a foot of very cold water. When they came back, Mickey reluctantly being pulled along, tail swishing, nose in the air and ears laid back, my father was extremely angry with me.

"How many times have I told you, the first rule is, never let go of the reins?"

"But he pulled me off over his head."

"That's no excuse. There is no excuse for letting go of the reins. You can fall off, fine. Everybody does that. But you must never let go of your pony. I want you to remember that, always."

It was a long way. It got dark well before we got there. I was wet all over, and shaking when I got off. Bridget's mummy came out to greet us, saw the state I was in, and set about my poor father.

"Do you realise she is only just six years old? You are not a fit person to look after a child. If anybody gets to hear about it, she could be taken away from you. I've a good mind to tell someone."

Terrified she would tell someone, I was led off by Bridget's Nanny, to a hot bath and a speedy recovery.

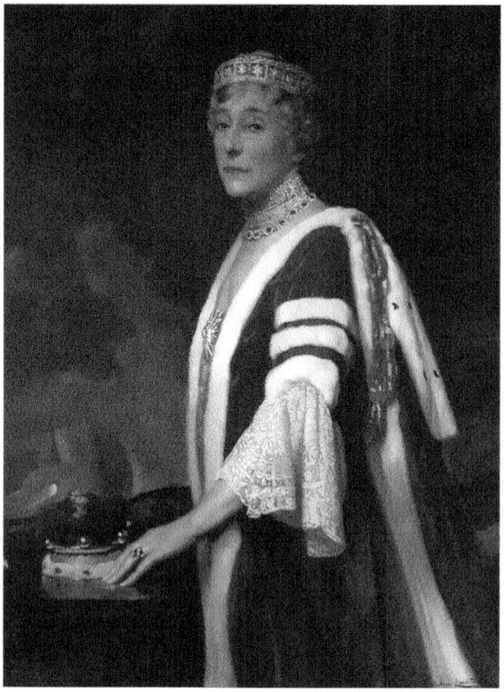

Portrait In Somerleyton dining room of Nick Crossley's grandmother, Dowager Lady Somerleyton, who complained at Christmas breakfast.

That was the Christmas my father and I spent at Somerleyton. He brought me there a week before, and went away to work, only arriving himself late on Christmas Eve, after Nick and I had gone up to the nurseries to bed. He was one of the last to go upstairs after dinner, having been talking for hours to his host over whisky, and then he discovered he only had three blankets on his bed. The house was now dark and quiet, so he crossed the corridor to another bedroom (there must be at least 20 principal bedrooms in Somerleyton: it was used as a hospital for wounded soldiers in the First World War), and helped himself to the blankets off that bed. He folded several of them so that they were doubled, and tucked in the biggest one tightly all round, put his overcoat on top of that, got into bed and fell asleep.

In the morning he went down to breakfast with all the other Christmas guests. We children had breakfast with Nanny up in the nursery. But grown-ups had breakfast in the dining room, where one wall was covered in two enormous paintings. The one I loathed was of a gory early 19th century battle scene from the Napoleonic Wars with soldiers shooting at each other, cannonballs flying and all of them, it seemed, dying or about to die in every kind of bloody agony. It was sickening, and if I was going to eat there, I always had to sit facing the other way.

When I was much older, I discovered that breakfasts at Somerleyton were magnificent. There were silver chafing dishes on the sideboard hotplate with porridge (and cream), and all the important bacon-and-eggs things: and kidneys and sometimes kippers. A footman served the guests.

On Christmas morning my father sat down beside Frank. Then old Lady Somerleyton, Frank's widowed mother, aged well into her 80s, came into the dining room.

Her daughter-in-law kissed her and asked: "Did you sleep well? And what would you like for breakfast?"

"No," she replied. "I did not sleep well. I had the most terrifying experience in the middle of the night."

"What was it? I didn't hear anything in the night. Did you have a nightmare?"

"Well, I thought at first it was a dreadful dream, but now I feel sure it was real."

All the other guests were now gazing at her with interest.

She went on, "I had been sound asleep for ages and then I woke to hear the door creaking open, footsteps padding across the floor, and deep breathing. Whoever it was (it must have been a man, he was so strong), came up to the bed and leaned over me. He pulled at the sheets, and then whispered in my ear: 'One, two, three. . .' and with a loud groan he wrenched all the blankets off me, and went away with them. I was very frightened and very cold, and after that I am sorry to say I could not get to sleep again."

Her daughter-in-law was horrified, and asked the footman to send upstairs to look for the missing blankets.

Realising discovery was imminent, my father was forced to admit that he had committed the crime. He grovelled before old Lady Somerleyton, and said he had no idea she was in the bed.

She snorted, "You could have looked."

Chapter 6
Hitler's Moustache

My father said, "Come and listen to this, it's important," when I was almost 6 years old, in September 1939. I remember sitting on his knee in his half-moon backed mauve armchair listening to the Prime Minister. We had a brown wooden wireless with an arched top. It had a little light inside, and took a long time to warm up, whistling as it did, but when it had, we could hear Neville Chamberlain, the Prime Minister, saying in a stilted voice that we were going to war with Germany. My father said, "I shall have to go and fight".

I had no understanding of what that meant. I think I supposed that some days instead of going to the hospital he would 'go and fight'. I had no idea where. In fact he volunteered to fight in the war during the first few months, but it took quite a long time before the army wanted him. He joined the Royal Army Medical Corps, and perhaps at first there were only a few wounded soldiers, and the army could use the regular army doctors and did not yet need the volunteers.

In the waiting months our home became very different. Chef and a boy called Boots seem to have been wanted straight away, and left: I suppose they volunteered too. We were told to dig for victory, and I watched with extreme interest as our gardener, Rose, who was too old to fight, dug an air-raid shelter, called an 'Anderson Shelter', on my father's instructions. It was very small, but still an enormous improvement on my own efforts to reach Australia in my sandpit.

"Will you get to Australia?" I asked, watching Rose.

"It will get very hot before we get there," he replied. "I can't feel any heat yet, can you?"

I felt the cold, wet earth. "No, not yet."

The shelter had steps made of cut earth, and went so deep it went lower than the earthworms, but if it rained it filled with water, and then the earthworms fell in and drowned. It only had a corrugated iron roof, level with the rest of the garden, weighed down with sacks of earth. We never used it.

I was telling a bit of this story once to someone who now lives in the house we did, in Newmarket Road, Norwich. He said, "How extraordinary that all the family pets had Christian names, like Stephen and Gretchen, while the servants were addressed by their surnames", and I am ashamed to say that as it was part of my childhood, I had never really considered the extraordinariness of the matter. And, even odder, now I do come to think of it, is that some servants were simply called by their job titles, as Chef, who cooked of course, and Boots, who among many other menial tasks, cleaned shoes.

We learned the chromatic howling sound of the air-raid warning, and the wail of the all-clear. When the siren went off in the night, we all went and sat in the hall in our dressing gowns, and warmed our hands on mugs of cocoa wondering what would happen next, but nothing did.

We had to have blackout curtains, so that the Germans, flying by our house, could not see in and shoot us. The shops had run out of black material and only had brown, which my nursery governess Dickie used to line all the curtains. I worried a lot about this, thinking it would not be called 'blackout' if brown was good enough, and perhaps the Germans would see enough through the brown to have a shot at us anyway. I tried to imagine bullets coming through the stained-glass panels of the front door, and how would the Germans be able to get their aeroplanes low enough to do that.

Two young Hungarian maids came to replace the menservants. They were sisters, spoke hardly any English, and had wavy long blonde hair. They made extraordinary strudel pastry: standing opposite each other they put the pastry together and pulled it apart further and further until it was the size of a tablecloth and so very thin you could see through it. As soon as it got a tiny hole they folded it all up again. On Sundays they wore big bright red skirts and colourfully embroidered white aprons and blouses: their Hungarian national dress. They cried easily and often, because they were homesick.

Roper, who was also too old to fight, told them that in the last war there was not enough water for anyone to wash their hair, and in this coming war there would soon be none either. Sadly, that news made them chop each other's golden hair off short. They made a very rough job of it, and looked horrible. Roper got a rocket from my father for making up nonsense.

I was most afraid, when Dickie and I took Gretchen for walks on a lead down Unthank Road, that people would throw stones at her as Roper had warned when we got her. I peered apprehensively around during our walks, wondering how I would protect her, but thankfully, despite my terror, it never happened. So Roper was wrong there too.

But Roper was very nice to me. He used to play 'Fly away Peter, fly away Paul; come back Peter, come back Paul' with me, making two little caps of silver paper from cigarette packets that fitted on the tips of his fingers disappear and reappear when he said the magic words. And Chef made me a hippopotamus from a potato with small potato legs that fitted into slots in its tummy, and a long-legged giraffe from a carrot, the tip of the carrot for its head and the rest for its body, using long fire-lighting spills for both its neck and its long legs. Roper could stand these on the dining room table, put my father's silk hat (his top hat for hunting) over them, and simply by magic make them vanish and come back again. I believed he really could do magic.

Before all this, when I was still only four, when I was not yet allowed a pony, I was given the smallest of two-wheeled bikes for a child, called a fairy bike. Riding a tricycle was easy, but a two-wheeled bike defeated me, until Roper spent day after day running about on the lawn holding me up and saying "Now pedal, Miss Alison, pedal really hard!" I would never have learned to ride it without him. So although I knew my father thought he was stupid, I knew he was clever, and I liked him.

As part of the early war effort all the people we knew got hens. We got a dozen knowing-looking Rhode Island Reds strutting round on yellow legs, their feathers the colour of the burnt sienna paint in my watercolour box. They fascinated my father, and he and I went out every morning to their dusty cage, the door so low that only I could get in, to collect the eggs. I had to telephone all his friends to see how many eggs they had got, and the day we got a dozen he was absolutely triumphant.

Early in the war Denmark was overrun by the Germans, and Dickie and I heard it on the news hour by hour. She was terribly upset, and knelt by her bed and prayed aloud for her country, and cried. She wanted to go back to Denmark, but did not think she could get there now. I certainly did not want her to go, and though I did not say so, I hoped the Germans would stay there, and stop her leaving.

Dickie taught me to knit. She knitted the Danish way, with the thread over her left first finger: much faster than the English system where you must move your whole hand forward every time you make a stitch. I still wonder why the English have not realised the benefit of the 'Continental' style, and taken to it. I could only knit plain stitch, at first.

Dickie adopted a submarine, and we knitted for the sailors, in a dark blue and very greasy wool. Our hands were blue, like the Jumblies, and smelled very strongly of sheep.

> Far and few, far and few,
>
> Are the lands where the Jumblies live;
>
> Their heads are green and their hands are blue
>
> And they went to sea in a Sieve. (*Edward Lear*)

She made jerseys, and long thigh-length stockings. I tried to make a scarf, but it had many mistakes in, some of which could not be sorted out by Dickie. I did wonder what my sailor made of his crooked scarf full of holes. I also wondered how the sailors kept the long stockings up. Did they wear suspenders, like Dickie, or Liberty bodices with white rubber buttons, like me? Dickie did not know the answer to that. We only had our adopted submarine for about three months. Then it was sunk. I cannot have understood the meaning of this and that probably all the sailors drowned, and I suppose Dickie was protecting me, kindly avoiding telling me such bad news. All I thought was that it was an awful waste of knitting.

Once, on Dickie's day off, the secretary said she would take me for my afternoon walk. I rode my fairy bike, pedalling along the pavement beside her.

The secretary was wearing high heels, and had difficulty keeping up with me. We went to Heigham Park, not far from home, where there were flower beds to ride round on many little gravel paths. Dickie used to sit down on a bench to watch me ride, and wait for me to tire. But this poor secretary kept puffing along behind me, her high-heeled shoes, now a serious disadvantage, tipping her over on her ankles. I got bored with her, and pedalled really hard, reaching a nice wide gravel drive in another part of the park behind a hedge, where she could no longer see me. When I got back to the park gates, she was not sitting on a bench waiting for me. So I set off for home.

Dickie and I had done it so many times I knew the way well. But as I was pedalling along on the pavement, to my surprise a policeman came and pedalled very slowly beside me. He wore a helmet, and his blue uniform, and was so enormous that my eyes were level with his huge shiny boots slowly circling. He said to me, "Now where are you going to, Miss?" I knew policemen should ride on the road, not the pavement, so I said "I'm going home. Why are you riding on the pavement? You're not supposed to, you know."

He replied, "Can I come with you, to your home?"

I said "If you want to, you can," and started to pedal really hard. He could keep up easily no matter how fast I went, and I nearly knocked him off his bike when I turned right across his handlebars straight into our drive.

There was a scene going on at home. The policeman and I stood beside our bicycles outside the front door, and in the hall the secretary was crying her eyes out, and my father was looking very fierce. He asked me how I had dared to run away. I said I didn't run away. The policeman reported that when he found me I said I was going home. That made matters no better, and I was sent to my room. Later, when Dickie came back, she said that I had caused everybody the most terrible worry, and that I must say sorry to the secretary and to my father. I did say sorry, because I had to, even though I did not understand why they should be worried. I knew the way home. What was the fuss about?

Friends of my father came to stay. Some were also waiting to be called up for the war. I enjoyed being talked to seriously, as if I was a grown up, by John Barratt, a young man who loved children, and we always talked and listened to each other like equals. He never teased me, or made fun of me, and I did so like him for that.

Two more friends, called Duncan Begbie and Charlie Scrope, who had been asked to leave their lodgings at extremely short notice for 'bad behaviour', were rescued by my father and also came to live with us. Duncan was dark and handsome, with straight black hair slicked back from his forehead, and a deep speaking voice like the engine of a very expensive car. He smoked a meerschaum pipe that I thought made him smell horrible. Charlie always read the sports pages of the *Daily Mail* at breakfast and took as keen an interest as my father did in horse racing.

Harold Cassel, though pleasant to me, seemed much more distant. Tall and good-looking, he performed a wonderful trick for us. When the chows did not need Evelyn's cottage by the sea at Mundesley, sometimes the rest of the Barclay family and friends of theirs used it for holidays. On the beach, Harold used to walk on his hands into the sea until only his feet were showing above the water. All children badgered him endlessly to do this.

And then I heard Harold ask my father at breakfast one day, "Tommy, if you are taking Pinkie out tonight, would you mind very much if I take out Ione?" I think my father must have pretty well decided on Pinkie by then, because he

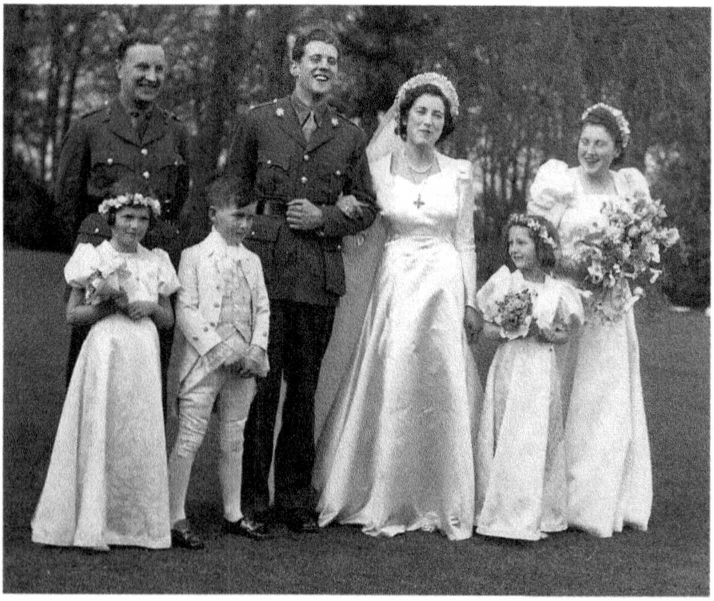

Harold and Ione's wedding, 1940, at Colney Hall, the Barclay's home. Nick is the page, Diana Birkbeck (far left) and Alison are bridesmaids. Back row: Best Man, Harold Cassell, Ione Barclay, Ursula Barclay.

seemed perfectly happy with this, and before the war started properly Harold, wearing his officer's army uniform, married Ione, in the little church with the round tower at Colney. Ione, with her delicate skin and black hair, wore a long very pale pink dress, and I thought then that she was the most beautiful woman I had ever seen. Nick was a page boy, and I was one of their bridesmaids.

I am surprised that I never asked why my father and Pinkie did not get married at the same time. The answer, if I had been told it truthfully, would have helped me understand the grim state of my father and mother's marriage.

Not long before, Ione had taken me to the pantomime, where there was a very frightening devil who wore a scintillating green and purple body stocking, and matching balaclava. I was horrified by him, and wanted to go home. But at the very end, just before the curtain came down, there was an explosion and a lot of smoke came up out of the floor, and the devil shot up through the hole. Then he faced the audience and sang a most unlikely song for a devil. I knew it well. He sang 'There'll always be an England. . .'. I was so frightened and confused that I wet my knickers.

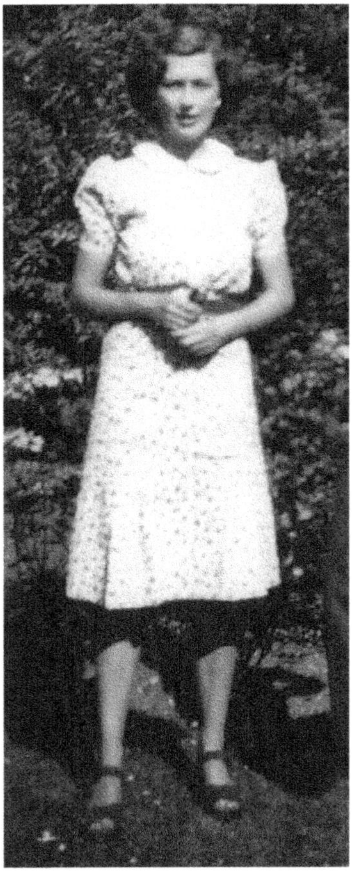

Pinkie (Rosemary Dering Bulwer) as she was when she and Tommy got engaged in 1940.

Dickie and I sang 'Run rabbit, run rabbit, run, run, run', and 'Pack up your troubles in your old kit bag' and 'Hang out your washing on the Siegfried Line if the Siegfried Line's still there'. I knew that along with 'There'll always be an England', these were war songs, but I had absolutely no idea what the war was about. And like everyone else, I suppose, I did not know how long it might last.

My father happily explained to me that although doctors are not supposed to fall in love with their patients, Pinkie was so lovely he could not help it. They met when she came to see him because she had broken her collarbone falling off her horse. She had a classically lovely face, a smile that demanded a response, a silky complexion, and soft brown hair. My eye was drawn to a kind of luminous quality that shone from her; somehow the way I imagined the Virgin Mary would look, with her halo. She was indeed heart-stoppingly beautiful. She used to take me out sometimes, and never minded when I always wanted to be taken to the Castle Museum in Norwich to see the stuffed animals, most of them with Indian ink labels saying they had been shot by Barclays or Somerleytons. Grand shooting expeditions had been undertaken by Somerleytons and Barclays before the First World War, and the skinned and stuffed results decorated Somerleyton and Colney, and filled the Castle Museum. Apart from the polar bears and lions, she used to show me the set scene of the salt marshes in North Norfolk, and helped me to see all the camouflaged birds and waited patiently till I found their eggs.

Before Harold had married Ione, my father became engaged to Pinkie. He gave her a superb emerald engagement ring. The prospect of their marriage delighted me, Pinkie had a wonderful grace about her, she was loving and kind and generous. We would be a proper family: my father would have a wife, and at last I would have a mother.

This stage of the war that was not a war came to a close in late summer. I remember John Barratt coming to the nursery in his new uniform to say goodbye to me because he was going away to the war. I had not seen an army uniform so close up, and was shocked at the difference it made to someone I knew so well. I hardly recognised him. John was near tears, and said "I've got to go away to get something for you. I promise when I come back I'll bring you a present. I'll bring you Hitler's moustache". It seemed a funny sort of present to me. I asked Dickie how he was going to get the moustache.

"Kill Hitler and cut it off, I suppose," she said.

I would never have believed that gentle John Barratt could make such a horrible suggestion.

Chapter 7
The Pony Trap

My Mickey Mouse now had a harness and trap; a Governess cart, it was called. It had been all newly done up and painted yellow and green. Pinkie was going to take me to stay with her at Cawston, a village about ten miles from Norwich, and we were going to go together in the Governess cart, with Gretchen. We set off from Norwich early one summer morning in 1940, and had a picnic on the grass verge by the road on the way. Pinkie knew all about horses, and was concerned for little Mickey. She said he could not possibly trot all the way, and sometimes we let him walk, and sometimes to spare him our weight, we got out and walked beside him. We got to Cawston just as it was getting dark.

I absolutely had not expected what happened next. I thought my father would be there when we arrived, but he was not. I thought he would surely come in a few days to take me home. But he was not there, and I waited, but he never came. He had gone to the war, Pinkie told me. He had never said that he would go away, that he might just vanish, and I was absolutely devastated when he did. I was six-and-a-half.

"Why didn't he say goodbye? He should have. John Barratt said goodbye."

"He kissed you goodbye, Darling."

"Yes, but he's always doing that. He didn't say a proper goodbye. Where is the war, Pinkie?"

"He has gone to Leeds, another town in England, for the Army to train him. Then when they want him, they will send him abroad to another country to fight. If they don't want him for a bit, he will get leave, and come and see us."

"What country? Will he go to Germany?"

"No, not Germany, but he might be sent to Palestine, and there I suppose he might be quite close to Bethlehem."

Bethlehem was in the Bible.

"Will he live in a stable? With a donkey and a bullock? Is Hitler in Bethlehem?"

"He may have to live in a tent. Hitler is still in Germany."

"He won't like it in a tent. He needs a lot of blankets. And where is Dickie? Isn't she going to look after me?"

"She is trying to go back to Denmark."

My father had been in exactly the same position as his friend Harold: he had fallen in love, got engaged, joined the army, but while he was still living at home in Norwich, he did not marry Pinkie. It is odd how children do not pick up clues. I did not wonder why.

"When will you and Daddy get married?"

"When the war is over."

"When are we going home?"

"When the war is over."

I thought and wondered about why my father had not told me he was going away. He should have done. I remembered I did not tell him I was going to run away on my fairy bike from the secretary, but then I did not do that on purpose. She could not keep up. I would have told him if I had really been going away. But he had meant to go. I was sad about him and angry with him for that disloyalty. I felt utterly bereft, and very afraid. How could I suddenly have lost my father, and Dickie, with no warning at all? I seemed to have fallen into a deep black whirling hole like the 'wall of death' ride that I had once seen at a funfair in Yarmouth. I had a high-pitched hum in my ears. I was not hungry and felt sick at the thought of food. I did not want to talk to anyone, even Pinkie. I could not sleep, and in bed at night I cuddled Gretchen, my plump German sausage dog, and cried. Pinkie said that my cat Panda had been given to the nextdoor neighbours for the war, and we could have him back when it was over. Gretchen and Mickey seemed to be the only familiar things I had left.

Of course, it was not like that all of the time. I liked exploring the enormous house, and Pinkie's bedroom in particular, because she had beautiful watercolours of wild geese painted by Peter Scott, who she said was a young man living in a lighthouse on the Norfolk coast because he loved waterfowl, and lived among them, just like that scene in the Castle Museum. She promised to take me to see the coast, at Blakeney or Cley, but we never went, because we had not enough petrol to go the eight miles there and back just for fun, and it was too far for the pony trap. Pinkie's care for me, and understanding, were a real help, but from time to time, with no warning, I was blacked out and ravaged with pain and tears, and homesickness, and longing for my father.

For strange reasons, for instance because they were other people's very grand homes in wartime need of evacuees, or boarding schools for girls, I seem to have spent much of my childhood in enormous stately homes that were on the cusp of disaster. They were no longer in use as places to live for the rich families that built them. Once outstandingly elegant, built in choice sites with lakes and woods and spacious parkland, their glories were much diminished: the war was making them shabby, and in danger of destruction beyond repair. Dry rot, leaking roofs and dangerous old electric wiring threatened them.

When I was not depressed and frightened, I liked walking on my own in the huge grounds of Cawston: woodland and heath, with the glorious scent of heather and pine trees warming in the sun, a string of five lakes, and lawns growing into long hay because it was part of the war effort not to cut them, and anyway, the gardeners had joined up.

It took some time, but in the end it seemed Pinkie leaned over the edge of the abyss and took my hand. Little by little, with all her gentle affection, she helped me climb out. She had my bed moved into her room. We did a lot of things together. We went blackberrying and then made jelly. We went looking for red squirrels, and for grebes and Egyptian geese on the lakes. We caught some newts and looked at them in a jam jar, and then put them back. We listened to stonechats. She taught me to put the trap harness on Mickey, and helped me to catch him. He was so elated at having a field of his own for the first time, instead

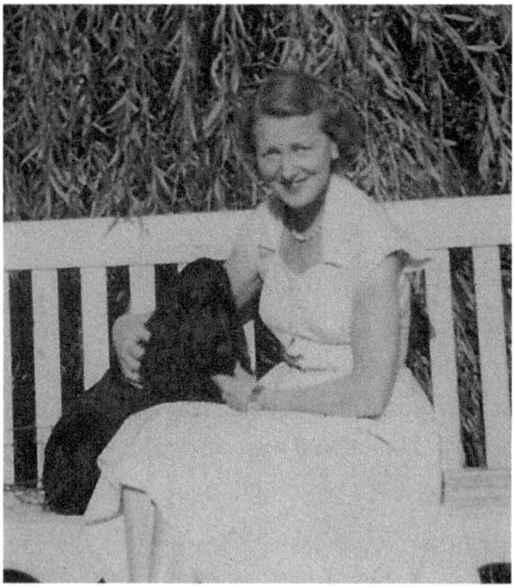
Pinkie and her black cocker spaniel Jonathan.

of living in a stable, that, in no mood to be caught, he high-tailed it round the field as soon as he saw us. Pinkie had a way with all animals, and I loved that about her. She knew how to catch a pony, how to hold a rabbit kindly (not by its ears), how to care for a hen sitting on eggs, how to listen to the nightjar in summer churring away beneath a pyracantha bush, how to open the nest-box of a blue-tit so carefully that we could count the ten tiny baby birds and close it again so quickly and gently that the mother bird would not desert (we waited at a safe distance to see her return), and how to find the tiny domed cobweb nest of a goldcrest. We took Gretchen and Jonathan, her black cocker spaniel, out for a walk every day. She pointed out that for a dog, going for a walk with a human, must be like walking with a blind person, since we obviously lacked a major sense so well-developed in dogs: scent. Together we chanted Chesterton's 'And goodness only knowses, the noselessness of man', as we watched Jonathan tearing from side to side of the path, nose down, exuberant stump tail apparently propelling him.

One day, Gretchen came into season. Pinkie explained she was ready to have puppies. So a dachshund mate was found for her, and she went to spend the night with him. Gretchen did not seem any different to me, and maybe we would never have known she was in this state if it was not for Jonathan, poor Jonathan, who was beside himself with worry and desire, clicking up and down the wooden floors all day, howling all night. After she came back, Gretchen was shut in our room to keep Jonathan away. We heard a bumping buzzing sound and did not guess that it was Jonathan scratching about a quarter of the paint off the door trying to get in. He was then shut in the log shed, but was out in a minute or two. So, Pinkie asked the Misses Clutterbuck, middle-aged sisters who ran a riding school and were well known for their devotion to ponies and dogs, if they would keep Gretchen for a few days until her season subsided. We took her in the pony trap, and she looked at us with misery as she was shut in a dog kennel with a wire run. But the following morning, a worried Miss Clutterbuck telephoned Pinkie to say she was so terribly sorry, but during the night a strange dog had bitten his way through the wire, and she found him in the kennel with Gretchen, with a big grin on his face.

"Is he a spaniel?"

"Yes, yes, a black cocker spaniel."

"Oh dear," said Pinkie. "Blast."

It was half a mile down our drive, and then two miles down the road to the Clutterbucks, and as far as we knew, Jonathan had never been there. Quite a long time later, Gretchen had ten puppies, one born dead. Four of them were dachshunds. Five of them were black long-coated cocker spaniels with very short legs. It seemed to us sad enough for them to have short legs, so we could not bear to have their tails cut off. They were so long and low to the ground they looked like long flying ribbons of black silk. We found homes for all of them, and even the Misses Clutterbuck, assuaging their guilt, took one.

I spent a lot of time in the holidays riding alone on Cawston Heath. There were lots of tracks made by rabbits and foxes to ride along. During that summer there was a heath fire that refused to die down. It crept along the ground, invisible in the day and a wiggly line of red at night, but when it reached a group of fir trees suddenly the dark sky roared and crackled and curling plumes of red flame reached for the sky. It left the heath covered in soft grey ash, and Pinkie asked me to take care riding near it, because although all seemed normal, beneath the ground the heather roots were still burning, helped by air in the rabbit tunnels. If I saw smoke coming out of a rabbit hole, I turned for home and cantered back. The fire could go round behind you in this way, and cut you off from a safe retreat.

My desperation subsided. I cannot remember how long it took, a few weeks probably. I loved Pinkie for her honesty and gentleness and her caring and kindness towards me. She had an absolute sense of right and wrong, and of how you should always err on the right, or kind, side. She said, "If you're ever not sure what to do, always think how it would be the other way round. What you would like other people to do to you? Do that. That will work best."

That was the golden rule. She treated me as if she might have been my mother, and I was terribly pleased to have a mother at last. I also learned that people thought bombs would fall on Norwich, and that we would be safer in Cawston. It was called 'being evacuated'. We were officially 'evacuees'.

Cawston Manor was huge, and Pinkie and her sister Bunny looked after between six and ten evacuees in one wing of it. The other two wings were an orthopaedic hospital for children: patients evacuated from the dangers of wartime Norwich. The only real danger that Norwich suffered was a direct hit on Caley's chocolate factory (perhaps the Germans thought, looking down on it, that it might be making something worse for them than chocolate) and the blissful smell of hot and burning chocolate could be detected as far as Aylsham, 10 miles from Norwich, for weeks and tempting weeks.

Cawston Manor was the recently built Elizabethan-style home of a self-raising flour magnate, who had decided rather unpatriotically to spend the war in Egypt. The last thing he did before he left, and the Manor was requisitioned, was to order a dozen peacocks. They arrived unexpectedly in a crate one day, and the gamekeeper just let them go in the grounds. I had never seen such beautiful birds. It was my job to stop them stealing the hens' food, but they were cunning, fast and hungry, and they often won. The males with their iridescent blue neck feathers and their tails full of eyes amazed me (as no doubt they did their dull hens), parading about the garden walls and screaming. They did survive the war, I think, because I went back many years later, and there was a peacock strutting the walls in the old way, just as I remember them. Neither the self-raising flour magnate nor his descendants lived there any more. No one there now could remember when the birds had arrived.

Food rationing had set in properly while we were at Cawston. We each had a saucer with a tiny square of butter on it, which was meant to last a week. Mine never did. I was aware that when we liked some sort of food, custard, say, the grown-ups often said they did not want their custard, and gave it to us. Meat was in short supply, but I never liked meat, and although I was made to eat some I hope some grown-up ate the rest for me.

One day the gamekeeper came to the front door and made us a present of some eels he had trapped. I had never seen eels, and was not sure I would like to eat them. We had converted what was once the downstairs gentlemen's lavatory, called the lobby, into our kitchen. It had two separate rooms for lavatories, with wide mahogany seats and chains with china pulls. Pinkie and Bunny cooked for us all on a small smelly oil stove that sometimes went wrong and filled the lobby, and covered the walls, floor and people, with black oil smuts, leaving Pinkie and Bunny in tears. The washing up was done in two wide marble basins with gold taps in which the men had once washed their hands, and the floor was made of big black and white marble tiles. The gamekeeper put the sack of eels on the kitchen floor, and it rose up and down like a concertina on its end, because the eels were alive. Bunny opened the sack and they all slithered out, looking like wet snakes with ears. They were highly active, and about three feet long. They whipped around the floor, and were so slippery that even if you grabbed one they whistled through your hands, which were left full of slime. They were impossible to hold. The gamekeeper was telephoned, and came back to catch them, but could not. So we were sent away, and he got a hammer, and hit them with it to kill them. They were very nasty to eat: just mouthfuls of bones, but the worst thing was that the gamekeeper had smashed the marble floor to pieces with his hammer. We hoped the flour magnate when he came back after the war would not notice the piece of old linoleum where his lovely floor had been.

My father did come home on leave twice while we were at Cawston, but each time it was just for a day and a night. Pinkie was radiant with happiness to see him, but sadly for me it seemed sudden and unreal. It just reminded me of how much I missed him. In his uniform, he seemed like a shadow or a ghost of himself: he made me feel shy. He was not there long enough to be really good for me, although Pinkie seemed to glow with pleasure all the time he was with us. Each time he came he had another pip on the shoulder of his uniform, which I was asked to admire though I could not see why. Anyway, they seemed to give him great satisfaction. He obviously felt sad leaving us, and I did not like to ask him why he had not said a proper goodbye.

In the other two wings of the Manor there were children with orthopaedic problems, who had once been my father's patients. They mostly seemed in every way normal, except that, poor children, their bones were rotten and crumbling with tuberculosis, or their muscles were paralysed by having had polio, both terrible medical scourges of the time. We often went and talked to them. Some, strapped on their backs, were wheeled out into the sun in the mornings. All they could see was the sky. Once they told us there was a new aeroplane, and would we ask the pilot who lived with us what it was? An RAF fighter pilot called Philip and his wife and children were living with us at that time, and we asked him, and he said no, there was no new plane. We said the boys know it, and it has a different engine noise from a Spitfire or a Hurricane. He looked astonished, and in the end admitted it was true, and he was amazed they knew it. It was a deadly secret, called a Mosquito, and we must all swear never to tell anyone. We kept the secret, though we did make him come and tell the boys.

There were at least six other evacuated children with us, and we went the two miles to school, past the five lakes and under green arches of trees overhanging the road, on our own in the pony trap. We were, quite rightly, not allowed to hit Mickey, so we had a long stick with a tin can full of stones hanging from the end, and we very quietly reached it out and held it just above his ears, and then shook it loudly. To our satisfaction, that speeded him up. With a lift of his head, he cantered a few steps, then trotted much faster for a bit. We seldom met any other traffic on the road. Petrol was so severely rationed, no one could use their car. We used to leave Mickey in Aylsham, the little market town, standing in the square outside the International Stores, not even tied up, for the whole morning.

Then we ran through the churchyard down to Miss Ivens' school, with our gas masks bumping on our backs. Mine was very smart, and had a red case. It smelt disgustingly rubbery and, when we practised wearing them, I wondered how long I could have borne to wear it in a gas attack. We sat in four rows at Miss Ivens', but she only taught the front row. Once you had been taught you turned round and taught the person behind you, and so on to the back of the room. This was a good way to learn. You cannot teach anything if you do not know it thoroughly, and by the time we turned round, we did. And Miss Ivens got a rest after every bout of teaching. I remember teaching Andrew Buxton, a boy who was evacuated with us and who sat in the row behind me, how to write little 'm' and little 'n' and big 'M' and big 'N'. Very important letters, these; as it says in the catechism 'What is your name, N or M?' Andrew had four sisters living with their parents in their big house near Norwich, but he, the son and heir, was the only one who was evacuated. When I asked why, I was told that boys were more important than girls. I wondered how that could be, and felt very glad that I, a girl, had been evacuated to live with Pinkie.

One of the letters written by my father during the war to his sister Ann has a strange request. He asks her if she would like to go and live with Pinkie and me at Cawston, bringing her two sons - my cousins.

'I wondered how you were placed and whether there was any chance of you joining Pinkie at Cawston Manor (with family). Bunny is being called up in May or June, Andrew Buxton, one of the children, is leaving and at the moment it looks as if Pinkie will be short of both children and help. Of course, the whole thing may be quite out of the question. . . Cawston is an absolutely beautiful place, three miles from Heydon. The children would have a glorious time. Woods, lake, pony etc. However. . . I am not asking you to do it and I know and you know that there are some things not mentioned in this which you spoke of in your letter to me. I should quite understand if you found it impossible and I am only writing in case it is what you would prefer. But it looks as if Pinkie will have to give up Alison otherwise and she has had such a hard time with me and everything that it seems dreadful, cruel on her, especially as she and Alison adore each other. I enclose a page of a letter from Pinkie. Please burn it. I copied the bit at the top from the page before.'

Why was Aunt Ann to burn the page of the letter from Pinkie? What were the things that he knew and she knew that were not mentioned? What was the hard time Pinkie had had with him that was so dreadful, cruel on her? I did not know what any of that meant when Aunt Ann's son, my cousin John, sent his mother's old letters to me and I first read them, a few years ago. In one thing my father was absolutely right, of course: Pinkie and I did adore each other.

He talks about Pinkie needing more evacuees to look after, and this must refer to the fact that as they are not married the War Office will not recognise that Pinkie has any right to look after me alone, as if I were her daughter, and not be called up. And he had volunteered to join up, and so not be with us.

At Cawston, and indeed all the time I lived with Pinkie, we had such freedom as I had never even dreamed of, and I loved it. In the holidays, after breakfast, we were let out of the house (there were about five of us children then), well wrapped up in coats and pixie hoods, to do whatever we liked. Pixie hoods, by the way, were very easy to make: you just knitted two similar squares of wool, each the size of your head. You put the two together and sewed up one side. Then you went on round the corner and sewed up the next side. At the corner of the two open sides you fixed two ribbons. When you put the hood on, the sewed-up corner stood out from the back of your head like a pixie's hat. They were very comforting hats because they kept your ears so nice and warm.

One of us had been lent a grown-up's watch, and we had to come back by 1 o'clock. We walked all over the place: through fields, woods, streams and farm tracks, and we had enough time to go quite far. One day we found a farm about two miles off, which had big barrels on their sides propped up on bricks. They had taps sticking out of them. We turned on a tap and black sticky stuff trickled out. It smelt nice, so we tasted it, and it was molasses, or black treacle, which the farmer used to make silage. Sweets and sugar were of course rationed, and we longed for sweet things. So we used to take it in turn to lie under the tap with our mouths open, while another one turned the tap on and off. It was delicious, but when the grown-ups were brushing our hair after our bath in the evening they asked us how we got our hair so sticky on our walks? We replied, "I don't know".

I thought the two children and the wife of Philip, the pilot who lived with us, were very lucky to be evacuated all together as a family. He was a fighter pilot in the Royal Air Force, flying a Spitfire from one of the local aerodromes. He used to go out in the evenings to fly. One morning he did not come back, and at lunchtime the aerodrome telephoned to say he had been shot down and was missing. There was just a faint hope that he had used his parachute and landed safely and been taken prisoner of war by the Germans. Pinkie and I prayed and prayed for him. Philip's wife cried, and waited in anguish for news. She endlessly dipped her teaspoon into her coffee cup, and touched the tip of it on the edge of the cup to drain it. 'Tink, tink, tink', the teaspoon went, trying to drown her agony. The children did not want to talk about it, and went very quiet.

I found it hard to believe that someone who had been there for supper the night before could be killed before breakfast the next day, but it was true: in the end they heard he was dead.

Chapter 8
Holy Water

In the Summer of 1942, for the second evacuation, we went to Pinkie's village, Heydon, even further from the bombs. To this day Heydon is a perfect unspoilt rural idyll. There is no traffic in the village, because it is not on the way to anywhere. It is a dead end. There are lovely old houses, made of soft dusty red brick, a bow-windowed shop and a pub set around a green. All the houses look out over the green, so everyone can see what goes on there. There is one of the famous, elegant, flint and stone North Norfolk churches overlooking it. Nestling beneath the church is a row of tiny almshouses, called Widows' Row, where very old people in the village lived, and we used to be sent over to them taking firewood and kindling, and jam, and to ask if there was anything they wanted. They did not seem to be very good at looking after themselves, they were so old, but at least they did not have to be dragged off to the workhouse. Inside the church we used to dare each other to drink the holy water for christenings, which we found in a green wine bottle in the vestry. It was labelled, by hand in faded blue-black ink, 'Jordan Water'. It tasted of tadpoles.

I was later christened with this water in Heydon church when I was nine. Pinkie said, "They forgot to do it when you were born because your mother was so ill that they had to spend all their time looking after her".

So I had had a mother, after all. I wondered whether to ask if my mother had got better, but then I supposed that she could not have, or I would have her instead of Pinkie. I thought my mother must now be in heaven (which once I called feather). I was extremely happy with Pinkie. She was all I wanted. I never asked the question.

I always thought my names were Alison Betty, but Pinkie said, "Why not be christened Alison Elizabeth, because Betty is only a nickname for Elizabeth, which is a proper name?" So that is what I became.

Heydon is much used now by television companies when they need to show an ideal English country village. I feel most uncomfortable when I see it on the screen: the scene of some of my happiest childhood memories suddenly filled with plainclothes police looking for murderers.

I lived with Pinkie at Heydon, along with her mother, her five grown-up siblings (Bunny was one of them) and a Nanny, and her older sister Fur's children, Mary Anne and William, and the baby Timothy, whose father had gone to fight; and of course, Mickey and Gretchen. Gretchen was happiest at Heydon: they had big wood fires there. To stop the logs burning too fast, the heap of white wood ash was never cleared away until the summer. Every night Gretchen put herself to bed on the edge of the fire in the lovely warm ash. She did get a few small burns when she lay on a glowing ember, but nothing persuaded her to sleep anywhere else. I was eight, a few months older than Mary Anne, and about two years older than William, who fell seriously in love with me. The poor boy asked me if he could marry me when he grew up. Mary Anne and I were merciless to him once we knew of his desire. We insisted that if he was one day to become my bridegroom, he could practice for it by being our groom now. We made him clean and saddle-soap the ponies' tack, and clean out the stables. Horse turds are called 'tadners' in Norfolk, and we buttoned him into a child's mackintosh so tight he could hardly breathe (which was his groom's uniform) and ordered him to pick up tadners and put them in the barrow. We inspected his work with scorn, always finding something wrong with it. Wretched William: how we abused love.

I am pleased to say, when I met him again when we were in our 60s, William was enjoying a long and very happy marriage.

William had a wicked, clever little dappled grey Shetland pony called Threepenny Bit. Mary Anne and I kept 'deciding' to ride in the Park, and thus drag William along with us. We knew that Threepenny Bit would immediately run away with William, and deliberately gallop beneath the low branches of the sweet chestnut trees, painfully scraping his rider off his back. William had awful bashes on his head and face. He was very brave about it and it took some weeks before his mother, Fur, discovered the cause of them.

William was given a new pony, Brownie, better looking than either of ours, and so, now very jealous, we humiliated him by blindfolding him and making him ride her back-to-front until she bucked and he fell off on the village green where everyone could see.

He once announced his name, on the megaphone, at the start of a bending race at a Pony Club gymkhana as 'William Hanslip Bulwer Long' (which after all was his proper name). We never allowed him to forget it, and thereafter always addressed him, loudly, with the full mouthful of his name. He was brave and agile, and we once dared him to hang by his knees from the bar across the well on the green. We sometimes helped to wind the handle on this well to bring up a bucket of water for an old woman in Widows' Row. We had not considered what the consequences of this dare might be. It is a very deep well, you can hardly see the water at the bottom, and if this had gone wrong and William had fallen in he would definitely have been killed. His mother saw it from the house, and came out white with fear for her son, and anger at us, and gently helped him off the bar and brought him in. Mary Anne and I were shut separately in our bedrooms, for a whole day, for this crime against William but Mary Anne escaped by climbing out of her window on the first floor, hanging on to the windowsill by her fingertips, and dropping onto the grass below, which meant she had to be shut in for another whole day.

William finally got the better of us. There was a tiny stream that led down from the green to the Grange, with huge *Gunnera* plants in it, prickly leaves bigger than an umbrella, growing with their feet in the water, and there were yellow azaleas with an exciting musky foxy smell. I am surprised that I have never found any scent for sale based on the smell of those yellow azaleas: perhaps it is a bit too exciting. One day we had a peeing competition across the stream. Mary Anne and I squatted down and leaned right back so that our pee would go in an arc, and hopefully reach the other side. We failed. William just stood there and with a happy grin, aimed, peeing on the far side effortlessly. We gave him rather more respect after that.

Lovely Elizabethan Heydon Hall had been closed up for the duration of the war, because it was huge, damp and cold, and without servants it would have been impossible to keep up, or heat. Occasionally we went there, and the grown-ups undid the shutters, and we took away extra mugs for village fetes, or flower vases for the church. Instead we all lived in the rambling old Dower House, which looked out over the village green.

Life was exciting and full of fun and things to do every day. We spent much of our time playing with animals, the least of which were ladybirds, which we made fly away, 'Your house is on fire and your children are gone', from the tips of our fingers. The Norfolk name for a ladybird is 'Busy-Busy-Barneybee'. Betsy the bull terrier, maddened by us howling at her and egging her on, tore round the walled rose garden crashing into rose bushes and garden chairs, doing a great deal of damage because she was so muscular and heavy. There was a litter of spaniel puppies, whose tails were docked on their second day of life by the gardener, who bit them off. This was said to be the best way, because in your mouth you can feel the space between the tail bones, and make a neat job of it. I woke up in the middle of the night thinking about it and wondering how anybody could have the strength of purpose to do it. Every morning we went down to the game larder, a room with a brick floor and zinc mesh windows, and many hooks in the ceiling. We were looking for ducks that had fallen to the floor. Pinkie's younger brothers, who shot them, hung the ducks up on a hook through their tails, and when they were rotten enough to be very tender eating, with a full rich taste, they dropped to the floor and we took them to the kitchen.

In the park and the farmland all round there were sheep with happy lambs, and cows and calves, and horses everywhere. Horses were just about the only form of transport, and we spent much of every day grooming or riding our ponies. We snipped the hairs off their fetlocks with a pair of Nanny's nail scissors. We endlessly practised plaiting their manes and tails, or thinning them out, 'pulling' it is called: we twisted one or two hairs round a finger, and tugged them out. Our fingers hurt terribly, but we did not mind. We wanted our ponies to look like thoroughbreds, and worked endlessly for that effect. Alas, our ponies not being thoroughbreds, we never achieved it. In particular William's tiny dappled grey Shetland always looked big-bellied, short-legged and far too hairy, both in the winter and summer.

The rose beds in the walled garden at the back of the house, with the roses that Betsy crashed into, were dressed with horse manure. Young Timothy was harnessed into his pram to rest in the fresh air there in the mornings. The tadners round the roses were completely dried out, and once we gave one to him saying "It's a lovely bun, Timothy, eat it up". He was obediently eating it when Nanny came out to pick him up, and serious sanctions were imposed on us: I cannot remember for sure, but probably not being allowed to ride for a whole day.

I remember Heydon for picnics, and learning to swim in the muddy deer park lake, and for everyone helping with the harvest. As the horse and cutter went round the field, starting at the outside, the rabbits moved secretly inward, until there was only a small patch of corn left in the centre. A friend used to come over to Heydon bringing two sleek whippets, and every time a rabbit bolted in panic, the whippets caught it. This was supposed to reduce the rabbit population, although they never seemed to be any fewer. But it did mean that every family who helped with harvest got a few rabbits to eat. If any farm then had a tractor, which I do not remember, it could not have been used, because there was no fuel for it. We children helped by riding the huge Shires, dappled grey Percherons and chestnut Suffolk Punches, as they pulled the wagons. They only understood a broad Norfolk accent, and in this we shouted "Hold tight!" when we wanted them to move on to the next stook. One man on the ground with a pitchfork piked the bundles of corn up to another man on the wagon, and he arranged them neatly and rose higher and higher as they did. 'Hold tight' was meant to be an instruction to the man above to hang on as we were going to move, but the horses understood it as 'Go'. The stooks were made into a stack with all the grain facing in and the cut ends on the outside. The stacks waited for the threshing machine, which visited each farm in turn to thresh the grain off the stalks. By the time the threshing machine got to them, the stacks could be full of rats, and as the stack was taken down the rats ran out and the farmers' terriers, growling and yapping, grabbed them one by one.

We had various chores to do, as part of our war effort. Once a week we took the laundry hamper in the pony cart about two miles through the park, down to the train at Corpusty, and brought back the clean sheets. We had to take the very fat puffing dog, Peggy, which belonged to an ancient widow who lived in a tiny house in Widows' Row, for a walk on a long linen line every day. We spent hours hanging about watching the blacksmith at work shoeing the big

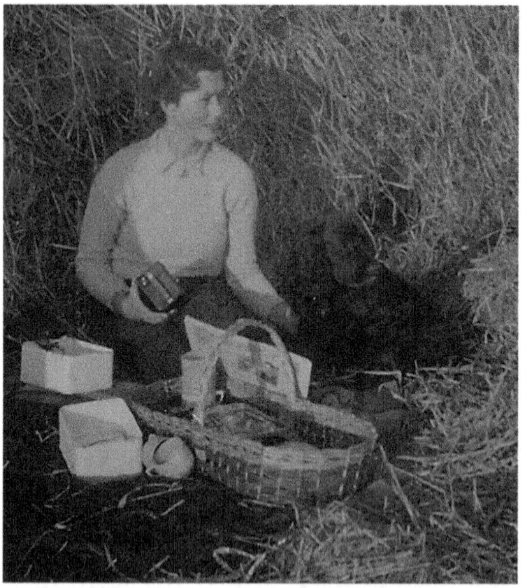
Pinkie and her spaniel Jonathan with a picnic at Heydon.

farm horses, hoping to be allowed to pump the bellows. I liked the smell of the blue smoke that rose from the horses' hooves as he tried the hot shoes on them. Later, watching my father operate, I noticed when he sawed bone it smelt exactly the same as burned hoof. But all we ever really wanted to do was ride our ponies, or just mess about with them. Mickey was so absurdly tame that we could put a tablecloth over him, tell him to 'stand', and then all three of us could sit on the ground underneath him, eating our tea. He had a party trick of which I was particularly proud. Sitting on him bareback, I could lean forward over his withers till I was nearly whispering in his ears, and say, quietly, "Hup, Mickey, hup!" This made him rear up till he was standing on his hind legs like any circus horse, and he could hold this position for several seconds. Then I just let go and slid off over his tail, which was great fun, and shocked the grown-ups until they knew about it, because they thought I had fallen off from a height and might have hurt myself. Every bit of that pony was mine, and I was his.

There was hardly any petrol in the war, but Pinkie and her sister Bunny could get a little because they went night-nursing in the local hospital and, once a month, with the petrol they had saved, they took a car stuffed with neighbours on a shopping trip to Aylsham.

The whole village of Heydon belonged to all of Pinkie's relations. Her Aunt Bee was very old and deaf and lived in the Grange. The Grange had an out-building, the coach house, and in it was stored a very pretty wickerwork bath chair. I think it must have been used by a relative a generation older than even Aunt Bee, who seemed then to me to be as old as anyone can get. It had two front wheels like a miniature Governess cart, and a third small wheel out in front. A long iron stalk came up from this wheel, with handlebars, so it could be steered. I thought it would be great fun to use it as a one-person pony trap, so after brooding on it for some time, Mary Anne, William and I harnessed Mickey up to it. We put on his blinkered bridle, and his collar and traces, but did not bother with the rest because we could see nothing to fix it to. I got in, shook the reins, clicked at him to start him, and shouted "Trot". Away we went: the first bit uphill through the village, going beautifully. Mary Anne and William were left behind, looking impressed. I was very proud of myself and Mickey, and hoped everyone was watching.

But then we went through the big gates into the park, and Mickey slowed down, and as we had omitted the breeching, which is that part of the harness that acts like a brake, the little front wheel went right between his hind legs. My face was buried in his tail. He was shocked. He bolted.

It was madly exciting. Tears poured from my eyes as we careered and careened around the park, crashing into tall sweet chestnut trees and iron estate fencing, and the wickerwork broke all around me. Bit by bit the whole thing fell apart, and I fell out of it, or through it, onto the ground. Some time later we picked up Mickey, grazing, and slowly dragging the ruins of the Bath chair, on its side. It was beyond repair.

I was really sorry for having smashed up the beautiful chair. But apologising to profoundly deaf Aunt Bee through her ear trumpet at the top of my voice, with Mary Anne and William giggling behind the door, was sickeningly humiliating. Not for the first time in my life, I had to make an apology. First to Noons Barclay, for calling her a twerp, then to Aunt Bee for the ruined beautiful wheel chair. Later on I had to apologise to Pinkie's Uncle Walter, for deliberately stamping on his young growing leeks. Awful.

The only thing I did like about the wireless was the 9 o'clock evening news. On light summer nights, when we could not get to sleep, if we were awake long enough to hear the booms of Big Ben, we could creep out of bed and go to the nursery and sit with Nanny, whose real job was to look after Timothy. But we could not say a word. Nanny made us a cup of cocoa, and brushed our hair, and the news was so boring we would probably be asleep before it was over. It did mean that when you went to bed you were not shut away for a whole 12-hour stretch.

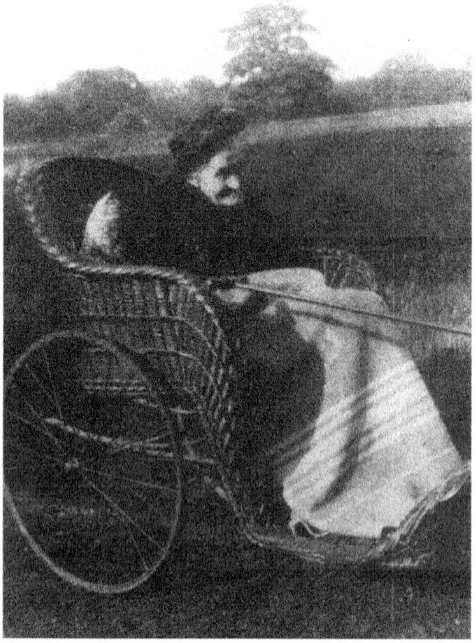

Aunt Bee's bath chair (used in this photograph by the Heydon game-keeper's wife) to which Alison harnessed her pony, Mickey Mouse.

We loved riding our ponies, and hated Sundays, when we were not allowed to ride, and Pinkie's brothers were not allowed to shoot. Sunday was a day of rest for animals, and a day of boredom for children. We went to Sunday school, which Pinkie taught. Then we went to church, and in the evening Pinkie read us Bible stories. I am grateful now for boring Sundays, because the beautiful English of the King James Bible, and Cranmer's Book of Common Prayer, ring in my ears, and I realise that these are no longer familiar to most people. I do wish I had read them to my children for the poetry, but I never did, probably because I was then by no means sure I believed in God, and did not want to tell them lies. On weekdays, Pinkie read us the books we wanted to hear: Black Beauty, over and over again, and the Jungle Books, and Finn, the Tale of a Dog. We never tired of these.

Mary Anne and William said that when they kissed their parents their mother had a furry face, so they called her 'Fur', and their father had a prickly face, so they called him 'Prick'. They really did, and indeed that is how they were addressed by all of us. It must be admitted that Prick's name was mostly pronounced 'Preek', which was only slightly less of a giggle. Their mother's name was Molly, and Prick was Boy, but these names were never used. Once or twice, Prick came home on leave, and taught us riding. He was a Brigadier in the Royal Norfolk Regiment, I think. He made us cross our stirrups over our saddles, so that we bumped at the trot, then we had to go in a figure of eight, exposed to view in the middle of the village green, and Prick shouted, "By the right, wheel" and other military commands. We seldom got it right, which made him so impatient with us that he became quite furious. He would have been a good soldier, and a bad enemy. I was very frightened of him.

It was while we were at Heydon that I noticed that Pinkie was not wearing her engagement ring. It was magnificent, and she did not have it on. I held her hand and asked her where it was. She said that she had dropped it, and damaged it.

"Emeralds are supposed to be unlucky," she said, "probably because emeralds are rather delicate, and are easily damaged. My lovely emerald has a flaw in it. I am afraid it may crack completely and fall out of its setting."

"Where is it?" I asked. "You haven't lost it?"

Pinkie went to her handkerchief drawer, and took it out to show me. The emerald was set in a square of diamonds, and I could see the crack in it.

"I am sure no one could be found to mend it during the war, but afterwards I will take it to a jeweller in London, and see if he can do something. He may have to cut the stone down a bit, which is a shame."

I thought it was a shame too, but I thought little more about it. Everything had to wait till after the war.

Meantime, my father in the war seemed to be having a wonderful time. His letters told us he had plenty of time to buy a horse and go off riding and trying to hunt jackals (no good, they will not run away from dogs) and buying grapefruit and oranges, which we could not get in England, for the Mess. There was a kind of wartime letter that had been photographed to make it as small as a postage stamp so more could be sent on an aeroplane at one time. Then when it got to England it was enlarged again so it could be read. We had no oranges in the war, but in one of these aerographs from Palestine he said that he had sent us a crate of them. It did not arrive because the boat it had been put on was sunk by the Germans. So he sent us another, but that boat was sunk too, so we never got any. I could not really remember what oranges tasted like. Pinkie felt sad for all the sailors who had gone down with the ships, and we said prayers for them. There were no bananas during the war, either, but we always wanted to be given 'banana' sandwiches made with mashed parsnips with banana essence in them. William's favourite hymn was:

We love the place O Lord,
Wherein thine honour dwells

William thought 'thine honour' was 'thy nana', and short for banana, and that when we got to Heaven there would be God's huge banana for us all to eat.

Chapter 9
The Mermaid

My father spent the war in Egypt, Palestine, North Africa and Italy. I did worry that he might suddenly die, like Philip. But I knew, probably Pinkie told me, that his 'fighting' was different. He worked in base hospitals, a long way behind the fighting front, dealing with injured soldiers who had already had First Aid, and now needed more substantial treatment. He would be far from the enemy. He was not at the same risk as a fighter pilot.

My father's letters to his sister, my Aunt Ann, are not terribly happy: more about making the best of a bad job. He wrote her stilted, inarticulate letters. Probably no one who has not been involved in a war, even if not in the forefront of the battle, can really understand how disorienting, depressing and demoralising such a situation can be.

In July 1943 my father writes to Aunt Ann from Cairo: 'It would appear that you have been complaining to Pinkie that I write so seldom. Well, it's true but the same, precisely, to you, my dear. And it is harder far for the exiles to write home as news is scarce, censorship strict and perspiration profuse.' And, further on, 'Yet, one has no regrets, for in looking after these men one is contributing, and without being soppy I can say that they are fine men to look after. Pinkie is wonderful as ever and writes all the time. I couldn't do without her letters and she has looked after Alison wonderfully – truly I am very lucky.'

In the first three letters to Ann he declares, 'I will write to Mother soon'.

In December 1943, the last letter, he writes: 'Pinkie and Alison are quite all right. The latter writes me such prim little letters now in a very neat hand. Alison sweeter than ever – also Pinkie, I need hardly say. Well, I am a bit fed up, as you might expect, the only salvation being that I am very busy indeed, doing a lot of operating and also there is quite a bit of administration. Riding, regularly, and bathing and tennis, squash and cricket – all make life almost tolerable – and the food is adequate. Also, riding in hunter trials and show jumps and point-to-points. I have never been fitter and weigh a stone less. But nothing makes up for exile, and to wilfully choose this as our life, as regular service do – is an indication of a love of adventure which is not in me.' Finally he writes: 'I have heard from Mother and written to her'. And he ends, 'Forgive this rather dull, grousing letter'.

While my father was having what was later described as a 'good war', what was happening to us?

Aunt Ann did not come to Cawston. But in 1943 when I was ten years old we were evacuated again and Pinkie, Mickey, Gretchen and I went to stay in Bolwick Hall in Norfolk near Marsham, with Pinkie's Uncle Walter, who seemed to me to be so old he might at any moment die, though in fact he was only 68. If you had a big house that was not full during the war, the Army could come and requisition it and fill it with soldiers, who everyone said would do it no end of harm. But if you kept evacuees or refugees in your house, the army left it alone. I expect Uncle Walter did not want soldiers. I lived at Bolwick with Pinkie, Gretchen and Mickey, and other refugees: her friends Diana and Rosemary whose husbands were away fighting, and their children. Sometimes, when the blitz (the bombing in London) was particularly bad, some of Uncle Walter's great-nephews and nieces were evacuated and came to stay too. Because Pinkie, Diana and Rosemary were looking after some refugee children at Bolwick, that was probably enough to prevent Pinkie being called up, so she did not have to give me up.

Bolwick Hall was a handsome 18th century grey brick country house set in parkland with tall elm trees shading the Old English park cattle. It had great big sash windows letting in a lot of light, so much so that if the carafes of water were left on the dining room table between meals on sunny days, these round-bellied vessels focussed the sun's rays and burned a small black hole in the mahogany table. As the sun went round, the burning moved, and tiny C-shaped blackened ditches could be found all over the table. Uncle Walter got very cross if he found another. There was a portrait of the great Quaker prison-reformer, Elizabeth

Fry, on the wall in the dining room, wearing a rather unattractive cap. She is the one who graced the British five pound notes from 2002–2016. The portrait no doubt hung there because she was related to Uncle Walter and all the four Norfolk Quaker banking families: Buxtons, like Uncle Walter; Barclays, like Ione, Noons and Evelyn; Birkbecks, with whom I did lessons; and Gurneys.

Food was in short supply at this stage of the war, and we had high tea with boiled eggs instead of supper. The smell of burning methylated spirits always reminds me of wartime high tea, because on the table stood a delicate silver kettle balanced in a silver rack above a methylated spirit flame, gently hissing. In bright sunlight the flame was barely visible: it seemed to be just moving air. Uncle Walter tipped hot water from the kettle into the teapot to top it up. Children had milk from Home Farm (the closest Bolwick farm to the Hall) and not tea, which was thought not good for us, and anyway it was rationed. Afterwards we all went to sit in front of the fire in the little sitting room because that was the only warm place, and there the grown-ups listened to the wireless for the news, and mended clothes, and cut them down to size for us, and unravelled old jerseys, knitting them up again as socks and jerseys and pixie hoods for us.

The dogs, Jonathan and Gretchen, snored on the mat in front of the fire all day long. Uncle Walter went off to his study, where I suppose he might have had a fire, but I cannot remember. He was very hardy, so he probably just wore more clothes. We had no fires in any other rooms, so they were only used in summer. There was a black line round the bath that showed how deep we were allowed to have the water, and two of us children had to be bathed together to save hot water. The bath itself was huge and the metal cold, and it had a plug like a long pipe that reached from the height of the taps down to the plughole. I always felt very cold in the bath, because although my bottom was sitting in hot water, most of me stuck up into the ice-cold steamy air.

Even our bones felt cold in the frosts of winter, and the rubber hot-water bottles had all gone rotten (it was called 'perished') and could not be replaced. We children were allowed hot-water bottles, but they were the stone ones, which burned our bleeding chilblained feet, though at least the heat lasted nearly all night. We had painful chilblains on most of our fingers and toes, that burst, and the frozen flesh beneath them was reluctant and slow to heal.

A handsome staircase with spirally carved banisters and great big wooden hanging knobs descended to the hall, a hall so large that dances could have been held in it. A green baize door at the back of the hall swung both ways to let the servants to and fro with trays, and beyond it was a wide plain wooden back staircase. These Bolwick staircases are still the standard for me. Whenever I read about a particular staircase in a book, for example there has been a murder on the stairs, or the heroine in her wedding dress comes down to greet her guests, it is one of these that in my mind I apply to it.

The other warm place, of course, was the kitchen through the baize door, with the Aga in it. But neither dogs nor children were popular there, because we tried to pinch food as it came from the oven and was set out to cool. We were quite hungry much of the time. Our favourite supper was called 'savoury rice', which was just fried cooked rice with a rasher or two of bacon chopped up in it, and a few currants. Given a choice, we always asked for that. We valued the sweetness of the currants above all else. In the winter, there was a fire in the Servants' Hall on Sunday evenings, and we children went there and sang hymns accompanied by a housemaid on the wheezing harmonium.

The elm trees in the park rocked in the winds of spring to the cawing of rooks, squabbling over nesting twigs. Uncle Walter had a gun room into which we children were never allowed, though we peered in whenever we got the chance. He seemed to have all four walls covered in locked glass cases full of guns: he could probably have equipped a small platoon, except that these were shotguns, suitable for killing birds, not soldiers. In late spring he shot up through the branches at the rooks in their nests. The babies fell to the ground and lay there pathetically calling. I picked one up and put it in an empty aviary in the walled garden. I dug up handfuls of earthworms for it. Uncle Walter found it two days later and wrung its neck. I was angry that he could do such a cruel thing to a helpless baby bird, but he said: "I don't want rooks. Why do you think I shoot them?" So I went out in my gumboots straight after high tea and carefully walked up and down on two rows of young leeks Uncle Walter was growing in the vegetable garden. I could hear them snapping and scrunching under my feet. I had small brown gumboots, and they could tell it was me from the tracks. Pinkie made me go to his study and say sorry to him, but I was not sorry inside: I thought it served him right.

The lawn on the east side of the house went down to the lake, where there was moored a delightful tiny, almost toy, canvas canoe. I was allowed to use it if I took great care of it. The lake was fed by the Mermaid stream, and under a footbridge over the Mermaid I saw a kingfisher fly out of a small hole. I told Pinkie I thought I might have seen a kingfisher's nest hole. She said that if I was very gentle I could probably get my skinny hand and arm right in, and pull out one of the babies to look at.

"But make sure you put it back quickly," she said. "Think how you are frightening it, and worrying its mother."

Next time I put my hand and arm right up to my armpit in the disgusting slimy tunnel, lined with rotting bones of little fish like sticklebacks, and pulled out an ugly baby kingfisher, all grey quills and monstrous beak. I quickly put it back again, and sat quite still in the canoe to watch the flash of blue and silver as the kingfishers dived for more fish. I was astonished that something so nasty and smelly could grow up to be so skilled and brilliant: a better version, I thought, of Hans Christian Andersen's ugly duckling. Swans did nest on an island in the lake, and I thought their soft grey babies were beautiful, not ugly at all.

On the bank of the Mermaid, beneath the birch trees, in autumn there were the red toadstools, the ones with little flecks of white on their caps. Uncle Walter was good at tapestry, and he had sewed all the tapestry dining room chair seats with patterns of his own design, of the interesting wild plants at Bolwick. His one of the fly agarics (those red toadstools) looked so natural, you could imagine picking them.

At the other end of the lake stood the mill, its huge wheel gone now, perhaps to be melted down for guns: I am not sure. Next to it there was the racquets court with leaking roof and green slimy floor. No one played racquets there. The water here was very deep, with a very long drop from the overflow to the continuation of the Mermaid below. It was dark under the trees, and felt spooky and I was frightened of the deep water, somehow imagining that it could draw me down, and I especially disliked the steady 'tock, tock' noise of the underground ram, the job of which was to drive water up to the house. It reminded me of the crocodile who swallowed the clock in Peter Pan. In this part of the stream, under the stones, I caught 'miller's thumbs', strange lumpy brown fish with

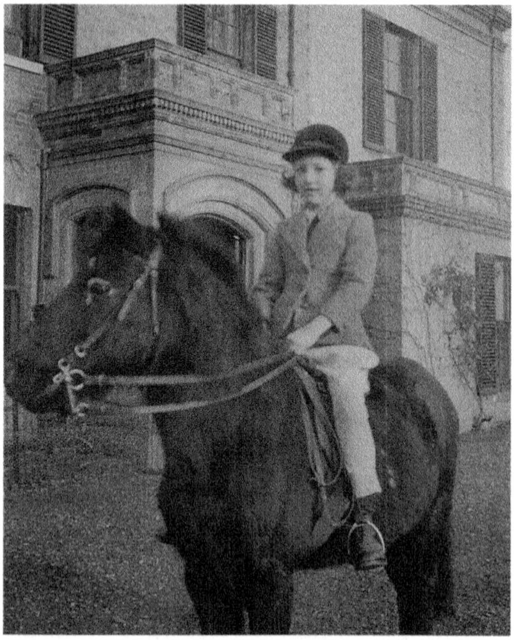

Alison on Mickey Mouse, her beloved first pony. Outside Bolwick Hall, about 1942.

big heads, which sadly never survived even a day in an aquarium.

A pair of barn owls nested in the stables. As I climbed the ladder to the hay loft to get Mickey some hay, there by the trap door sat the four babies, shuffling from one foot to another, and staring with enormous eyes, hissing and sizzling at me with disapproval. The smell of the hay was comforting and warm, but even so it took some courage to go up there and face the angry owlets.

In summertime, after a long ride in the rain, I led Mickey, sweating, into an enormous stable, built for a horse the size of my father's huge hunter, Caravan: far too big in every dimension for tiny Mickey. There were no hunters at Bolwick during the war, of course, so Mickey could have it: indeed he had to have it, because if left out to grass he ate so much and grew so fat he got laminitis, which gave him swollen sore feet. I took off his saddle and bridle, stroked his neck and nose, made a wisp (like a thick piece of rope twisted up on itself) of some of the golden pile of oat straw lying in one corner, and rubbed all the steaming sweaty patches dry.

I poured a cold bucket of water in his trough, reached up with a pitchfork to put plenty of hay in his rack, and gave him a handful of cow cake in the manger. He put his nose down to sniff his bedding, wandered about so I had to follow him round with the dandy brush, stretched out his hind legs like a greyhound, and urinated. A well-built stable like this, with mahogany doors and sides and iron railings on top, had a good central drain down which the urine disappeared leaving only a warm wet smell.

This was the first time he had had to be put in the stable. After I left him I thought about what he would have made of it, and although I had looked after him properly as I had been taught, I wondered what he himself would say about it, if he could. It was Pinkie who taught me that if you are looking after an animal you will often understand it and care for it better, if sometimes you put yourself in its shoes, so to speak, and try to think like it does.

"I haven't been in here before. There isn't anything here for me: just a bit of straw. I am tired now, and hungry. I need to roll on grass and eat and eat and eat it. That's right, take off my heavy saddle, and get that bit out of my mouth. I want to go out to the field now, but you have shut the half door and made this a prison. The edge of the water trough is so high that it digs into my neck and I can hardly swallow. And how do you expect me to get hay out of that rack without standing on my hind legs? There is no need to rub and brush me. Feed me. You have given me just a handful of cow cake, is that it? I can grab a mouthful and then pull my head out of the trough to gobble them, and they spill on the ground, but I can eat them there more easily than in that neck-breaking manger. I want you to go away. Stop stroking me. I don't like my head touched. Perhaps you'll go if I pee. Aha, there you go."

The Old English Park Cattle were white with black noses, ears, knees and tail tips, and had a few black spots down their backs. Some of the rabbits we kept were called Old English too, and had the same colouring. We used to go to Home Farm and climb up and sit on the high wooden wall of the bull's stall, and wing acorns at him. He had curly hair and such a thick neck that he could not look up and see where we were. He did get very angry, and snorted loudly and pawed the ground, and we were told to stop it because it was cruel and dangerous. "Think what would happen if one of you falls in," the old farm workers said.

As part of Uncle Walter's war effort we kept rabbits. I had a pet one, a tiny little chocolate coloured Havana rabbit. She had bulging eyes and a constantly twitching whiskered nose, and smelled very sweet. She was never to be eaten, but all the others were for food, and I felt extremely sorry for them. In winter, the farm delivered stalks of kale for the rabbits. Our fingers froze cutting them up lengthways into quarters so that the rabbits could eat the translucent green pith. Even their chisel teeth were not capable of grinding their way through the outer fibre. I was allowed to take my rabbit up to the farm to be mated, and told I could watch as long as I did not talk about it at high tea, when Uncle Walter joined us. I never saw anything, because no mating happened, but I always wondered why I was not allowed to talk about it. Every afternoon in summer we went for walks down the country lanes with a handcart, picking food for rabbits. In summertime now I never see a fine piece of cow parsley, or hogweed, without thinking how much a rabbit would like it.

A couple of times, as we walked down the lanes, the stallion came by. I found this thrilling: the stallion was a huge bay Shire horse being led by a short man in a fawn coat and breeches. The horse wore a blinkered bridle and a leading rein, and his mane and tail were plaited with ribbons. He had a great fat arched neck, and as he proudly walked, swinging his legs with their curtains of long black hair, we could feel the ground shake beneath his hooves. We had to push the handcarts onto the verge, and stand very still when he came by, so as not to frighten him, because if he did take fright, his tiny groom would not have been able to hold him. He was being walked from farm to farm in the district, to do his duty serving the farm carthorse mares. He probably weighed a ton, and my heart pounded as he went by.

Some days we went on our walks past a cottage where a very old, dirty, smelly, bearded and long-haired man called Abraham lived. Pinkie and Diana went to see him, to see if he was all right, and he came to the door and shouted rudely at us. Eventually it was decided that he was no longer fit to look after himself and live on his own. He would be better off in the workhouse at Aylsham. Every time we saw him he shouted, "I'm not going to the workhouse, I'm not". But one day they came with an ambulance and took him by force, and everyone in the village could hear him screaming and bellowing in misery and rage. I could not understand how they could use force to take away a man who had done nobody any harm, and lock him up in the workhouse. The thought of that cruelty to him upset me as much as the wringing of the baby rook's neck.

I rode Mickey two miles across country to do lessons with the neighbours' governess, at Rippon Hall. In November, I rode past earthy fields where German and Italian prisoners of war were cutting the leaves and roots off sugar beet, in the frost, with bare hands. People said it was a backbreaking job, and were glad we had the prisoners to do it. I used to think that if my father got taken prisoner, he might have to work with sugar beet, and I knew he would not like that.The prisoners always smiled and waved at Mickey and me, as we went trotting by.

The Birkbecks with whom I did lessons with were three sisters. Diana, the youngest, had been a bridesmaid with me at Ione Barclay's wedding. They were extremely tough girls: nothing frightened them. Known collectively all over Norfolk as 'The Boos', they were not only fearless, but in later years, extremely pretty: a devastating combination. Louie, their governess, wanted to teach us everything, but the only thing we wanted to learn was drawing and painting. We used to bring Mickey through the French windows into the school room, tie him to the fat wooden foot of an upholstered armchair, and then draw and paint him. Louie would suggest algebra, and we would shout "No, no, let's take our easels and do landscape drawing," and Louie came with us on our ponies and taught us perspective, and good ways to draw trees. I do not think the parent Birkbecks paid much attention to what exactly Louie was teaching us, and I really do not remember learning anything but drawing with her, but she made us do it well, in pencil and charcoal, making linocuts, using pastels, and watercolours and oil paints. This seemed to me quite the nicest sort of learning, and I was very happy doing it.

Opposite the front door of Rippon Hall there was a cedar of Lebanon, and attached to a high branch was a long chain that went under the middle of a seesaw, a seesaw that was just a plain very long plank of wood. One other girl did lessons with us. We called her Bittern, because her father was a naturalist, and these rare birds lived in the reeds on a broad he owned. We were told the birds made an odd booming call, but I had never heard it. Neither Bittern nor I were anywhere near as tough and ruthless as The Boos. They used to put the two of us on either end of the seesaw and rotate it until it was too high for them to reach above their heads, and the chains were clanking and knotting themselves in anger as the seesaw rose. Then they let go, and the seesaw started to turn, slowly at first. Every time it came to a knot in the chain there was a tremendous jump, and as it gathered speed we were clinging on desperately to the plank with our hands and knees: the world swung by in a blur until the chains were undone and the seesaw started to wind up again, with the threatening chains knotting above us. The Boos really enjoyed it, laughing uproariously. I always felt physically sick, and sometimes when I got off I was sick. As I lay in bed at night worrying about it, I remembered my father saying "Never show anyone, or a horse or a dog, that you are afraid, or it will be worse for you. Hold your head up, laugh, show courage, and you will be all right". I knew what to do, but I found it very hard to do it. It was a fair training, though. You can take anything, if you set your mind to it, and tell yourself it is not going to go on for ever.

We had rabbits at Rippon too, but these were pet Angora rabbits. They have the softest, fluffiest fur of any mammal (it flies up your nose and makes you sneeze madly) and they have temperaments that are anything but soft. Each one has to be brushed for ten minutes morning and evening, or their fur becomes hard, lumpy knots pulling at their skin. If they do have knots, the only way to deal with them is to cut them off, infinitely slowly, almost one hair at a time, with a pair of nail scissors. As they were groomed, the Boos' Angora rabbits tried their mightiest to kill us. The poor things lived in a state of permanent apprehension, terror and rage at being hurt by the hair pulling, and if not firmly held, they galloped at us, bit deeply, scratched and viciously kicked us. Apparently they are usually kept by nuns, and perhaps nuns are more patient and kinder than we were, though I bet the rabbits are still pretty fierce with them. When she grew up, Bittern herself became a nun, and I sometimes wonder if her decision had anything to do with the skills she had learned in trying to make friends with, and soothe, furious Angora rabbits. The Boos gripped their rabbits tight and laughed at their fury. I, less brave, got seriously bitten and scratched.

Before they kept Angoras, the Boos had black pet rabbits, some of which had escaped, and with no gardeners to prevent them had established themselves in a great warren in the lawn, which was pocked with rabbit holes. There, rabbits were shot early every morning by the Boos' father, Christo, and brought indoors for the pot. The Boos had seen one or two shot ones with black fur, and made it a rule that in no circumstances would we children eat them. At lunchtime with the grown-ups we sat silently staring at our empty place mats, our lower lips stuck out in disapproval. "It would be like eating our own children," the Boos announced. We did not go hungry, though. Wartime rationing and shortages did not prevent us from getting sweetcorn or globe artichokes from the walled garden to begin with, and sago pudding with milk from their farm and stewed apple from their own trees afterwards. Christo kept gundogs, and the Rippon Hall kitchen smelt disgustingly of the stockpot that lived permanently in the simmering oven of their Aga, into which all plates were scraped after meals, making sour-smelling stock to flavour the dogs' biscuits.

The Boos were excellent riders, and on my first day there they took away my saddle, saying: "You'll never ride properly with that. Must learn to ride bareback, if you want to be any good."

They were so right. If you want to learn to ride, start bareback. You can feel every movement of the warm horse beneath you, and although it is slithery and slippery, you very quickly learn to keep your balance on it, to curve your lower back outwards slightly and sit back on your haunches: go with it and become one with it. You will fall off more often at first, of course, but falling off is easy, bareback. There is no danger of getting a foot tangled up in the stirrups and being dragged along, head bumping on the ground. After a bit, you do not fall off any more. The horse can buck and shy and rear up and paw the air, and you stay on. If you want to win a bending race, nipping in and out of the poles with a quick turn at the end before you bend back, you will do it much faster bareback. Now you can really ride, and it is a skill you will never forget.

Outside his study, Uncle Walter had a framed miniature plaster cast of the Elgin marbles, and I used to look longingly at it and wish Mickey was a bit less stumpy and a bit more like one of those spirited little Greek horses. But the Greeks rode bareback, I could see, and so I knew they were brilliant riders. I wanted to ride like them, and if only the summer would get warm enough, I would like to try it like them, naked. I never tried, of course. With Uncle Walter just the other side of the study wall, I knew that would cause trouble.

I used to hate the wireless. All it had was boring news about battles and bombs. The grown-ups listened to it for a whole hour every lunchtime, and they said shut up to us because they wanted to hear. I once asked them if there was any news on the radio before the war, and if so, what was it about? They looked puzzled, and said they could not really remember, but they thought it was about weddings and sports and things. Sometimes the grown-ups told each other that Hitler had laid another egg last night, and they said where. We knew perfectly well they were talking about bombs, and did not want to frighten us.

Because of the big sandy coastline of Norfolk, and the important aerodromes around, it was thought that Hitler might invade there, and pillboxes had been built on the coast and in the fields from which the Home Guard was going to defend us if the Germans came. We children were told never to go inside a pillbox, in case the Germans had already arrived, and were holed up inside one. As I rode past them, I used to imagine a frightened German running out. How would I know he was a German? Not sure. But Mickey and I would do our bit and gallop after him, and grab him by the collar and hold him down until the Home Guard turned up to arrest him. I could not be certain, with Mickey being so small, that I could have reached up to the man's collar, but, if I had a saddle, I would have stood up in my stirrups and had a damn good try. Imagining myself doing things like this I thought I would be helping with the war effort, helping to win the war like my father, and helping to bring him home again.

We were warned of things called 'anti-personnel mines', which the Germans, when they came, might lay under tufts of grass on the ground. They were hidden, and we had no idea how to find them or tell that they were there, but we did know that if you stepped on one you would be blown up. I worried about them as we cantered down the road edges on the way to Aylsham. The thought of my adored Mickey being blown up gave me terrible nightmares.

There were some big aerodromes near Bolwick, because Norfolk is close to Germany, and very flat (Noel Coward was right). After we children had gone to bed, we could hear a loud groaning noise, and if we looked out of the window we could see the grown-ups standing on the lawn counting the hundreds and hundreds of huge bombers called Flying Fortresses and Liberators, darkening the evening sky, going over to bomb Germany at night. It was summertime, and we heard them flying back, very low over the house, just as it was getting light. If we looked out of the window then, there were the grown ups-again, in their slippers and dressing gowns, on the dewy lawn, counting them back, to see how many had been shot down.

In summertime too, we could use the drawing room, because it was not unbearably cold and darkened with the shutters and curtains drawn as it was in winter. On some weekends, Canadian airmen from the nearby aerodromes took 36-hour leave at Bolwick (it was part of the war effort), and one man in particular could play the piano well, so we stood round it in the drawing room in the long summer evenings, singing hymns and songs. I particularly remember 'Coming in on a wing and a prayer':

Though there's one engine gone,
We can still carry on,
Coming in on a wing and a prayer.

We shared our rations with the airmen. They got bacon and eggs for breakfast, for instance, but they said we should not do it because they could get plenty on the air base. We thought it was right to treat them, because they had only these two days' holiday from flying, and their work was dangerous, and they might be shot down. Having seen the devastation that the shooting down of Philip at Cawston caused, I was very frightened for those airmen, and I am sure that Pinkie and the other grown-ups knew how fragile their lives were, and we prayed they would always fly home safely.

When the war moved to Italy, my father was put in charge of a big base hospital in Naples. He brought back from the war a few little faded photographs of himself sitting on his horse and buying many barrels of wine, and sometimes pigs, for the Mess. He often had to work hard, but sometimes the war went quiet and there was nothing to do, so he had a local cobbler make for him a leather head harness, so that he could strap two or three books on top of his head. Then he swam out into the Bay of Naples to a flat rock and lay in the scorching sun with little waves lapping around him and read, and if the hospital needed him, they hoisted a big yellow flag and he swam back.

In the Easter after I became nine, in 1943, I was absolutely horrified to be told by Pinkie that I was to be sent in the summer term to a boarding school. My father had said I must go, Pinkie told me.

"But why, why must I go?" I kept asking. "I don't want to go."

At this school we all wore purple. The headmistress wore a purple coat and skirt, and had purple hair; well, actually, white hair dyed mauve. We had to wear purple tunics, purple and silver striped ties (which I could never tie), and purple bloomers, knickers with long legs with elastic in them, which we wore tightly rolled up our thighs, probably encouraging varicose veins in the process. Wearing this uniform I did not feel like Alison Elizabeth Brittain. I was just a purple girl and had no longer any sense of who I was. I lived in a dormitory, and worked in a class full of purple girls. I did not know any of them, either. The school was in Horwood House, in Buckinghamshire.

The black abyss was back, and now there was no one to pull me out. As I lay sleepless in bed in the dormitory, I physically missed Pinkie's voice and touch. I missed the soft cuddliness and doggy smell of my Gretchen, and the glossy new summer coat of Mickey. I realised I had no person or animal left to love, and there was no one to love me. I had been used to being good with Pinkie, and doing what she asked me, because we loved each other, and it was easy. But now that I had no one, I felt quite certain that the only way to survive on my own was, at all costs, to avoid doing what the bossy teachers told me to do. I would do what they wanted only if I wanted to. Otherwise, in order to preserve myself, I would suit myself. Of course, now I understand why this turned out to be a most unproductive attitude, but then I could not help it.

What did I learn at that school? I learnt to put 'i' before 'e' except after 'c', and where apostrophes go, and a great deal of Palgrave's Golden Treasury. We had to run the gauntlet of senior girls on the way down to breakfast. They wrote you down for a punishment, a 'lateness point', if you had failed to strip your bed, or clean your teeth, or polish your shoes, or clean your nails. I got four lateness points on my way down, and another for being late for breakfast, every day. For five lateness points, you got a punishment. So I had to learn a poem for this punishment every day, and some of them I am glad I did. We could choose to learn anything we liked from Palgrave's Golden Treasury. I probably learned nearly half of it, and much of it has stayed with me. And then in despair one day because I seemed so deserving of punishments, and thus unable to allow anyone to get the better of me and so improve, I remember reciting to the duty mistress:

> Alfred Lord Tennyson:
>
> Break, break, break,
>
> On thy cold grey stones, O sea!
>
> And I would that my tongue could utter
>
> The thoughts that arise in me.

And she stopped me there, and asked "Why did you choose that one?"

The usual answer I would have given, of course, would be "I don't know", but I disgraced myself by bursting into tears and blurting out: "Because I can't bear it here, and I can't tell anyone."

And after that I did not seem to have to spend so much of my time doing punishments. But I still felt completely abandoned in that school. Every day except Sunday we queued up for letters, but I never had any. None from my father, none even from Pinkie. It seemed so unlike them both, I wondered what had happened to them. I did get a blue and purple picture postcard of the mountains in Ireland from my Uncle Douglas in the Navy, and on it was written: 'Ireland is like a saucer, a hollow in the middle full of bog, and mountains round the edge'. It was the only post I got all the time I was there, and I kept it under my pillow and read it often, because it did show that someone outside knew I was there.

Horwood House, in Buckinghamshire, was another large country house, probably being saved from the depredations of the army by being used as a boarding school for girls evacuated from Upper Chine, in the Isle of Wight, which was considered to be in danger of invasion by Hitler. Old girls made new girls climb a rope onto a high branch of a cedar tree, and jump off. It was a horrifying drop, and landing hurt all the bones in your body, and made you bite your tongue till it bled, even though the ground is quite soft beneath a cedar. A few years ago I went to look at it. The tree was still there, but that branch had been cut off. From the scar on the trunk I should say that the drop was at least 15 feet.

There were ornamental lily ponds, with yew hedges around them. On hot days we were made to sit on the stone edges, with our feet in the water. A teacher was in charge of us, but she just sat in a chair, and knitted. We new girls had to offer up our big toes to classmates who made slits in them with the razor blades we used to sharpen our pencils. Then we had to put our feet back in the water, and the trail of blood soon attracted the goldfish, which came and sucked the wounds. It did not hurt, because the water was cold enough to numb our feet, but I remember thinking how interesting that goldfish like blood so much, and what a strange feeling it was, having them sucking your toes. But there was one poor little new girl, called Ursula, who had terrible nightmares about it, and screamed in her sleep. We had to wake her up and reassure her, "Ursula, Ursula, look at your toes. Look, no fish. See, they aren't there? No fish at all. Don't worry about it any more." I bet she did not tell her parents, because they would not have understood, and might not have believed her.

Then one day to my utter joy Pinkie came to see me. I was allowed to go and meet her off the train at the little Halt at the bottom of the Park. It was wonderful to be hugged to her soft bosom, and to smell again her delicious smell. She only had an hour before she had to catch the only train back, so we sat in the grass, and had a picnic she had brought, and talked. I pleaded, "Please, please, take me back with you to Heydon," and she said she could not, but that the headmistress had written to my father saying I should leave the school at the end of term. What a relief! But then she said that I had to be evacuated again and go to live with my aunts in Dublin.

"But I don't want to," I said. "No! I won't go unless you come."

"I know you don't," said Pinkie, "but I can't come, and I'm afraid your father says you have to go." I really did not want to go. I was used to Pinkie now, I thought of her as my mother, and I loved and trusted her, and she loved me. I could not think why she had not fought harder for me, with my father. I had learned that the person I was with was infinitely more important than any place I happened to be. I would willingly have gone to Ireland or anywhere else with Pinkie, but not alone. I only knew one of my aunts, Aunt Ann, wife of Uncle Douglas the postcard sender, and I could hardly even remember her.

I stayed in the park for hours, till it was dark, after the train chugged slowly away with Pinkie: I simply could not bear to go back to the school. When I turned up after supper they were very cross because they had been looking for me. But all I was thinking about was how could I stop being made to go to Ireland?

I had one last forlorn hope. If only the war could be over, then my father would come and take me home with him and marry Pinkie. I knew how I would know that the war was over. I remember hoping, wishing and praying that, some time in the next few days, in spite of the horror of it, John Barratt would turn up, waving Hitler's moustache.

Chapter 10
Slugs and Snails

In the Autumn of 1943, when term ended at Horwood House, Pinkie came with me on the train to Holyhead and put me alone on the boat to Ireland, and asked some nuns to look after me. I was absolutely choking at saying goodbye to her, and could not really understand why I had to go. I am glad I did not know then that my father would never marry Pinkie, and that she would never mother me again. I cannot imagine how I could have coped with that. As soon as I was on that boat I felt desperately lonely and sad and homesick for Pinkie and Mary Anne and William and Gretchen and Mickey and Jonathan and Heydon. I am afraid that if I had known that I would never really see Pinkie again, I think I would have jumped overboard. I tried to comfort myself by thinking and praying that the war would soon be over, that my father would come back, and that we would all be together again. I never stopped loving her, and never in the rest of my life did I find anyone else whom I could love and trust enough to accept as my mother.

The nuns on the boat sat on deck on hard wooden slatted benches in the biting wind, and did nothing but pray silently, pulling their rosaries through their fingers, blue with lack of circulation. I decided not to be a nun. They said nothing to me and seemed very dull, so when I had finished praying for the war to be over I left them and went exploring the boat. I went down and down the stairs and found a kitchen where two black cooks in chef's hats were frying eggs. These were the first black people I had ever seen and we quickly became friends. They seemed to have a great many eggs; eggs were rationed in England, but they said there were plenty in Ireland, and these were Irish eggs. There was a huge square pan with 30 eggs in rows sputtering in it. One chef just kept breaking them in, and they were cooked by the time the other one took them out. They explained to me how quick you have to be to cook eggs perfectly. I spent the rest of the journey practicing breaking eggs for them, and helping clear up when we had finished. When we arrived in Ireland, I was the last person to go through Customs. Aunt Ann who had come to collect me was worried that she could not find me. It was 1943 in late autumn, and I was still only ten years old then, and I had brought a pet slug with me in a jam jar. I proudly showed it to the Customs man who said I could not bring it into the country. So I said I did not want to go to Ireland either, and please could I go back on the boat? My aunt at last found me, in floods of tears, stamping my foot and shrieking at the Customs man that it was jolly well *my* slug and he was not having it. In the end he let me keep it.

My Aunts had plenty of children. I had 16 cousins in Dublin. I went to and fro between three families of aunts and their children. One more aunt, Phyllis, would not have me, because she was having another baby, which she said was enough.

In Dublin, although I missed my pony Mickey very much indeed, I heard that he was given to William, and later to one of Mary Ann and William's brothers, David, who was born with achondroplasia and so stayed small and never grew out of Mickey. They were very happy together. I missed Gretchen too, but she was well looked after, because she, lucky dog, stayed the rest of the war with Pinkie.

My Aunt Ann was my guardian, and officially I lived with her and her two sons, James and John. Uncle Douglas (who had so kindly sent me the postcard at boarding school) was not at home. He had volunteered to be a chaplain in the navy, and was on the ships plying the seas round the North Cape of Norway to Archangel and Murmansk in Russia: the Russian Convoys. His ship, HMS Trinidad, was badly damaged, like a great many others, but he was quickly rescued. The rescue had to be fast, or the swimmer died of cold: those seas were freezing cold at the best of times, and solid ice in winter. The only thing he hung onto as he jumped overboard to be rescued was his portable typewriter, which was completely ruined by the salt water, so, as he told us later, he need not have bothered.

My father heard about it, and wrote to Ann: 'Please write to me and tell me about your life and everything. You must have had a nerve-wracking time after Douglas left. I sent all sorts of messages to you from various places on the way out, as I heard about the Trinidad then, but later, I heard from Pinkie that Douglas was all right'. In one of his letters from North Africa to Aunt Ann, written some time before I arrived in Ireland, my father suddenly announces, apropos of nothing, 'I am busy learning Italian'. All the letters sent home by soldiers during the war were censored to make sure that if they fell into enemy hands, they gave nothing away that the War Office did not want the Germans to know. Writing he was 'learning Italian' is him getting round the censor. He intends that Ann shall interpret this remark as 'I am being posted to Italy'.

I am not certain that Ann would have interpreted it correctly. At that time Uncle Douglas was waiting on HMS Trinidad somewhere in Northern Ireland to be sent off to Murmansk. When he went, Aunt Ann stayed on in tiny Lavender Cottage in Lancing, Sussex, where Douglas had trained for holy orders. He sent Ann a telegram. She was so distressed on getting it, that she immediately telephoned Mabel, asking if she could come and stay with her in Dublin because she had had worrying news.

"Of course you can. Come at once."

So Aunt Ann caught the next boat over, and Mabel fetched her off the ship.

"So what is this terrible news you've had?"

"It's Douglas, he sent me a telegram. He's being posted to the Galatians on 22nd May: he's going to have to go and fight."

Reaching her house in Leeson Park, Mabel said: "Can I see the telegram?"

She read it, and said, "Let's get an atlas. I think St Paul wrote letters to the Galatians. Let's see where Douglas is going."

So they looked at the telegram again, and it said 'GALATIANS V.22'.

"That's not a place where Douglas is being sent," said Mabel. "He's not going to the Galatians, wherever they may be (they probably don't exist today) on May 22nd. It's a text, isn't it? Now we need a Bible. He wants you to look it up."

So Aunt Ann, feeling a bit small and stupid, but highly relieved to be among family again, looked it up:

> 'But the fruit of the Spirit is love, joy, peace, longsuffering, gentleness, good ness, faith, meekness, temperance. . .'

It was a list of virtues. Douglas had just taken holy orders, and was telling her how pleased he was that he had done so. He thought it had been good for him, and was grateful to Ann for letting him do it. He was not telling her where he was going: he was telling her he loved her. She stayed on in Dublin after that.

The house in Anglesea Road where we lived looked out over a rugby ground, and we watched the matches out of my bedroom window. Games like rugby and football were still going on in Ireland, though they had ceased in wartime England. At the bottom of our garden ran the Dodder, the river that powered the bakers with the pleasant names of Johnston, Mooney and O'Brien.

My cousin John, six years younger than me, was the darling of the family. He had had tuberculosis, and though he had now recovered, he was always given the best of everything, and made a great pet. Needless to say, James and I were jealous of him and used to think of ways of tormenting him. The river was very shallow, and James and I could wade across it, but John's gumboots were too short, and we took much delight in holding both his hands to help him across, and then when his boots filled with water, delivering him back to Nanny for a scolding.

We lived with Nanny in the nursery in the dark basement, and the kitchen was the front basement room, with a big black range, and Nora the cook. Nora, in her blue apron that exactly matched her eyes, was young, shapely, blonde and pretty, and even we knew that the milkman fancied her. He had a pony and cart with two milk churns on it, and came down the area steps to meet Nora with the blue and white striped jugs. He had dippers which held one pint and half a pint, and when he had given Nora her order, he took a special little dipper and gave her a bit more, with a wide grin, "For the fairies".

When we were having breakfast in the nursery, Nanny once left the room. James and I were messing about with the things on the table, and I took a butter pat (in Aunt Ann's house, butter was always presented in pats, made by Nora with two reeded wooden bats) and put it on the end of my knife, and bent the blade back and flicked it away, and it flew up and stuck on the ceiling. Delighted, James immediately imitated me, and in a minute we had all the butter pats up there.

"Don't look up," I hissed, "when Nanny comes back. However much you want to, we mustn't look at the ceiling, or she'll guess."

We kept our nerve, and did not look, and Nanny seemed not to notice anything although we were frantically trying to suppress giggles, when suddenly the warmth up at ceiling level got to the butter and a pat came down and landed with a nasty yellow squelch, the softened grease oozing into the tablecloth. I had to own up as being the one who had thought of it, and had to go to Aunt Ann for a talking to, because Nanny was threatening to leave. As far as I was concerned she could leave when she liked.

James and I were supposed to walk to school, but sometimes we used our pocket money to go on the bus. We became excellent at imitating the bus conductor's tuberculous cough. "Er-hm", we went, "Er-hm, er-hm, aargh-hm, aargh-hm, oich-hm, oich-hm, oich-hm," and then with much effort we forced the imaginary phlegm up our throats and spat it out: "coihhggha". We thought this was terribly funny, but Aunt Ann did not. What were we doing, where had we learnt such a disgusting thing? We said "I don't know."

Eric was a laundering uncle, and Dico a dry cleaning one. Sometimes I stayed at Carrickmines with Aunt Doris and Uncle Dico, who was in charge of the dry cleaning part of the Swastika Laundry. He had a most impressive wartime car. Before breakfast he went out and lit two anthracite stoves in the boot. After breakfast he blew them hotter, until a large black balloon on the roof was filled with gas. Then, leaving a rather nasty smell behind him, he set off in a stately fashion for the dry-cleaners.

Aunt Doris had a Basenji dog, called Trigger. He was chestnut and white, very bouncy, with a curious tail stiffly curled over his back that was impossible to uncurl. Aunt Doris was particularly proud of the fact that he was silent, and unable to bark. Her oldest son Philip said: "Come on, Alison, it's got to be possible to make Trigger bark," and I agreed. We barked at him furiously, with no result, though he became quite excited.

After various other attempts, we finally found a way to make him bark, nearly. I gripped him between my knees, one hand holding his collar, the other his muzzle. Philip then applied the nozzle of a bicycle pump to the Basenji's ear and pumped like mad. I am afraid children can be horrible, and we were no exception. I feel very sorry about it now, but then we got great satisfaction from hearing that poor dog frantically trying to howl.

If it surprises me now that a laundry and a dry cleaners should make a whole family so prosperous and well established, I must remember the main reason, not obvious today. It was not just that Dublin was damp, and Grandpa had a Protestant work ethic. We forget, in these days of washing machines, that washing by hand the clothes and bed linen of a family once took a whole week. If you remember the song 'Dashing Away with a Smoothing Iron', it takes the singer's darling a whole week to wash her clothes:

> T'was on a Monday morning,
> When I beheld my darling,
> She looked so neat and charming,
> In every high degree.
> She looked so neat and nimble, O,
> A-washing of her linen, O.
> Dashing away with a smoothing iron,
> Dashing away with a smoothing iron,
> She stole my heart away.

She hangs the clothes on Tuesday, starches on Wednesday, irons on Thursday, folds on Friday, airs them on Saturday and finally gets to wear them, and steal his heart away, on Sunday. In damp old Dublin the pleasure of simply packing up the dirty clothes and receiving a parcel of clean dry ones must have done away with an awful lot of drudgery. It has got to have been a huge lifestyle improvement, and it will surely have quickly caught on.

Besides this, of course, my grandfather must have known all about the Magdalen Laundries. Until he brought his machinery to Dublin, all laundry in Ireland was either done at home or was done by wretched women who had become pregnant with no husbands to support them, and were made to live in convents (frankly, they were very tough workhouses). They were in such disgrace they were only allowed to see their children for an hour a day – they were made to work long hours washing laundry by hand. Many mothers and many, many children died. Their work paid for their being looked after during late pregnancy, birth, and caring for their babies for up to three years after they were thrown out by their families for immorality. After the three years, often without their mothers' being told or legally signing any agreement, their babies were given to American families for adoption in return for a large donation to the nuns. It was very cruel. My protestant grandfather cannot have been unaware of this system, and this I suppose was a reason that he chose to introduce kinder more considerate work for his 'laundrymaids'.

In spite of my father's sneering at 'being in trade' and 'taking in other people dirty washing for a living', my grandfather's strangely-named laundry was actually a very kind and progressive institution.

Aunt Doris's daughter Happy, a little older than me, told me one day that she knew something about my mother that her mother had told her, but had made her promise she never would tell me.

"What is it?" I asked.

"I'm not going to tell you. Ha, ha", sang Happy.

When I got back to Aunt Ann, I asked her what Happy knew about my mother that she would not tell me.

"Oh take no notice of Happy, Darling," said Aunt Ann. "She is just trying to tease you. But your father is coming home on leave soon, and if it worries you, you can ask him."

I wondered about my mother, of course I did. What did Aunt Doris know about her that she had told Happy? Was there a way to find out? The more I thought about it the more I knew that all the ways to that piece of information were closed off, so I simply had to put my mother to the back of my mind, and plan that if ever I got a chance to find out, I would. It made things easier. It actually was the only way. I obviously did not have a mother so that was that. I knew very well that my father, who had been away so long that I only remembered him indistinctly, was the last person I dared ask.

Although the grown-up Aunts were as nice as they could be to me, I felt really lonely and lost for that year in Dublin during the war. I had no special person to love, and no one seemed to be there to love and care specially for me.

My father was telephoning to Dublin on a very crackly line from the war in Italy. He had seen the wartime film of 'Henry V' and was very taken with it. He asked me to learn some speeches from the play, and my aunt gave me a marked copy. I can recite them to this day. The play was about the only good thing in Dublin.

"O that we now had here
But one . . ."

"That's right, go on."

"Ten thousand of those men in England
That do no work today!"

"Good. Do you know the whole speech?"

"Yes nearly." I got to the end:

"And gentlemen in England now a-bed
Shall think themselves accursed they were not here,
And hold their manhoods cheap whiles any speaks
That fought with us upon St. Crispin's Day."

"Well done. For all that I think you should have riding lessons. There's a riding school outside Dublin run by a man called Duggan, who wins everything. You'd have to get there on your bicycle. Could you do that?"

"Oh yes I could I could. Can I go today?"

It was a long hot uphill bicycle ride to the riding school. Mr Duggan looked at me. He was of the family that had given the Duggan Cup presented at the Dublin Horse Show and won three times by my grandfather's van horse 'Swastika Rose'. I was ten years old, as thin as string, with huge grown up teeth. "What do you want to ride?" he asked. "We don't really have ponies. How about this?" he said, leading out of its stable a tall strong heavy horse. It had large hooves, an ugly head with a roman nose, was as fat as butter, and its nature was every inch that of a horse. As soon as it had its freedom, it wanted to gallop. It was a lovely pale cream colour, with dark lower legs and a coarse black mane and tail. The colour was dun, and once I was up on it I saw that it had a bold black stripe down its back from the base of its mane under the saddle to the top of its tail. Mr Duggan had a track laid out on the edge of his ground and we went up there and galloped round and round it. My horse galumphed along, whacking his tail up and down with joy, tears streamed from my eyes and I loved it. It was a rough ride, but once a week I bicycled up to the school, and had another go.

Mr Duggan said dun was a primitive colour, and it was a primitive horse, which was just as well because it had been perfect in the battle scene in 'Henry V'. "Some of it was filmed here in Ireland, you see. We all galloped downhill in full armour."

My horse was famous. It had been in a film. It was meant to be primitive and ugly. I learned to appreciate its enthusiastic nature and its happy, flared-nostril, half-whinnying greeting on seeing me. Shakespeare, and the dun horse with his black stripe, were the only saving graces of Dublin.

My father came to get me just as the war was ending. He took my cousin James and me to Leopardstown races in a jaunting car. We were wildly excited at the ride. I could see that none of the race-horses had a stripe down their backs, I supposed that meant they were not primitive horses.

I asked if there were leopards in the little town outside Dublin.

"I don't know," my father said. "Look it up."

It turned out that 'leopard' was a corruption of 'leper' and as in the Bible, lepers were made to live outside the city. This was Leperstown not Leopardstown. There were no leopards there.

When I was 20 years old, one of my Dublin aunts (one with only sons) gave me some advice. She told me three things she thought I ought to know about men. The first was a lesson she gave me in how to make white sauce. She said once you could do that you could cook, and that men could never master white sauce, so they had some respect for your skill. Secondly she said you must always wear a coat with a nipped-in waist. Men did not like those tent-shaped coats at all, so if you wanted them to like you, you must wear one that went in at the middle. Finally, she announced that you must never ever mention defecation to a man. Apparently it really upset them. I said "But surely they do it too?" She replied, "Yes they do, but you must never talk about it".

I had another big bouncy aunt who advised me, also when I was 20, always to wear a 'Rollon', a kind of elastic tubular corset you pulled up over your bottom that had suspenders dangling from it. "It is not nice", she said, "to show that you have two buttocks. Just one is much better." With these pieces of feminine advice I was set off to make my way in the world.

At first I liked staying with my oldest aunt, my father's red-headed older sister, Aunt Mabel. She was positive, confident and affectionate. She never made you feel guilty about anything. Punishment was rare, encouragement and enthusiasm everything. She could keep order if she wanted to, but most of the time she let everybody do what they wanted. She played the piano well, and at family parties she sang very funny Gilbert and Sullivan songs, and we all sang the choruses. It was family lore that she never set foot out of bed in the mornings until the maid, Marcella, had brought her a gin and tonic on a silver salver. I do not know if it was every morning, but I certainly did see Marcella do it.

I wanted to play cricket in the garden with her two sons and their friends, and eventually they let me, on two conditions. One, that I may not bowl, because girls were no good at that, and two, that I was the one who had to go next door and tell them the boys had hit a six and sent a ball through their downstairs lavatory window: the boys were sorry and would pay to have it mended. Aunt Mabel was not furious with them: she just put stoppages on their pocket money until it was paid for.

Aunt Mabel was lovely to live with, but her husband Fitz, a barrister, was a horrible blight. He was far too keen on saying goodnight. He used to give me the same direct look that Evelyn Barclay had done at his dining table, and when I kissed the grown-ups downstairs before going up to bed he squeezed my bottom, which I, now aged ten, hated. He used to come upstairs to go to bed before Aunt Mabel, and peep into my room, which was the dressing room next to theirs, with a communicating door, and blow me a goodnight kiss. I thought he need not bother, because he had said goodnight already. After a few nights, he came into my room in his blue and white striped pyjamas to kiss me goodnight again. First it was just a kiss on my forehead, then it was him sitting on the bed, and then in the end, him lying beneath the eiderdown but on top of the blankets with me squashed underneath. His stomach stuck out, as hard as a rugger ball, it had no give in it. It stuck into me pressing on my chest and squashing my guts out to the sides, when he lay on top of me, and I thought I would suffocate. Eventually he wiggled and grunted and wiggled and grunted and wiggled on top of me, and kissed me with his huge fat tongue in my mouth, nearly choking me. I found it terribly hard to breathe, partly because he was heavy, and partly because I had to breathe in exactly when he did, and out when he did. I could not bear to breathe in the horrible smell of the brandy and ginger ale he drank on his breath. He had reached this stage of kissing by very slow degrees, and I could not think how I had come to let him, or when I should have stopped him. He said our goodnights were our special secret. He used to say, "I am kissing you goodnight just like your father would if he was here. I'm doing it for him."

I certainly could not possibly imagine my father ever saying goodnight like that, and I did really hope he would not try to do it when he got back.

After many nights of anguish, I finally discovered how to get rid of him. I just had to get enough breath to say "Aunt Mabel's coming upstairs" and he would leap off the bed and scurry next door to their bedroom. It did not matter if she did not come: he did not come back again that night.

Luckily I never stayed with any Aunt and Uncle for long (I apparently had an upsetting effect on their Nannies), so Uncle Fitz never progressed beyond the kissing and wiggling.

Some time later, staying again with Aunt Doris, Uncle Dico, Philip and the Basenji, my cousin Happy asked me: "Do you know the facts of life?"

"No", I said. "What are they?"

So she told me, ending with a phrase I shall never forget, ". . . and then he shoves it well and truly up inside you".

"Oh that's horrible: I don't believe you," I said. "You made that up."

"Oh no I didn't," she said. "Mummy told me, and it's true, it really is true."

"Come on", I said. "It can't be. Not Aunt Mabel, *not* Uncle Fitz?"

"Yes," she said, "Even them."

It seems to me now rather surprising, another odd childhood failure to pick up an obvious clue, that at the time I did not equate Uncle Fitz's bedtime manners with the facts of life.

When he came back from the war, some time later, one of the things my father asked me was: "Did Fitz ever lay a finger on you? Because if he did, I'll kill him."

So, it dawned on me, my father knew about Fitz's goodnight proclivities. How did he know it, I wondered? But did he really want to kill him for that? *Kill him*? My father could be trusted to follow through with his threats. If he said he would do something, he did it. I knew he might kill people, because he had told me that he had tried to once, to a patient in great pain who was not going to get better. He did it with morphine, I knew. I asked who he had killed and he told me about a Scotsman in his hospital in Italy who had been terribly injured by a landmine. He had had both his legs and one arm blown off, and was cruelly burned. My father did what he could for him in theatre, and late that night went to see him and gave him a massive injection of morphine. He knew it would put him out of his pain, and he hoped it would kill him. The next morning, on his ward round, a bound and bandaged body was still in the bed, and my father was shocked that sister had not yet removed the corpse. He walked up to the bed, just to check, and said "Hello Sergeant, how are you?" and through the bandages that covered even his mouth, his patient said clearly "Champion". He did recover and was invalided home, but he was an exceptionally tough man. My father said he found his recovery so shocking, that he never tried it again. "I didn't kill him," he said. "I only tried to." However, he thought he was trying to help the wounded Scotsman, but he would not have felt at all like helping Fitz. Quite the reverse. He could get hold of morphine if he wanted it, he had the means to hand, and I was afraid that if you have tried something once. . . maybe you will try again.

I thought that what Uncle Fitz did was unnecessary, uncomfortable, unpleasant and really very rude. I could not easily stop him because he was a grown-up, and Aunt Ann had said it was nice of him to have me to stay. But I knew he felt bad about it because I could so easily get rid of him by saying I heard Aunt Mabel. I certainly did not think that he should die for it.

I still thought that although it was nasty, and puzzling (because he seemed to like me very much indeed at night, and simply gave me a direct unblinking stare during the day), it was not necessary that he should be executed by my father.

It did sound as if my father meant his threat to kill Fitz, and I thought of what would happen if he did. Aunt Mabel would be devastated. She doted on Fitz, and would never, ever believe any ill of him. When Fitz was old and ill with prostate cancer, she used to say "Amn't I lucky that God has given him to me for so long?" She would certainly say that my father and I were liars. The Police would come and ask me if it was true, and would I be able to tell them? What exactly would they want to know? Then they would take my father away and maybe put him in prison, or even have him hanged, and I might not see him again either for a long time, or for ever. I could not bear to let any of that happen. So I decided to tell the absolute truth: "No," I said, "Uncle Fitz never laid a finger on me".

I was not asked if he laid anything more than a finger; not if, for instance, he had laid himself on me, and so I did not have to say that he did.

My father said "Good", and Uncle Fitz lived. I am sure many paedophiles (a word I did not know then: we girls were aware of them of course and called them 'dirty old men') 'get away with it' because their victims are quite capable of imagining what will happen if they tell, and think that that result would be worse than just putting up with it.

Later on, in our 20s, several of my girl cousins and I got together and reminisced, and we found out that Uncle Fitz had had a go at each of us in turn. Sadly, I heard later that one girl cousin was terribly traumatised and upset by it.

Now, in my old age, I have been talking to one of my female cousins. Yes, she said, she hated Uncle Fitz: he was horrible. When she was seven or eight he used to back her into corners and feel her up. And then her sister struck up. "And you complained, didn't you? You went to Aunt Mabel and told her."

"I don't remember really, did I?"

"Yes, you told me you did, and what Aunt Mabel said."

"What did she say?"

"She said, 'You sit there, and I'll get Marcella to come and bring you a glass of milk and a biscuit. She'll stay with you till I get back'. And about 20 minutes later she came back with Uncle Fitz, Aunt Doris and Uncle Dico. They all sat down on chairs around you and stared at you and Mabel said 'Now listen, it is quite natural for children to have big imaginations, and to make up stories to tell. Every child does it, at some time. And usually, they are just stories, and it doesn't matter. But sometimes, although the children don't mean to, telling such stories can do an awful lot of harm. You know perfectly well, Darling, that that story you told me about Uncle Fitz is a complete fib. You just made it up. It did not happen. But you are, I'm afraid, a very bad girl to go making up stories like that. It is wicked to say such things, and you must never ever tell such cruel untruths again'. And you told me they all sat round and agreed with her, and gave you frightening looks."

On hearing this, I must say I have changed my mind. I wish now I had told the truth to my father, put the fat in the fire, and let them get on and sort out the mess. I doubt if my father would have killed Fitz, or that it would have got as far as the police, or a court of law, but hopefully Uncle Fitz might have had such a fright as to stop him, at least for a while. Fitz was a barrister, and I bet barristers get struck off for that. I am told that paedophiles are very rarely able to stop altogether, which is a great shame for them and their victims, but it would have been better if we girl cousins had been able to grow up without Fitz's nasty fiddlings. This particular cousin's mother and father were at the time in the midst of a dramatic marital bust up, and I think she was probably sent to stay with Mabel and Fitz for respite from the trauma going on at home. Hence Mabel's decision to go for the glass of milk and the biscuit, and the need to understand that she was under such stress that she was driven to making up wicked lies.

What long-term harm did Fitz do to me? That is a hard question to answer because I cannot be sure how different I would have felt if he had done nothing. I have always thought that kind of kissing with the man's tongue in my mouth absolutely revolting and done my best to avoid it. If I have been denied one of the forms of love-making, I have found plenty of others, and I can get along with that. And I have been much warier, I hope, than the Aunts were, about trying to make sure (not always successfully) that situations were avoided where my own daughters might have been vulnerable.

But did Aunt Mabel not actually know what Fitz was doing? Had she never suspected him? She must have done. Mabel was a doctor: one of the first women to get a medical degree from Trinity College, Dublin. She was able to save her marriage by refusing to believe anything bad about Fitz, but even so I find it hard to believe that she did not know what was going on. If she had had any suspicions, she certainly knew I was only ten years old, that Fitz went up to bed before she did, that there was a connecting door between our bedrooms. And she did nothing about it.

There were six of us girl cousins. I know that three of us were abused by Fitz, and one by another uncle. One spent her childhood years in Dar-es-Salaam, and escaped. Out of the five who could have been, four were abused. What on earth were our aunts thinking of, that they could not protect us? One cousin agrees with me that they must have thought that nice chaps could show affection for little nieces, but that would be as far as it went. It would be disloyal to their marriages to think anything else. If they suspected, they immediately repressed the thought. Actually, they dared not know. I must assume that they never confronted the facts full on, never dared consider what might be happening. Otherwise, how could they be forgiven? I am afraid that such behaviour needs to be told.

If we do not know about such things, that can happen right under our noses, how can they be prevented? What children say is worth listening to, however unlikely it seems, and should be believed until proved otherwise. Denying it, even to save a marriage, cannot be right.

Looking back now, I can see why, at the time he asked me, I decided not to tell my father about Uncle Fitz's despicable bed-time manners. I did not know, then, of the cruelty to my other girl cousins: in particular, of the lies forced down the throat of one of them. I have to say that of the painful things that happened to me during the war, Uncle Fitz's good nights come very low down the scale. My father, my closest friend, disappearing at the beginning of the war; and my trusted nursery governess Dickie doing the same; Philip the pilot suddenly going missing one night; the shuddering cold and chilblains of Bolwick; my terror of the seesaw swing at the Birkbecks'; finding myself at that purple boarding school where I could do nothing right; losing Pinkie, Gretchen and Mickey when I was sent to Ireland; and, above all, realising that I had lost Pinkie for ever at the end of the war. These were all in their way ten times worse than Fitz's nasty fumblings. From what I know now, of course, I think I should have told. But that is because Fitz just sat there allowing his wife to persuade my cousin that she was a liar, when he knew how wrong that was. That was utterly wicked, and I do not really care what sort of an explosion exposing him might have caused (no of course not death, I am certain: my father would not have risked it). I can believe that little girls can be terribly traumatised by being raped by grown up men, but fortunately in my case it was not rape, just more of a nuisance and embarrassment than it was horrifying.

Chapter 11
Leopardstown Races

None of the cousins saw much of their parents. They were all looked after by Nannies. These Nannies were very strict and unloving. The reason they did not like us, the Nannies said, was because they were Catholics and they wanted Ireland for the Irish. For their holidays they used to bicycle to the West of Ireland to learn to speak Irish. They did not like Protestants or the English, and I was both. I disliked them back. My cousin Happy remembers her Nanny telling her that one day she would murder us in our beds, and Ireland would be free. "Did you tell your parents?" I asked. "No," said Happy, "I did not. I thought that might make them do it."

We used to sing 'God Save The King' at the end of the Sunday service at the protestant Church of Ireland in Dublin during the war, grown-ups and children squashed closely into the pew in the fusty mothball smell of Sunday clothes. My cousin John was extremely clever at putting his penny on the collection plate, and nicking half a crown instead. He claims he was taught this trick by our cousin George, who was about six at the time. George said, "You mustn't take more than one coin, or they rattle and then the man sees you. So go for the biggest, the half-crown." James and I did not like John for this, and we told Aunt Ann. I suppose we might have guessed that she would appear to have difficulty believing it.

In Dublin, all sorts of things were available which could not be obtained in England. I saved up my sixpence-a-week pocket money and bought my father a packet of razor blades, the ones with only one sharp side, which he always used, and that were not for sale in England. Good steel was needed for munitions. I bought Pinkie two hairnets, because she liked her hair to dry in a net, so that

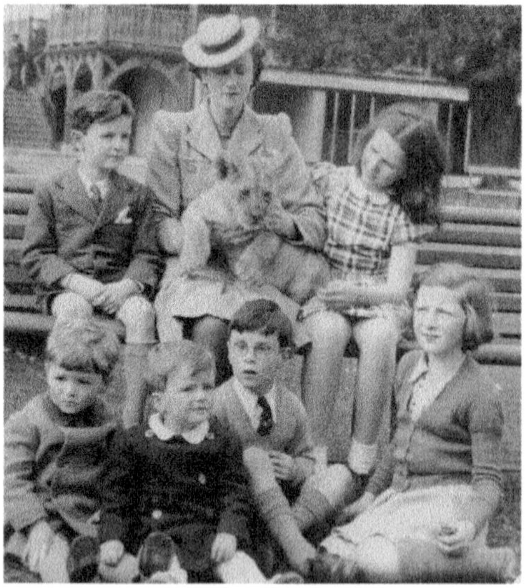

A lion cub at the Phoenix Park Zoo, Dublin, with Aunt Ann Graham and six Irish cousins. The cub may be a descendant of Mitzi and Fritz from Colney Hall, Norfolk. Back row: Richard FitzSimon, Aunt Ann, Penelope Wall Morris. Front row: John Graham, George Wall Morris. James Graham, Judy Brittain.

it came out smooth and gently curly. You could not get hairnets in England either. I asked Aunt Ann to send these gifts to them. When I asked my father about the razor blades after the war he said he never got them, but he did not need them anyway, because the soldiers could get anything they wanted. And I suppose that Pinkie never got her hairnets either. I am afraid Aunt Ann must have suppressed them.

Pinkie had been much better at helping and encouraging me to write letters to my father than Aunt Ann was, although I did maintain some contact with him. It was sometimes possible for him to telephone us in Dublin, and talk on a faint and crackly line, and I was filled with excitement and joy when he did. He told us that in Italy he made great friends with a patient, a war photographer who got blown up by a mortar bomb. When the photographer, Baron, arrived from the field dressing station, at the big base hospital in Naples, his right arm was hanging useless at his side, the bones of his shoulder joint shattered. He was told, "I'm afraid we're going to have to amputate this arm, it's never going to be any use to you. I'm sorry." But Baron pleaded, "Please, please don't. I'm a photographer [he was an official war photographer then]. Even if the nerves are all ruined, and the joint cannot be mended, I don't want the arm cut off. Isn't there any way my arm could be made to be of a little use? I know it won't ever be a proper arm, but I need a limb for steadying a camera."

So it was left dangling, supported by a sling, and the understanding was that when the war was over Baron would come and stay with us, and my father would do an operation to give him a bent but rigid arm. Because of the arm, Baron was then invalided out, and spent the last bit of the war advising on the making of the film of Shakespeare's Henry V, directed by Laurence Olivier.

Baron took many of the photographs in this book. He was a very close friend of Prince Philip in the war. Tired of the usual beautifully dressed and posed royal photographs, after the war Prince Philip, now married to the Queen, advised on Baron's appointment to be a new, modern Royal Photographer. Given one hour to take pictures, he took one assistant with him and, chatting away, he snapped away reel after reel so that he took more than 200 pictures in one session. "There's got to be a good one among them," he said, "and I have plenty of time to go through them afterwards and choose the best." One of his assistants was Antony Armstrong Jones, later Princess Margaret's husband.

So my father re-read the play, and was terribly excited by it. He loved the story, so apposite for the war, but he also adored the words. I was now 10, and he wanted me to learn some of the speeches. If he got through to us on the telephone, he would ask, "How much do you know now?" and I would start: "O that we now had here but one ten thousand of those men in England that do no work today."

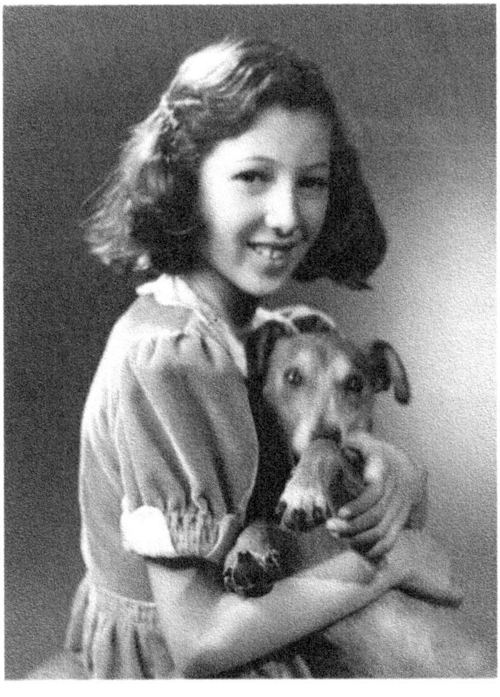

Alison aged 14. Photograph by Baron, celebrated society photographer, close friend of Tommy Brittain and also of Prince Philip.

I did not understand all of it then, but I am so grateful that he made me learn so much. Our telephone conversations often consisted of long quotations from Shakespeare, and knowing some of it so well, I have had a lifetime of pleasure out of it.

And then, wonderfully, he was invalided out of the army. He had jaundice. There he was, brilliant yellow, especially the so-called whites of his eyes, talking with an embarrassing loud harsh English accent (I did not realise, of course, that by now I spoke with a soft Irish one). I felt wildly excited and pleased: it was so lovely to see him and to have the punch of that exciting male company again. I asked him, "When are we going home?"

He replied, "When the war is over. It nearly is, and next time I come it will be, and then we'll go home together."

So then I asked, "When we get home, when are you going to marry Pinkie?" I knew that he and Pinkie had been engaged from just before the war started, when I had been five, rising six, and now I was 10.

"Never," he replied.

I felt stunned, as if I had been hit, my hair prickling up and down the back of my head, and cold with shock.

"What?" I asked, horrified. "Why not?"

"She wrote me a 'Dear John'."

"What is a 'Dear John'?"

There was a long pause. "It's a letter from a girl to a soldier saying she's fallen in love with somebody else and that she's breaking off the engagement."

"That must be a mistake, a dreadful mistake. You're called Tommy, not John, and Pinkie called you Peter, her rock, after the apostle Peter. It can't have been for you. Of course not, if it said 'Dear John'. Can't you read her writing? Maybe you were too ill."

"No, I bloody wasn't ill then, and yes I could read her writing, and she meant it."

"I can't believe it," I said. "She loved you, she loves you, I know she does, and I love her and I miss her terribly. I want you to marry her."

"Well, I'm not going to, so shut up about it."

"Why did she write it?"

He looked out of the window. "She said she had fallen in love with an airman she had met at a dance, at a dance, and she was going to marry him not me. She sent the ring back."

Going to dances in Norfolk was part of the war effort. Every woman old enough to go to dances and not yet married went. The dances were held at air force bases, and Pinkie and Bunny, and later at Bolwick, Pinkie and Diana, went to the nearest one, wobbling along in their long dresses on their bicycles, about once a fortnight. Diana, who I later heard left her husband during the war, was particularly keen on going to dances and insisted on Pinkie coming to keep her company. It kept the airmen cheerful, and helped them to win the war, they said.

"What did you do with the ring?"

"Threw it in the sea in the Bay of Naples." His yellow face looked bleak with pain, and he said: "'See Naples and die'."

What on earth had gone wrong? It seemed beyond belief that Pinkie, so loving and loyal, could possibly have fallen in love with someone else. I refused to accept it. In desperation, I defended her.

"Look, Pinkie never stopped doing things for the war effort. She looked after refugees like me, she worked as a night nurse, and gave blood, and she taught our Sunday school, and made jam with the Women's Institute and gave lifts to people who needed them and went with Bunny to dances and it was all part of the war effort. She had to go to dances. Everyone who could go did."

"Shut up, I said. I'm happy to tell you that before the letter reached me her airman was shot down over the sea and killed."

"Oh no! Poor Pinkie. How awful for her. But you could still marry her then?"

"Miss Pinkie Bulwer won't be marrying anyone in a hurry now."

"I still wish you would."

"Shut up."

Oh poor Pinkie. What pain she must have gone through. She would never have made such a decision lightly. She always seemed to me to have such a straight grasp of right and wrong, and to be so utterly loyal. It amazed me that she had fallen in love with another man, and I always wondered what could have made her do it. It was so completely uncharacteristic of her. Only now, in the middle of writing this, am I finally beginning to find out.

My father had been away for more than three years by then. His letters did not come very often. It was a cause of great excitement when we got one, about once a fortnight or a month, I suppose.

Although my father will have written lovely letters to Pinkie, it is well known that many wartime letters did not get through. No doubt after three years of such distant communication, the bond between them loosened. She may have feared he would never come back and marry her. She did not know him nearly as well as I did (they had never lived together) and it must have been hard for her to remember him. By now, of course, having spent three years with her, I knew Pinkie much better than he did, and I knew that for her, so honest and true and kind, her airman's death must have caused terrible grief.

My father never forgave her. Full of fury and despair he had fallen ill with hepatitis, got jaundiced and went bright yellow, and was invalided out of the army. He must have forbidden her to have any more to do with me, and insisted that I went to boarding school, and when that was a failure, to Ireland. I supposed that must be why I never got a letter at school from her. Her visit to me on the train at Horwood House school was probably clandestine. Travel was difficult and took a long time during the war, and it must have taken her a whole day or maybe two to come and go. She must have made the effort out of her kindness, and undoubted love, for me. I constantly grieved for the beloved mother I had had for all too short a time.

Mary Ann, Pinkie's niece, says today that she thinks she has seen a photograph among the family collection at Heydon Hall, of Pinkie in army uniform in Holland. It looks as if, eventually, Pinkie, having no evacuees to look after, was called up.

I was dreadfully sorry that my father's reaction seemed to have so little understanding: he was just bitter and cruel. After the war, if he ran into her, he simply turned his head away, and stalked past her. I saw him do it once on the stairs at a hunt ball, and felt sick in the pit of my stomach. I worried all my life about what could have caused such a breach, because the story I was told did not make sense. Pinkie would have had to have an extremely good reason to allow herself to fall in love with another man: she was about 26 then, and she would not have just been bowled over. As ever with my father, when something pained him, I could never ask the reason, but I could turn it to and fro in my head to see if I could make it out, or just hope that one day it would fall into my lap. Eventually, it did.

My father's reaction to bad news was always to up his game a bit. I should think the misery of jaundice must have been helped along by his shock and bitter regret, but by the time he got to Ireland he had picked himself up and was doing everything to the utmost, as usual.

I remember an argument he had with Aunt Ann, in which she insisted that there were people with principles which they would stick by always, and he cynically contradicted, saying: "Everyone has their price."

At that moment, my cousin James, aged eight, came into the drawing room with a jam jar full of slugs; slimy small black ones, and disgusting yellow ones twice the size (at that time we used to race slugs in the garden, starting all the runners in the centre of a paving slab, and seeing whose slug reached the edge first). My pet slug had by now got mixed with other Dublin garden slugs, and I no longer recognised it.

"James, what would it take to make you eat one of those slugs?" my father asked.

Round eyed and aghast, "I would never," James answered.

James only got threepence a week pocket money. My father pulled a ten shilling note out of his pocket.

"If I gave you ten shillings, would you eat one?" he asked.

James looked very awkward, and studied the jar.

"I'll eat a black one for ten shillings," he announced, "but I'd need a lot more to eat a yellow one."

Delighted, my father said to his sister, "There you are: that proves the point. Everyone has their price. I win." And he gave James the note and said he need not eat a slug. I envied James the money, but I was very fond of slugs, and am not sure what my price would have been.

My father was amazed at the quality and quantity of the food available in Ireland then. Rationing in England was very strict, especially for supplies of butter and meat, which were plentiful in Dublin. So he decided to send a pound of the best rump steak to all his friends in England. We went together to the butcher, who agreed to do it, and my father gave him the addresses and paid him enough to send it to about 20 friends once a fortnight till the war ended. Unfortunately, this was summertime, the meat took more than a week to arrive. When we got back to England after the war was over my father's friends were quite guarded in their thank-yous. They joked that they wondered how they had offended him, that he should decide to send them regular parcels of slimy-green, stinking, maggoty meat from Dublin.

The absolute highlight of his visit was when he took my cousin James and me to the Leopardstown races in a jaunting car. Having my father in such a state of high excitement and sheer whooping joy did start to drive away my disgust at Uncle Fitz's awful behaviour, and pushed a little into the background my misery at the loss of my adored Pinkie.

There was no rubber in the war. Perished hot water bottles leaked in your bed (I liked that word 'perished', and that it applied equally to hot water bottles and 'those who perish on the sea', like Uncle Douglas nearly did when the HMS Trinidad was torpedoed). And so there was no rubber for cart tyres. So they pulled the solid rubber rings from the wooden wheels, and cut them up into squares and nailed them on the other way round so that the thick pieces at the edges were now in the middle of the tyres. You sat outside in a jaunting car, and they made a buzzing sound and you could feel the vibration of their cut tyres, which added to our state of wild excitement at going to the races. It was a very different form of fresh air from that forced on us by our Nannies: I was bored to fury at the unavoidable dull daily afternoon walks along the pavements with the youngest in the pram, Nannie snapping at us to walk with one hand on the pram, and pick up our feet, and keep up, and not hang back.

There were so many coaches and jaunting cars on the road it seemed as if the whole of Dublin was going to the races. When we arrived my father gave us ten shillings each and said we could spend it all on Mars bars and eat them all at once if we wanted. Unable to believe our good fortune, we went at once to the man with the table of sweets, and duly invested. We saw edgy horses in the paddock, with jockeys lifted onto them, we heard galloping hooves and the brush and smack of horses jumping fences, heard the roar of the crowd at the winning post, and we saw horses steaming, their neat nostrils suddenly opened wide, with every vein on their bodies standing out, in the winning enclosure. At every excitement, we ate a Mars bar. We had just finished them by the time we got on the jaunting car to go home, and the swaying, rumbling motion, the excitement, and the five or six Mars Bars each that we had eaten, made us sick. Interestingly, we both noticed that vomited Mars Bars taste like soap. My father was very pleased with us, saying it did not matter at all, because they did not have to stop for us, or clean anything up, since we just did it over the side onto the road.

The Aunts strongly disapproved of everything: the races, the Mars bars, us being sick. They said it was completely disgraceful, and no way to treat children. But we could not possibly have been happier or more full of whizz, bounce and giggles. And I was happy indeed, thrilled, delighted, flying, to be in my father's exciting company again.

On his next visit, as he had promised, we went back to England together, and not long after, the war ended.

Chapter 12
The Life of Riley

On the way home from Ireland we spent ten days in London, in Claridge's Hotel. The hotel room, though large and grand, seemed quite like a prison to me, an 11-year-old, especially as my father had important people to see, and so I was told to stay there and read. I read all my father's books, some of them very grown-up and nasty. I read about prostitutes in South America in Vicky Baum's The Weeping Wood and was horrified at how cruel and painful that seemed. I decided not to tell my father I had read it, and never to become a prostitute or a nun. But then I took to exploring outside the room and found several good ways of avoiding boredom.

Once we got back to England, we found that things did not all return to normal at once after the war. But as I could not really remember what 'normal' had been, it did not matter to me. Even in Claridge's, you had to take your own eggs if you wanted one for breakfast. The breakfast kitchen on our floor had rows of eggs with their owners' names, titles, ranks and room numbers on them, and I was allowed to help the room service waiter find the right eggs to be cooked for their owners. Downstairs in the hum of chatter and clink of glasses in the dining room, a kind man in the orchestra who played the double bass let me sit, in my pale green velvet best dress, on a high stool beside him and pluck one of the strings when he said so. But what I will never forget about that visit was the terrifying bidet in the bathroom.

Still quite yellow and not very well, my father also had a stomach ulcer. This was to be cured by drinking whisky and cream. The drink came upstairs on a silver tray: a cut glass tumbler with a double whisky in it, and a glass jug of cream. Cream could be got in Claridge's, but not anywhere else in the country at that time. The glass looked dirty after use, lined with drying out cream. My father had his own supply of whisky, and if he wanted to reuse the glass, it had to be washed. I often did it for him in the bathroom basin, but one day I wanted to go to the lavatory at the same time, so, as I sat there, I upended the creamy tumbler on the nozzle in the middle of the bidet beside me, and turned the taps on. I did not know what a bidet was for. A tremendous jet of water shot out of the nozzle and drove the glass up to the ceiling, where it smashed and crashed all round me. I cowered under the shattering glass and for several soaking seconds I was too surprised to turn off the fountain. My father sent for another glass, and the room service man to clear up the mess. Aware of my embarrassment, he did not explain how it came about. Since then I have of course discovered the purpose of a bidet, but a huge sense of anxiety overwhelms me when I think about it, and I have never been able to persuade myself to try one.

Back home in Norfolk we could really feel that the war was over. The Germans had surrendered. Hitler was dead. The war in Japan seemed very far away. When, three months later, I heard that an atomic bomb had fallen on Hiroshima, I knew no better than to think, 'Good: that's that, then'. But my father insisted on taking me to Norwich to see a newsreel film of British soldiers relieving the concentration camp at Bergen-Belsen. Grown-ups were always telling me that I looked thin, but here were thin people nothing like me: I did not know it was possible to look like that. Suddenly I saw what 'skin and bone' really meant. And there were awful piles of naked dead bodies, stacked up like the sugar beet beside the road in Norfolk waiting for the lorries to take it off to the factory at Cantley. Judy's mother was shocked, and told my father that, at only 11, I was not old enough to be exposed to such horror. He simply said, "Next time it happens, we won't be here to stop it. She will."

I remembered how he had seemed to be so proud when he joined up and went away to fight. He obviously had a very different view of the war now.

But now there was no more war, we had a true sense of restoration, almost as there must have been when Charles II came to the throne after the dullness of the Commonwealth. There was a feeling of having earned a better life than anyone had had for five years, of new, different, exciting, extravagant times ahead.

My father always said "Money's for spending", and spent it lavishly. But I suppose that during the war the Army paid him some money he had no opportunity to spend. He wrote to his sister Ann that he was able to save his pay, with three exclamation marks, and offered to give her some. He owned shares in the Swastika Laundry. He had a great many private patients. He earned a very high income, and he must have had some cash saved up.

The first luxury we acquired was a new car, a beautiful Rolls Royce. There were no new cars made straight after the war, but the best of the old ones could be bought, and my father purred with pride at this acquisition. It was a 1936 Phantom III coupé with an aeroplane engine that did nine miles to the gallon. Navy blue and black, it had a full-size silver lady on the bonnet, and a hood that folded down like a sports car. I thought it was much too big, and the smell of leather inside made me sick.

One of the first journeys we made in it was to go to Heydon to fetch Gretchen. I guessed my father wanted to show off the Rolls to Pinkie.

"Will Pinkie be there?"

"She'd better bloody not be."

"I want to see her."

"Well you can't."

The door of the Dower House opened ajar, and I saw a hand: perhaps it was Pinkie's. Then Gretchen was pushed out. She looked rather indignant. Then she saw us, and rushed to greet us, leaping up and down, yipping with pleasure. She became a storm in our arms, wriggling and writhing so that neither of us could hold her. We could not set off till she stopped crying and calmed down. While we waited, I kept looking at the house, but Pinkie (if it was her) never came out. I do not think I understood till then how much my father's once affectionate feelings for her had now turned to hatred. Once he got really angry about something, he never forgave. He must, I suppose, have thought that the best way of humiliating her and punishing her was to arrive in his new Rolls Royce and arrange, probably with his secretary, that she was not even to come out and greet us. I know that the car will not have impressed her in the least. Cars were not something she admired and she disliked showing off.

My father's brass plate was still fixed to our brick gatepost: 'H. A. Brittain, M.A., M.Ch., F.R.C.S.'. The car turned in past the low brick wall that leaned inwards supporting the bank of earth inside, and the hedge of Portugal laurel behind it. We went round the gravel drive circling a bed of wallflowers and forget-me-nots, and stopped. Gretchen was squeaking with joy as she recognised where she was. She leapt out of the car and squatted on the lawn between the monkey-puzzle and the yellow-leaved Indian bean tree, said to have been the oldest Catalpa in England. Having left her mark on the lawn, she galloped up the steps, along the blue and red quarry tiles, and into the house, to renew her old acquaintance.

Our old house was a great late-Victorian chunk built of red bricks: part of the ribbon development on the Newmarket Road that led into Norwich. Other big ugly houses, similar in spirit but none of them exactly the same, sat either side of it and opposite it all along the road.

Gretchen went to visit room after room, sniffing furiously, in the order of which ones she had liked best. She looked for Chef, hopefully with a bit of cheese for her, in the kitchen. The stronger and smellier the cheese, the more she liked it. Gorgonzola was her favourite. The kitchen was dark, painted green and cream, with a black range in it that was never used except by the two Hungarian maids. There was no chef now, but when there had been chefs, they preferred to use a tough-looking four-ring gas cooker that sat in the corner. Whenever I hear of someone putting their head in a gas oven, it is always this one I see, and I still have no idea how you would put your head in and get the door shut.

Gretchen trotted into the larder and stood on her hind legs, better to smell what was on the shelves, covered in shiny green gingham oil-cloth. Then through to the scullery with its big rectangular china sink and the long wooden draining board, and her old place to lie beside the nice warm boiler. She came back to the hall, and whizzed into the dining room, gloomy with mahogany furniture, which had been the patients' waiting room in the afternoons. But you never knew, there might be crumbs from the table. Then she went across the hall again to the drawing room, where there were sometimes nuts, and little biscuits, and a log fire. Not today, sadly. No fire, nothing, just the heavy dark red velvet curtains and the grand piano squeezing the space.

Gretchen just stuck her nose into the consulting room where she knew she was not allowed. It had a hard bed behind a curtain in it, for looking

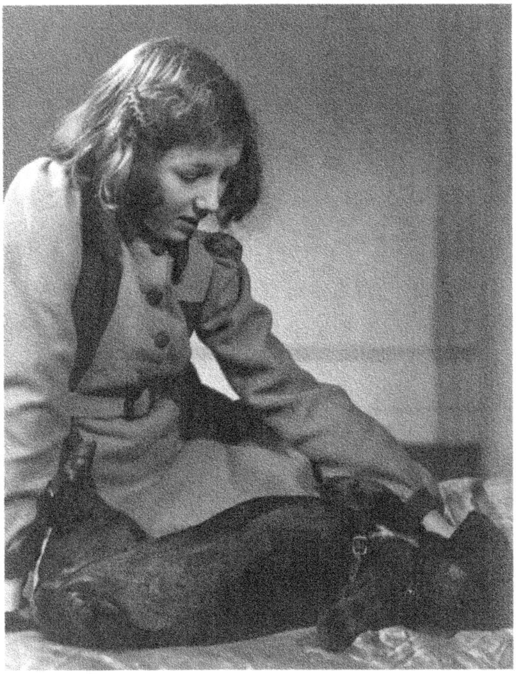

Gretchen. Much-loved sausage dog (dachshund) back in Norwich after she spent the war years in Heydon with Pinkie.

at patients, and on the desk stood a barograph, a framed photograph, and a solid silver inkwell and pen stand with 'To the doctor who made me walk again' engraved on it. My father hated that. He also had a disgusting life-size drawing of a skeleton trying to wrest a patient from a doctor, a gift from another grateful patient, which frightened me.

Gretchen galloped upstairs to the sitting room, looking for crisps or chocolate there, and jumped into the slightly threadbare armchair in which I had once sat on my father's knee listening to the broadcast announcing that we were at war. Before I could really remember, my father had had a dog called Stephen, a white scruffy Sealyham. Stephen was trained to jump onto any bit of furniture he was told to, and the dog never made a mistake. My Aunt Ann remembers staying in this house, and my father sitting in the armchair, reading a newspaper. He heard the clicking toes of Stephen coming into the room, and said, from behind the paper: "Coffee table, Stephen."

Aunt Ann looked up and saw that the table had a tray of old coffee things on it. Stephen was bracing himself, bouncing up and down, ears pricked, forcing himself to give it a go. He was stopped just in time.

I called Gretchen off the chair and she shot into my father's bedroom and got on the bed. I was quite cross with her and she leapt off, ignored the empty bedroom next door and went round the landing to my room where she stood on my bed wagging her tail and inviting me to get in with her. Never popular with the secretary, she skipped her room and thundered up the straight flight of stairs to the attics, long rooms with sloping ceilings and dormer windows. The room the servants slept in was of no interest, but my day nursery, with its coal fire and table on which meals were served to me and Dickie, pleased her very much and she settled down, home at last.

Later, she wanted to go out and I let her into the garden at the back. The house faced south, so on the north wall at the back there were almost no windows: the only one was protected with a mesh screen. On the lawn there, my father used to run up and down practising tennis with great vigour, against the wall. Further down the lawn stood Troy, a life-size wooden horse, on which he would sit on summer evenings practising his polo swings. Gretchen squatted down beneath Troy, then remembered that we sometimes had tea in the shade of the copper beech, but there was nothing there for her today. Away to the back was Rose's domain: the apple trees and the vegetable garden, with the air raid shelter, collapsing now, and paths lined with parsley. Only the remains of the chicken run seemed worth inspecting. She paid cursory attention to the garage, big enough for the two Vauxhall cars, Big Squirty and Little Squirty, which had been laid up on bricks at the start of the war. Big Squirty was sold, in favour of the Rolls, but the secretary, having got her going again, kept Little Squirty. Possibly the Rolls would not fit in the garage. Certainly, it never went there. When my father was at home it stood proudly, showing itself off, by the front door, always.

Having been empty for three years, the house had a disturbing unfamiliar smell of mould. It made me very happy to have Gretchen back to cuddle, with her dear doggy smell, strongest under her armpits and between her toes.

But this was our old house. To his intense pride and pleasure, as well as a new car, my father had also bought a new house, Witton House, five miles east of Norwich. To be accurate, it was new to us, but it was actually an old house in terrible condition. It had been thoroughly ruined by the army, which had had it for the duration of the war. Damp had ravaged it, and dry rot had invaded one whole wing, which had to be rebuilt. Judy came with me in the back seat to look at it for the first time. We sailed up the front drive to the pillared portico by the front door.

"You two can't come in. With the builders at work and scaffolding up all over the place, it's too dangerous. There's plenty outside to go and explore. When I want you, I'll blow the horn."

We got out and wandered round the orchard, as big as a small paddock, full of blossom and bees. It was May: lovely, promising early summer. From the bottom of the orchard we could see the house at a distance: a miniature Georgian country house, with a lovely big bay window the full height of the building, built of pale grey stock bricks, sitting on a terrace, as pretty as a peach. It was smaller than any of the grand houses I had lived in with Pinkie. It had a glass dome over the dramatic, wide 180°-curved staircase around which the whole house was built, and that lit the hall and stairs. In the cellar was the date, in Roman numerals, MDCCCXX, 1820. It was all built at the same date, all of a piece.

There was plenty outside to explore. We found a Nissan hut, and Judy told me that a huge country house near her, Kimberley Hall, had also been taken over by the army, and then while it was left vacant, all the many Nissan huts filled up with people needing somewhere to live. She said they were called 'squatters', a new word to me. When Lord Kimberley returned from South Africa after the war, he used to give shooting parties in which he and his friends drove round his estate in their cars on the new tarmac roads made by the army, and shot out the windows of the Nissan huts as they went by, to get rid of the squatters. Why Johnny Kimberley was not arrested for this no one knew. They said it could only happen in Norfolk.

We discovered three cottages, some stables, big garages, apple rooms, a harness room, clock tower, five greenhouses full of peach and nectarine trees and a grapevine. Judy lived in a beautiful very old house that had all these things, but not five greenhouses, and only one cottage. The further we went the more we found. Judy said that the three lawns, each one down a slope two feet lower than the next, must have been tennis courts: they were the right size. Later, when we had moved in, my father met someone at a party who told him that geese were the very thing for overgrown lawns: they ate grass, after all. So thirty geese were ordered, and within a fortnight they had eaten all the grass, and returned it to the ground in the form of squishy green droppings that the geese paddled out flat with their feet. The sun came out and dried them up, and then they cracked open like crazy paving. Much to the gardener's relief, thirty hungry geese were then sold, though it took a year for the tennis courts to recover.

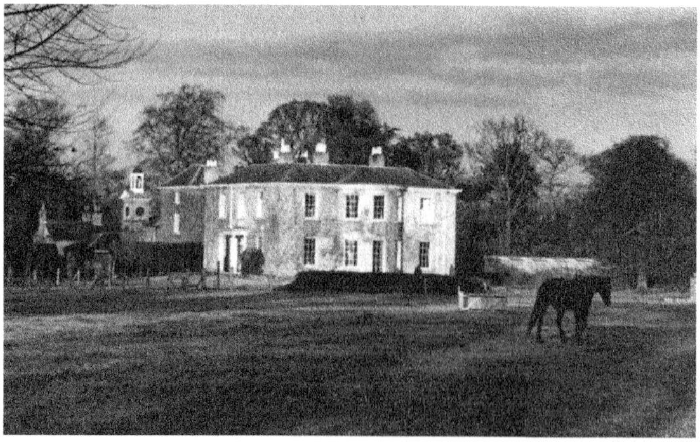

Witton House. Georgian house, dated 1820, located five miles from Norwich. Bought by Tommy at the end of the war. Years after Tommy sold it, it was burned down for the insurance money.

We were exploring the big walled vegetable garden when the gardener, Brister, who lived in the biggest cottage, came out of his potting shed and said, "Hello. Is one of you Miss Alison?" I replied, "Yes, and this is my friend Judy". He shook our hands, and said if we wanted to know anything, just ask him.

Judy's house had a large verandah whose glass ceiling dripped with pale purple wisteria blossom, hummed with bees and smelled gorgeous at this time of year. I wanted to know if we had one too, but Brister said no. However, as he led us round, showing us the ornamental water gardens, the little bowling-green with the old brick summer house, and the dried up lake with islands with trees on, I could see with satisfaction that we had plenty of wonderful things that her house lacked. There was an enormous Wellingtonia tree with a green woodpecker hammering on it, and a cedar of Lebanon. A huge magnolia with waxy scented white blossoms the size of pigeons leaned on the East wall all the way up the house. From the six big asparagus beds, Brister cut us a bunch of asparagus to take home. It wanted eating, he said. There was a great big meadow which seemed to run seamlessly from the tennis lawns and the sunken Dutch garden, and Brister led us up to it and showed us the huge ditch that formed its boundary.

"Do you know what that is?" he asked.

"Yes," we said. "It's a ha-ha."

"Quite right. And look, here is a great big air raid shelter built into it by the Army, big enough for all the soldiers that lived here to get into, and look" he said, pressing down the Bakelite switch, "it has electric light." Much good that would have been, I thought, if the Germans came and opened the door and found you there.

There was a shelter-belt of trees right round the gardens and meadow, with a path all the way through it. Later, jumps were put up across the path, and every morning in summer, when the horses were kept in the meadow, my father and I rode round it, jumping the jumps. In the shelter-belt was the saw-mill with its jagged circular saw that made that frightful whining, keening noise when it was working, Nearby, we found a dark brick-built underground ice house with a short entrance passage and no warning of the straight drop to the bottom (probably there was once a ladder). It had been filled with ice from the lake in winter, and used like a giant refrigerator for keeping meat for months. There were two more Nissan huts, and big signs declaring 'OUT OF BOUNDS' and 'LATRINES' which Judy and I decided might have meant lavatories, though we could not find any.

We heard the car horn and we rudely abandoned Brister, saying a quick good-bye, and not taking time to shake his hand and thank him for his trouble, which we felt bad about later. The engine was running, and we jumped in, and the car slid away with us, down the back drive.

As for the inside of the house, when we finally moved in, it smelled of new carpets and fresh paint. Gretchen immediately moved into the kitchen, and spent most of the rest of her life lying in front of the big cream Aga. Not for her the pretty dome over the wide curved staircase, the double drawing room, dining room, little library, cold dairies, pantries, and larder with slate shelves, or even the servants' hall. She utterly refused to go down the steps to the underground wine cellar, the home of many crawling toads.

My very favourite room was the smallest in the house. Behind the huge curve of the main staircase, under the rise of the stairs, in the back passage opposite the butler's pantry, the solid semi-circular wall had a tiny room. There was just space for a high stool, a shelf with a telephone, and it had a curved door that matched the wall it was set in. When that was shut no one could hear you and if you turned off the light no one could see you were there. I spent hours and hours in here gossiping with Judy and Sara, completely oblivious to the length of time I spent chattering to friends. Only the telephone bill gave me away, and often my furious father would snatch the door open off its pinger any time he passed, to make sure I was not in there.

Alas, I am not a naturally tidy person, and I never have been. I can do it all right if I have to, but in those early teenage years I felt it quite unnecessary to tidy my own bedroom. The floor was usually covered with clothes, shoes, boots, hard hat, dandy brushes, halters, bridle, saddlesoap, girths and other harnesses, papers and books. From time to time my father would step in, study the chaos on the whole floor very slowly, eyes sweeping from side to side, and then announce, "God help your bloody husband!"

Faced with tidying our bedroom now, I still remember him saying that as clear as day, and these days, if I do not say it, my husband, who has heard this story many times, says it for me.

Not one for interior design, my father was daunted by the need to furnish and decorate his exciting new house. He sent for Aunt Pat, an aunt in both senses in that she was his cousin, and they were lovers, to do it for him. Delightfully extravagant, Aunt Pat sent for tradesmen and antique dealers from all over Norfolk and Suffolk and from Bond Street in London. They arrived daily with pantechnicons full of furniture, Turkish carpets, looking glasses, and very expensive Genoese cut-velvet curtains that could be re-made to fit. There were Queen Anne walnut tallboys with curvy legs with claw and ball feet, and dressing tables and pretty stools to match. There was a Chippendale side table whose flame-patterned mahogany table top had been carved out half-an-inch lower than the raised edges so that it was all one beautiful piece of wood, not frame-edges carved separately and stuck on afterwards (much like a saucer, or Uncle Douglas's version of Ireland, I thought). Art dealers arrived and pictures were held up in different places all over the walls.

When he first came to Norwich my father had rooms in Tombland, just outside the cathedral close. He told me he bought a joint of meat on Saturday, and gave it to his landlady, who served it to him as a roast on Sunday, cold on

Monday, cold again on Tuesday. She would then make rissoles or cottage pie on Wednesday and Thursday, he had fish on Friday, and soup from the bone with sausages afterwards on Saturday, the day he bought another joint. In Tombland on the ground floor of the house where he had rooms, was an art dealer's shop, and my father succumbed, quite rightly, to temptation. He had bought several Norwich School paintings: four John Cromes looking up and down the Wensum river at dawn and dusk, and a lovely luminous little Stannard of Yarmouth beach with fishing boats. The dealer said that poor Stannard had moved to Yarmouth for the sea air, because he had tuberculosis, and died there in his 30s. My father, who had so many tuberculous patients, felt sorry for him. Many more pictures were bought now, some nice, one nasty: a treacly current one of a sad girl, almost of the big-tear-rolling-down-cheek kind, that Aunt Pat tried very hard to persuade him he did not want, and finally hung in an unused bedroom. He was as pleased as punch at becoming a country gentleman, and had some very happy times here.

A sturdy Irish cook came to us, who wore white false teeth that we could see were a huge improvement on the original ones when she showed us a photograph of herself as a young girl; and a brown-eyed thick eyebrowed hairy girl from the village came to do vegetables and washing up. A week or two later we got a housemaid and her husband the chauffeur-cum-butler, called Oliver Cromwell. When his wife wanted him, she used to shout, "Olli, Olli, where are you?" and we hoped the original Mrs Cromwell had once done the same. We addressed him as 'Cromwell', of course, and his wife was 'Doris'. Only cooks and housekeepers, married or not, had the honorary title of 'Mrs'. The head gardener, Brister, lived with his wife and daughter in the large cottage, and there were three other gardeners and a boy whose main purpose, my father said, was to make a tax loss.

My father had never tasted rook or moorhen pie, and hardly ever rabbit, that were used as extra protein food during rationing in the war (they were off ration), and we never had them now. We acquired two pigs, Hengist and Horsa, and a cow. This was an allowed way to get meat and milk during food rationing. The pigs lived near the sawmill, and stinking scraps were boiled up in a copper pot every day for them to eat. Only one pig per family was allowed, so one of these was ours, but the other belonged to Brister, in theory, but his family, at least two of them vegetarians, got very little of it, and I think we ate all the rest. Anyway, there was no shortage of pork, ham, bacon, sausages, brawn and lard in our house. The cow was purely theoretical. We never saw her. She was one of the neighbouring farmer's herd, and the farmer brought us five gallons of milk every morning, which was put in big flat earthenware dishes in the cool dairies, and skimmed with a shallow enamelled scoop pierced with many holes, for cream, in the evenings. The cook made the cream into butter, using a big glass jar with a handle and cogs to turn the wooden paddles: a sort of cross between hand beaters and a Kilner jar. It was very hard work, and made your arm ache. I sometimes took a turn and after all that paddling it was exciting and satisfactory to see the little flecks of gold starting to appear, and to know that at last the butter was coming. The buttermilk was fed to the pigs. We were all set up for the life of Riley.

My father's work was done at the hospital in the mornings, operating and doing ward rounds; then he had lunch at the Norfolk Club, played bridge there until he started seeing his private patients in his consulting rooms in Norwich at three, after which he did an evening round of seeing his patients in hospital, and came home for dinner. Unless, of course, it was a hunting day.

The Norfolk Club was for men, although women were allowed into one room at the front on the left. They were allowed to go in there and wait for their husbands to pick them up in the car. I often waited there for him, in the old-fashioned smell of gravy and roast potatoes and cigar smoke. He once took me to show me how you voted for new members of the Club. There was a table on which were boxes with the names of the proposed and seconded members. Each existing member was allowed two balls that could be put into any box. The balls were white or black. "Watch this," he said, and took two black balls and dropped them into the box of Duncan Begbie, the deep-voiced friend who had stayed in our house and been a friend of his before the war, but whom he now hated and despised.

"I have black-balled him," he said. "For two black balls he now won't get in, no matter how many white ones he gets."

"What did you black-ball him for, Daddy?"

"He didn't fight in the war, and other things," he said.

"What other things?"

"Never you mind."

I did not know what the 'other things' were then, and plainly I was not going to be told. But I think I may be able to guess, now.

Men's clubs, with no women, were thought quite normal then. In those days, not only could you not get into a club if you were a woman, but you could also not get in if you were 'in trade'.

Later, my father became a member of the Carlton Club, the Conservative club, in London. Once he left me in the car parked outside the club, saying "Women are not allowed in here at all. No waiting room. You'll have to stay in the car."

He took ages to return, and I wondered what men did in there, especially without women. A gorgeous head porter stood at the top of the steps by the front door, wearing a navy blue frock coat with gold buttons and frogging on it, and a top hat. I got out of the car to look through the windows, and see if I could see what went on, steadying myself with a hand on the railings.

The porter came down two steps and towered over me.

"Ladies are not allowed in here, Miss," he said.

"I know that," I answered. "I was only looking."

He was not having that.

"And ladies are not allowed to touch the railings either, Miss," he said.

I went back to the car and got in. I knew that membership of clubs gave my father satisfaction, and that it cost an awful lot of money. I could not see that the absurd grandeur and protection of the Carlton was worth having if you had to pay for it. It appeared to be men bestowing glory on themselves. I thought that you should not have to pay for honour: you should earn it.

Chapter 13
The Value of Hens

My father's sliding scale of fees, depending on whether you were a nun or a Bentley owner, had another variation. A private consultation cost five guineas, unless you paid cash, when it was five pounds. This cash all went into the bottom left-hand drawer of the secretary's desk in her office, and had a very specific purpose. Sometimes on Saturdays we drove to the consulting rooms, raided the drawer for betting money, and went off to the races at Newmarket.

There were a couple of good luck pointers on the way that told us if we would have a good day. The road to Newmarket went straight as a Roman road across Thetford common, but curving around it across the slightly contoured land, on one side and the other, lay the railway line. If we saw a train coming and could get the car up onto the bridge so that the train went under us, we would win. This necessitated either crawling along saying "Hurry up, bloody get *on* with it!" to the train, infuriating any driver behind us; or driving with utter disregard for safety, my father's right foot flat on the floor with the car windows rattling and shaking, in a frantic attempt to beat the distant train, so far ahead of us, and get up onto the bridge as it went under. That was the first good sign. The second was seeing the fat boy in Attleborough. In those days, just after the war, serious obesity was rare. But in the petrol station in Attleborough worked a young man in overalls with a big tummy, a big bottom, wide, wide thighs and little eyes, nose and mouth surrounded by a great fat face. His hands were little puffy extremities like mushrooms. You can see people as fat as that in any shopping street every day now, but then it was most remarkable. If you were exceptionally lucky, he filled your car with petrol, but our rule was that he did not have to, you just had to set eyes on him. We used to hang about in that garage for five or ten minutes, hoping to see him. It was almost worth missing the first race to do so. If the train went under us and we saw the fat boy, we were overjoyed. We knew we were right in the middle of a winning streak. There was a bit of a hold up at a junction near Barton Mills, but we never bothered with that, we took the shortcut. A lovely old red brick coaching inn with Flemish crow-stepped gables, called The Bull, had arches leading into and out of its courtyard, and several minutes could be saved by going straight through it and out onto the Newmarket road again. Elated, we charged into the Bull, juddering over the cobbles, startled open-mouthed waiters and cats and squawking chickens flying everywhere, and shot out the other side in triumph. The Bull at Barton Mills still exists, though now it is unfortunately called Ye Olde Bull Inn, and today it has glass doors across its arches, and little tables and chairs in the courtyard: we would make a terrible mess if we tried that one again. Whether in actual fact these predictions of good luck came true or not, I do not now remember, but I shall never forget the fun of notching the stick.

In Newmarket, in those early days of 1946, I learned the joy of judging a thoroughbred, of choosing a horse to bet on. I cannot tell you how to do it, it is something that comes with practice over the years. You take your chance standing in the paddock before the race, watching the horses being led around. You must concentrate very hard, you haven't got long, about 20 minutes usually; do not talk to anyone or look about you. You must look at each horse in turn, decide which you think will win, know its number and bet on it before the race starts. You know how long the race is, what the ground is like that day, what extra weight has been put on to handicap it and the age of the horse.

Importantly, what does it look like? Is it a nice shape? Not too long in the body, not too short in the leg? Has it a nicely arched neck and a firm swinging gait? If the going is wet and heavy, you want a big strong punchy horse. But a nippy little lightweight horse might win before it gets tired on a dry day when the ground is firm. Does it seem alert and pleased to be there, ears pointed forward, walking steadily, no jiggling about, no head tossing, tail swishing, no frothy sweat on its neck? Is it fit? Maybe not, if you see a 'poverty' mark, a C-shaped indentation downwards toward the back of each hind-quarter? Is it lithe and glossy, calm, steady and keen. . . yes or no, that's all you have time for, you must look at the others. After many days of racing you get the feel of it, for flat racing you can usually tell the best two or three horses, you will choose the winner from these. Over the sticks it is much harder to choose. You need to know the jockeys: their quality counts for a lot. If you have chosen the favourite, the odds will be rotten, so ask yourself if you really want to put money on; the price is big, the winnings small. The punter who wins usually has extensive experience of going to the races, and best of all has some inside knowledge. The person who I guess would win with great regularity, because she has been at it for so long, is Her Majesty the Queen. But although she has owned many winning horses, she does not bet.

My father loved race meetings. I could feel his spirit lift up as we walked in among the crowd, greeting friends, members' labels on our field glasses. As for choosing winners, I used to think he cheated. He carried up-to-date copies of *Raceform* or *Chaseform* that listed every detail of every horse. He did not have to study the horses themselves, he could just look them up. However, it has to be said that he did so enjoy it all that inevitably he spent a lot of time looking at horses. His heart was out there on the grass watching every race.

On the way home we always stopped in Prince of Wales Road in Norwich, to buy the racing copy of the *Eastern Daily Press* (the 'pink-un') to see how we had done.

Soon after we moved to the new house, Witton, I thought it would be lovely to have a pet bantam: I had found a little cage in one of the stables, and decided I could keep her in that. "Have you got any money to buy one? Because I'm going in to the Norfolk and Norwich for about an hour, and I'll take you with me and leave you at the cattle market, and you can see if you can find one. I'll pick you up at noon: you must have bought it by then."

The cattle market was large, noisy and stinking of cattle urine and dung. All the cattle were complaining, and every man seemed to be shouting, and beating poor puzzled beasts up and down the ramps of their lorries, and the railinged passages to their pens. When I found the place where chickens were sold, I could not find one hen on her own anywhere. They were all in cages in groups of three or more: usually two hens and a cock. And none of them were coming up for sale until 2 o'clock.

At noon my father found me, now in quite a state.

"I haven't got one," I wailed. "They aren't going to be sold till 2 o'clock. That's the hen I want," I said, showing him a little speckled one in a cage with two others. "But I don't want the others, I just want her."

"Well, have you asked her owner if you can buy her on her own?"

"No, I don't know who her owner is."

My father looked at the cage number, and the catalogue, and took me to the nearest pub. He asked if anyone in there knew where Mr Trowby was. Mr Trowby came away from the bar smiling and saying, "Yes?" He wore leather gaiters that buttoned up over his trousers and boots, and smoked a pipe.

"This is my daughter and she wants to ask you a question."

"Yes my darling?" he said, beaming at me. "What can I do for you?"

"I want to buy a bantam hen."

"Well, isn't that lucky? Because I've got three bantams in the sale."

"Yes, but I only want one of them, a special one, and Daddy can't wait."

"You come and show me which one you want, darling, and I'll see if I can sell her to you."

We went to the cage. I showed her to him. He pulled her out and gave her to me to hold, so beautifully speckled, soft, warm and plump, with nice little dark grey legs.

"There she is, my love, she's a real beauty, isn't she?"

"She's lovely," I replied, stroking her beautiful complicated feathers, each fawn feather laced with black. "She's just what I want. Will you sell her to me? Can I have her?"

He took her back, and dropped her into a sack. Then he handed me the sack, looked slyly at me and said, "It depends if you can afford her."

"Oh I hope so," I said, "I do hope so. How much does she cost?"

"How much money have you got?"

"23 shillings and ninepence."

"Well now, aren't you a lucky girl? Because that's exactly what she costs: 23 shillings and ninepence."

I gave him all the money I had, and walked away with the sack, near tears with joy. I had chosen the best bantam in the cattle market, and had had enough money to buy her.

In the car, my father said, "Let that be a lesson to you."

"How do you mean?"

"You must have paid five times as much as that hen is worth. I did not interfere because I wanted you to learn the lesson. Never, ever, tell anyone how much money you've got."

My father's early lesson in economics was lost on me. I opened the sack and peered in at my shy little hen, regarding me calmly now with one boot-button eye.

"Oh don't worry about it, Daddy. Please," I said. "I don't mind at all. You don't understand. I would far, far rather have this hen than 23 shillings and ninepence."

The move into the new house led to a great expansion in the good things of life. Now we could have not only a pet hen and strawberries and cream, but friends to stay, horses to ride, dinner parties and a very full social life.

He took an enormous interest in everything around him. If he asked a question he expected a good answer: short, sensible and true. Why did we keep two pigs?

Every family was allowed one pig in the war. Well, one for us and one for the gardener Brister. But Brister and his family were vegetarians. All right, two for us, presents for all our friends and Brister had all the fruit and vegetables he could grow, and was paid extra to look after the pigs. What shall we call them? Hengist and Horsa. Good names for pigs.

So by now my father was rich and famous. He was an item greatly sought after by hostesses, an eligible bachelor, and he was hugely in demand all over Norfolk to go to dinner parties. He was always very good company, full of jokes and laughter, invited everywhere. Unless he was giving a party himself, he was out most nights of the week. We used to play Gin Rummy together, and became very good at it. So, if he knew his hosts were going to play cards, he took me with him to be his partner. Because we had played together so much, and it was the essence of the game, we were able quite early on in any game to tell what cards the other held. So we often won. By now I got ten per cent of the winnings, real money for a change.

We were a tough team again, so close, we were each other's best friend. We had the intimacy of shared experience in everything we did together. We could, and did, talk to each other about nearly every subject. Except, of course, not about Pinkie. We were so close, and yet he could not talk about her. He never brought this subject up, and so neither did I: it was absolutely taboo. It was easier never to think about it, and I tried hard not to. Life became far more exciting than those dull Nanny-ruled Dublin days.

I found there were ferocious rules about going out to dinner. If anyone told a joke and everybody laughed, I was not to laugh too. I was not to let anyone know I understood the joke, which would certainly have been a rude one. And if I actually did not understand the joke I was to say nothing, keep a straight face, and I could ask what it meant in the car on the way home. I learnt quite a lot of rude jokes that way. I was not allowed to drink alcohol, and did not want to, disliking the taste. But guests did get extremely drunk at these parties. Whoops of loud laughter greeted any witticism, and really good ones received a ferocious banging of the gong in the hall (the houses where he went out to dinner all had gongs in those days). Sooner or later, the men all stood in the hall bent over with their hands on their knees, while the women tore downstairs shrieking, and leapfrogged over each man in turn in flashes of suspenders and fits of giggles.

Now became the era of aunts. Not just two girlfriends, like Pinkie and Ione before the war, my father now had them without number, and I always knew which they were, because I had to address them as 'Aunt So-and-so'. Nearly all of them were pretty, some of them were married, many of them tried to be nice to me and most of them got terribly drunk. So did my father, of course.

I remember a very grand woman walking unsteadily round at the end of a party giggling, and telling everyone: "I was a whore before I married." This seemed a very bold announcement to me, and when everyone had gone home, I asked my father, "Was Aunt So-and-so really a whore before she married?"

And he replied, "Oh, tut, did you hear that? Well, yes she was, but it was spelt H-O-A-R-E (her family owned a bank you see), not whore, not a prostitute."

Chapter 14
"Other Bugger's Effort"

Soon after returning from Dublin we went to visit an old friend, Nobby Clarke. We had a key to his consulting rooms in Harley Street from where Nobby was going to pick us up. When he did not turn up, my father started looking for a drink.

"Must have something here," he said. "Never known a consulting room with nothing to drink. Where is the bloody whisky?"

We searched every cupboard and drawer, and eventually all we came up with was a well-corked bottle of sherry. Finding only this one bottle of sherry had done nothing to improve my father's poor opinion of Nobby's abilities. He was always joking about it, usually to his face. They had remained close friends since they were medical students together, at Trinity College Dublin. There they always sat next to each other in examinations, and my father claimed that he had had to tell Nobby the answers to many of the questions in their final exams. And he also felt sure that if he had not written much of the paper for him too, Nobby would never have got the Fellowship examination of the Royal College of Surgeons of Ireland. Nobby got a knighthood in the end, and my father would have been delighted, and also mortified, to know it. That, mercifully, was long after he was dead.

"Christ! Sherry!" he now exclaimed with horror. "Is that all? Now where's the corkscrew?"

We turned the consulting rooms upside down, but there was no corkscrew there.

"Damn!" my father said. "We could snap the neck off, but it will make a frightful mess. There is another way to open a bottle. Takes a bit of time. If Nobby gets here before we get it open, well and good. If not, at least I'll have the sherry. You find some cushions."

I found some expensive looking cream silk ones on a sofa in the waiting room.

"Yup," he said. "Good. Put two or three on top of each other and hold them against the wall. Don't let go of them."

And so saying, he removed the foil and started to bang the bottom of the bottle, with both hands, onto the cushions I held against the wall.

"The force of the banging shoves the sherry against the cork," he shouted above the thumping, "and it eases the cork out. Hard work, though."

My arms ached, but so interesting was the task, and so urgent his need for sherry, that neither of us thought for a moment of the effect this pile-driving might be having on the neighbours. The neighbours in Harley Street are amongst the best paid doctors on earth: they pay a fortune to put up their brass plates here. At a very great price they care for rich patients with, as my father said, "Probably very little wrong with them, and much more money than sense."

The final bit of the cork, once he could get hold of it, was pulled out between his teeth, and we had just got it out, and were wondering whether he should put the sherry in a coffee mug or drink it straight from the bottle, when Nobby turned up, highly ruffled. He had a round, cherubic face, now bright red.

"The police are coming," he said. "They rang me, and told me I had a lunatic loose in the consulting rooms tearing them to pieces and I was to go straight here and they would join me. What have you done?"

"Well, if you'd turned up when you said you would, we would probably by now be having a drink in your flat," my father said, taking a huge glug from the neck of the bottle. "You ought to be ashamed of yourself, an Irishman, no whisky in your consulting rooms, no corkscrew, no glasses. Just this awful sherry." And he took another glug. "We had to get it open."

"That sherry was a present from a grateful patient," Nobby said, peeved. "So how did you get it open?"

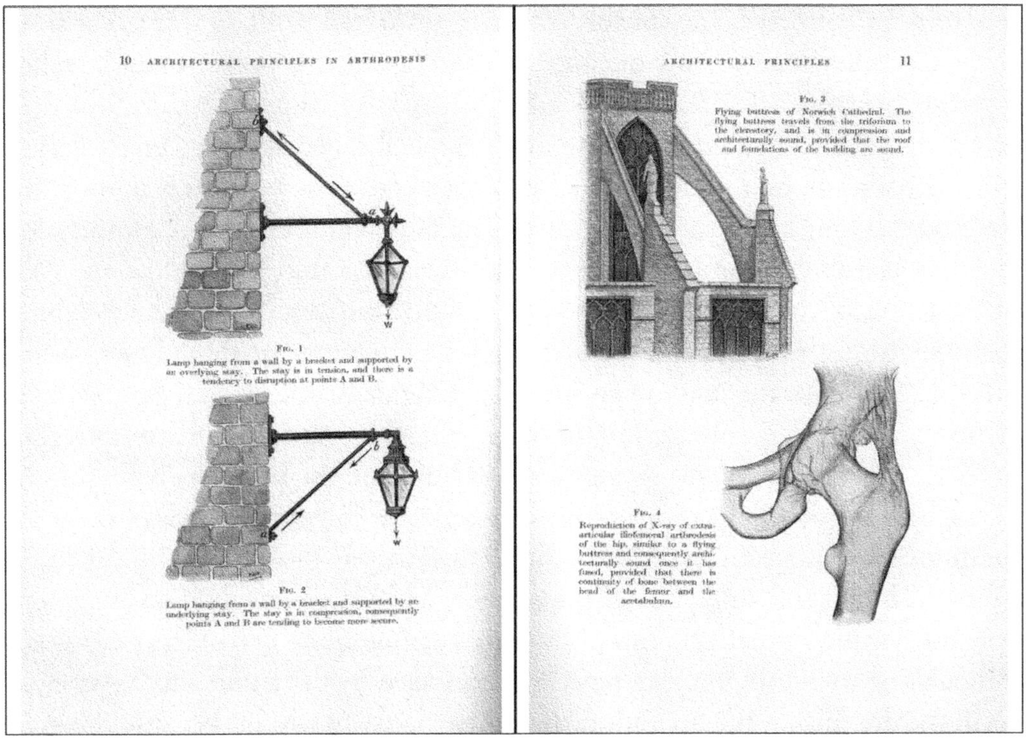
10 ARCHITECTURAL PRINCIPLES IN ARTHRODESIS

FIG. 1

Lamp hanging from a wall by a bracket and supported by an overlying stay. The stay is in tension, and there is a tendency to disruption at points A and B.

FIG. 2

Lamp hanging from a wall by a bracket and supported by an underlying stay. The stay is in compression, consequently points A and B are tending to become more secure.

ARCHITECTURAL PRINCIPLES 11

FIG. 3

Flying buttress of Norwich Cathedral. The flying buttress travels from the triforium to the clerestory, and is in compression and architecturally sound, provided that the roof and foundations of the building are sound.

FIG. 4

Reproduction of X-ray of extra-articular iliofemoral arthrodesis of the hip, similar to a flying buttress and consequently architecturally sound once it has fused, provided that there is continuity of bone between the head of the femur and the acetabulum.

An excerpt from 'Architectural Principles in Arthrodesis' by Tommy Brittain, showing the influence of the flying buttresses of Norwich Cathedral in his pioneering hip joint operation.

The principle of slamming the sherry against the cork was explained, and my father said, slightly apologetically, "We did use cushions to soften the blows."

Nobby giggled. "Well come on, quick, let's get out of here before the police arrive. I don't want to explain that to them."

My father now had a new operation of his own (thanks to Professor Girdlestone and the bathroom mirror). The inspiration for it came from the flying buttresses of Norwich Cathedral. His first lodgings (above the art dealer in Tombland), were just outside the cathedral close, and he used to go for runs round the close and gaze at the cathedral and think about its engineering. The top storey of windows, the clerestory, just under the roof, has as many windows as possible to lighten the top part of the walls. Then, when a heavy lead roof is placed on them, a huge outward thrust is imparted to these thin walls from above, and they tend to bow outwards and collapse. This pressure can be taken by flying buttresses that leap off the top of the walls taking the weight in a delicate arch attached to a free-standing pillar. A weight, usually some pretty carved stone decoration, on top of the pillar holds it steady. The buttresses support the clerestory so long as the roof and foundations are good. They are in compression and architecturally sound. This most beautiful solution inspired him. The neck of the femur of the human hip is a kind of flying buttress, taking the weight of the body from the pelvis and transferring it to the femur or thigh bone. When it breaks, becomes tuberculous, or in old age the ball and socket joint becomes arthritic, it causes its sufferer unremitting pain. If it were possible to get a graft in there, in compression, to strengthen and hold still the neck of the femur, the flying buttress of the hip, the problem would be solved. Nowadays there are titanium hip replacements, but the first solution was to fix the joint, giving it strength, but preventing painful movement. My father invented an ingenious operation to fix an arthritic hip joint with a strong bone graft. The graft was a difficult one to put in, its exact position controlled by instantaneous X-rays taken in theatre during the operation. It was particularly strong, because the graft was in compression between the pelvis and the top of the femur. This allowed a patient to walk again (but with a slight limp, because the joint was set slightly bent, so that the patient could both sit and stand) and to be completely free of pain. The limp could actually be concealed by a very determined patient: a friend of my father's who had fought in the First World War wanted to pass a medical to fight in the Second, but he had had an arthrodesis of his hip (my father's operation). He normally walked with a limp, but he practised for days in front of a long mirror, and also up and down a corridor with my father coaching him, and they were both proud of their work when the army accepted him. No previous attempts at this operation were successful, other kinds of grafts failed: patients had been crippled, in terrible pain, and those who broke the neck of the femur could never walk again and often died soon after, of pneumonia caused by the shock and forced inactivity.

My father said it was extraordinary and very satisfactory that the first thing that patients said, as soon as they came round from the anaesthetic, was: "I can't feel any pain".

As for titanium hip replacements that might get the joint moving again, and make it possible to walk normally with no limp, of course my father considered them as a solution. He told me, however, that from experience he knew that live bone against live bone grows and forms a strong bond, but live bone applied against metal eventually fails because the bone cells in contact with the metal die. He thought hip replacements would work briefly, but sooner rather than later would fail. He thought there would need to be frequent replacements, and there was limited room at the head of the femur for that. But much more than that, his most hated enemy, Kenneth McKee, the second orthopaedic surgeon at the Norfolk and Norwich Hospital, did want to try them. My father absolutely loathed McKee, and it was his children I had to beat on my ponies at gymkhanas and hunter trials in order to please my father. As far as he was concerned, anything that McKee thought was good, had to be bad and dangerous. This hatred was due to McKee having failed in a gentleman's agreement. He arrived at the beginning of the war, when my father had already volunteered, to take his place in a reserved occupation while my father fought. The agreement was that when you took on the private patients of another doctor who was fighting, after the war you gave the money you had made, or some of it anyway, to the returning doctor whose patients they had been. McKee gave none, and my father did not forgive.

My father needed to publish his work, and without much difficulty persuaded other orthopaedic surgeons to do his operation also, so he could gather sufficient numbers of patients to write it up. An orthopaedic friend of his, Bobby Burns, had invented an operation to cure slipped discs in the spine, and each of them, delighted with their two new inventions, helped each other out by doing the other's operation.

Gentle John Barratt was one of the last soldiers to return from the war. He was one of the three friends who came to pay rent. He came back from Burma in a terrible state, having been forced by the Japanese to work on the infamous railway line. He spent the whole war in the Far East, and was never anywhere near Hitler.

"Hello darling Alison," he said to me. "I am so sorry I let you down. I didn't keep my promise. I never got you Hitler's moustache."

I wondered what I would have done with it if he had got it. Nailed it up among the pony club gymkhana rosettes in the harness room, perhaps.

He was hardly recognisable, thin and gaunt, with terrible dysentery. He at least had survived, though many of his companions there had not. He had been a highly athletic man, and an excellent tennis player, and for some reason, after he had returned from the war and was recovering from his dysentery, he slipped a disc. So it was my father who operated on John, with such success that he was able to film him jumping our ha-ha (at least 14 feet across), and took the film on a lecture tour of America. Because of the new operation, and the book he had written about it, with the uninspiring title 'Architectural Principles in Arthrodesis', he was now in demand to give lectures all over the world, and coach loads of American surgeons came up to Norwich to watch him operate. The first edition of the book, by the way, which came out in 1941, had a title page dedicating it, in large gothic letters, 'To R.D.B.': Rosemary Dering Bulwer, Pinkie's proper names.

I still often talked to my father as he was getting up and having breakfast. I remember one morning he stood in his shirt and underpants gazing into the bathroom mirror. There was a strong smell of a burning match, and wax, as he lit a candle on the basin.

"You know when I went away to fight I was just a Captain?"

"A Captain. Were you?"

He held a long pair of medical forceps in the yellow flame, and black smoke guttered above it.

"Yes, but I've come back as a Lieutenant Colonel, with an OBE, and Mentioned in Dispatches."

"What does OBE stand for?"

"Other Bugger's Effort. The brave chap who should have got it gets killed. So someone who was just standing by gets it. One day I'll tell you why I really got it."

"Tell me now."

"No".

"And what is Mentioned in Dispatches?"

He stuck a comb upwards through one side of his moustache, next to his skin.

"They write a letter to the War Office, saying 'This, that and the other one got killed or wounded, and Major Brittain didn't, but he did try hard'."

"Now the war is over, does it matter?"

"No, not much."

He clamped the forceps onto the hairs sticking out through the comb, and twisted them upwards. There came the dark smell of burning hair.

"What *are* you doing, Daddy?"

"Curling my moustache."

"Why?"

"Because I'm a Lieutenant Colonel. If you're a Colonel in the British Army, and you grow a moustache, it should be curly. Mustn't look like Hitler."

He had black hair on his head, but his moustache was red. He pushed the hot hairs upwards with his fingers after he had taken away the forceps and comb, and turned round and glared at me.

"Do I look tough?"

I knew the right answer to that.

"Yes you do," I said, and he looked particularly pleased with himself.

Later, I heard him tell a friend of his why he had got his OBE. One day in his base hospital in Naples, an orderly came rushing into theatre saying: "We're in trouble. Major General Templer has been blown up in his jeep, and is quite severely wounded. His back is broken. He has been through two field dressing stations (where they did first aid), demanding that they deal with him at once. When they refused, and sent him on, he sacked the entire staff of the field dressing station. And the same again at the next one. And now he is coming here." "We'll take him as he comes," my father said, and went on operating.

When the General arrived, all the staff were fidgety with fear. My father examined his patient, and found his back broken in four places, and I think a

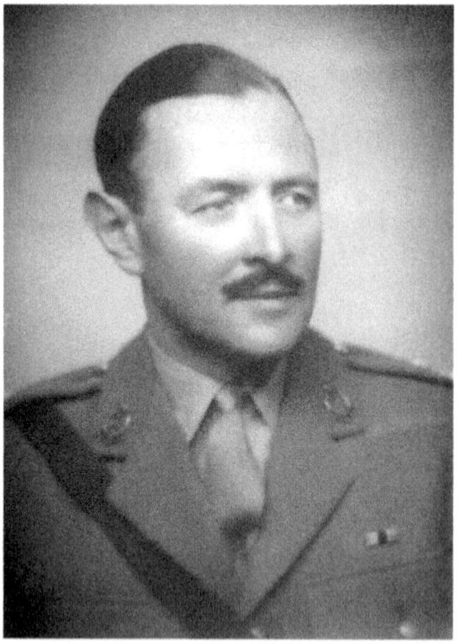

Tommy Brittain in the Army Medical Corps, "Do I Look Tough?" c. 1941.

femur was broken too. So he explained what was wrong to him, and said he would make him comfortable, and operate next morning. The General, as expected, announced that my father was sacked: "I shouldn't do that, if I were you, because then there will be no one to operate on you."

It had been three hours since the injuries had occurred, he had been examined, painfully, by two dressing stations, and was now in severe shock.

"You can sack me if you want, but under no circumstances will I operate on you tonight because it will be a waste of my time. You are in shock, and it will kill you."

The General backed down, was given morphine for the pain, and was in theatre the next morning. While he recovered, they became the best of friends: both appreciating the toughness of the other. Towards the end of his recovery, though still in plaster-of-Paris all over his torso, he told my father, formally, "At 1800 hours this evening Wren Officer [he named her] will come to my room. She will leave at 0800 the next morning. During that time, we will not be disturbed."

My father answered, "Sir".

And it all went according to plan, and my father got the OBE. I did ask the War Office what he got it for, and they would not tell me, so I shall have to believe the only version I have. Later, after the war was over, they remained great friends, and Field Marshall Sir Gerald Templer became Chief of the Imperial General Staff, head of the army.

The first time I watched him doing something to a patient, it was called a 'manipulation', not an operation, and it was done in the corridor outside theatre. The patient, a woman, wore a hospital nightdress and her knickers, and lay on a hospital trolley. My father and his registrar grabbed her, and I thought they would kill her. They took each limb in turn and bent and twisted all the joints, one by one, even her fingers and toes, as hard as they could. Then one of them held her down by the shoulders and the other pulled her legs up over her head till her ears were between her knees. They were both big strong men, and they turned her over and this time curled her spine backwards till her feet were by her ears. They huffed and grunted with the effort they were making, but the most awful thing was the way she groaned at the last two manoeuvres, as if in terrible agony.

"You must stop it, Daddy," I said. "You're hurting her."

"Shut up, or go away."

"Please stop it, now."

"I'll talk to you later. For God's sake, do as I tell you, go away."

In the car, on the way home, I asked "Were you trying to kill her?"

"Maybe," he said. "A bit."

"You were really hurting her. She was groaning in agony."

"No she wasn't. She was deeply, deeply anaesthetised. The groaning was just the air being squeezed out of her lungs."

"Why were you trying to kill her, Daddy?"

"When she wakes up I want her to feel as if an atom bomb has hit her. She makes a frightful fuss about everything. She can't move this, she can't move that: this hurts, that hurts." He grinned. "About now I bet it all hurts."

"But that's cruel, you know it is. Why did you do it? Will that make her better?"

"We were putting each of her joints through its full range of movement. When she comes to she will be a bit stiff and sore, but as that wears off she should find she is more mobile. And better still, she will stop complaining, because I am sure she won't want us to do that to her again. Do you want to be a doctor when you grow up?"

"No."

"Good. Women doctors are awful."

"Are they really?"

He smiled with satisfaction, and said "Horrible".

If he could come back now and discover that two of his granddaughters are doctors, it would actually be much more in character for him, instead of thinking them horrible, to be rather embarrassingly proud of them, and to bore everybody with news of their medical successes.

On a much later occasion I did say that although I did not want to be a doctor, I thought I would like to go to university.

"Oh for Christ's sake," he said, "whatever next? In God's name give that idea up quickly. You'd only become a bluestocking, and then no one will marry you. Stupid thought. All you need is to be able to play tennis, speak French and play bridge. And have a fine seat on a horse." I was never any good at tennis, or French, or bridge. I do have a good seat on a horse, but have never been able to afford one to sit on. I never went to university, and I did get married. Even so, I think he was wrong.

What today is known as alternative medicine, he always referred to as 'faith healing for the simple minded'. Physiotherapists were fine, he said. They could make all the difference to the result of an operation. You did the operation, but they got the patient going again. They were a knowledgeable and essential part of orthopaedic surgery. "However, there are utterly despicable charlatans, called 'Push-me-Pull-Yous', who have no proper training and have no idea what they are doing. They are extremely dangerous, and either they do more harm than good, or their patients get better in spite of them. They mostly deal with back pain. A lot of people get back pain, and usually there is nothing to show for it. You can't see anything on an X-ray."

He started to laugh.

"You remember the other day I came home from my consulting rooms walking on air, saying I'd had a wonderful day?"

"Yes. I thought you must have won on the horses. What was it?"

"Well, a fortnight before that, a woman came to see me with a pain in her back. Not a bad pain, couldn't see much, she could move about all right, walk and everything. She had a very slight slipped disc, which I thought would probably resolve on its own. You know, you can make a frightful muck of someone doing a slipped disc operation. Chisel slips a bit, and in you go, straight into the spinal cord, and then my God, the patient is paralysed from there downwards. That's the worst that can happen. But very occasionally it does. So you don't want to go doing this operation unless you really have to."

"Did she get better?"

"Ha, ha. That's the wonderful thing. Just as I was sending her off to take it easy and get better on her own, she said to me: 'I was wondering, Mr Brittain, if I should go and see a 'Push-Me-Pull-You' to whom I've been recommended?' Only she didn't say 'Push-Me-Pull-You', of course, she said osteopath. So I said 'I have already given you my advice, and I cannot possibly discuss whether you should visit an osteopath, but by all means if you want to, do so'."

"Did she?"

"Oh yes indeed she did, and with his so-called manipulations he wrenched her vertebrae apart and the disc slipped really badly. The day I came home walking on air she had just been brought to me in my consulting rooms *on a stretcher*. Hoo, hoo! And I operated on her a few days ago and she's fine now."

"Did you tell her it was the 'Push-Me-Pull-You's' fault?"

"No, of course not. It would have been most unprofessional. I didn't have to, did I? She won't be seeing one of those again, I bet, in the rest of her life."

We often discussed other medical matters.

Once, when we were driving along in the car, he told me the perfect way to commit suicide.

"A massive dose of insulin will kill you, but you've got a few minutes before it does. It starves your brain of the food it needs, and off you go. Quite painless, it seems."

"Do you swallow the insulin? Does it taste nasty?"

"No, no. You inject it. What you do is, you find a road on a steep hill with a T-junction at the bottom of it. There must be a house, or a substantial wall across the bottom. About 3 o'clock in the morning, when no one's around, you park at the top, with the engine running and the handbrake off, fill a big syringe with insulin, and inject it. You have time to throw the bottle and syringe away into the bushes where it won't be found. Then you rev up the engine, let in the clutch, and hurtle down hill hell for leather for the wall. That's it."

"Why don't you just drive into the wall?"

"Might just make an awful mess and not kill you, but in a minute or two, the insulin will. It starves your brain. As it kills you it is metabolised in the body, and no trace of it remains. And apart from the crash damage, there won't be a mark on you, so no one will know it's suicide."

"But what's the point of that? Once you're dead, what does it matter who knows?"

"It matters to the insurance company all right. If you've got life insurance, and they think you committed suicide, they won't pay out. So the people who were going to get it, don't."

"Why don't they know?"

Only if a very clever doctor does the post mortem, and suspects this method (it is very rare, or not often discovered), might he look carefully for the tiny hole from the injection. But they never do. Too hard."

"It must be awful driving deliberately at a wall."

"Well, you aren't going to do it unless you want to be dead, are you? So then it's simply nothing."

You would still have to be amazingly tough to do it, I thought. You would have to plan it all in advance, and keep your nerve while you set about it. No cry for help, this. No hoping that someone would find you and bring you back to life. If you had that much courage, I wondered why you did not want to live.

Chapter 15
The Operating Table

One summer evening in 1946 we went to the livery stables right in the middle of Norwich. "That's my new surprise," my father proudly declared. A stunning, glistening, slightly rangy bay horse with one wall eye was led up and down on the cobbles before us. "I bought him in Ireland, on advice, and he's just arrived, and what do you think?"

"Oh Daddy, he's gorgeous. Can I please ride him? What are you going to do with him?"

"Hunt him, and then ride him in a point-to-point, I hope."

We called him O'Hara, because he was Irish. His sire was a famous winning thoroughbred stallion called Steelpoint, all of whose progeny were well known for being very fast, and very mad. One of them was five lengths out in front coming up to the finish at Newmarket, and, to the astonishment of its unprepared jockey, suddenly decided to jump the white railings and take the shortcut back to its stable. Other progeny refused to pull up at the end of a race, and careered off for miles and miles over fields and farmland, quite out of control, jockeys simply taken for a ride. But if a Steelpoint horse got to the winning post, it usually passed it first.

O'Hara was the very devil to ride. He ran away with my father. He bolted with me. He tore away with riders much more experienced than either of us. But he went like the wind. My father hunted him, and if he fell off it took us days and days to find the horse. Then he entered him in a point-to-point, and lost two stone in weight, to give O'Hara a chance.

It was a three and a half mile race, and at the last fence there were two horses out in front jumping it side-by-side, one of them O'Hara. I saw them jump, but

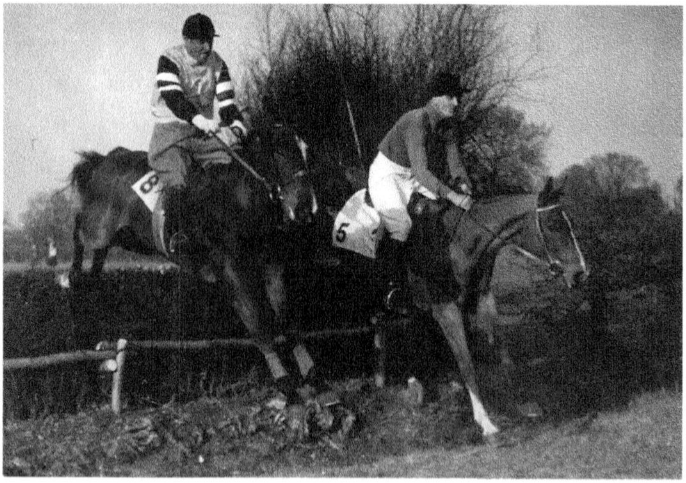

Tommy Brittain, nearest camera, riding O'Hara in the Norwich Staghounds point-to-point. Tommy Phillips is beside him: at the next fence both men fell off and were seriously injured.

could not see the other side, where my father fell off. He lost a stirrup, and with all his weight in the other one, the saddle slipped round, and that was that. It took a fortnight to find O'Hara, but that hardly mattered.

Ten minutes after the finish I saw my father, hatless, covered in mud, walking uncertainly over the field towards the car with his clenched fist under his chin.

His secretary drove him and me to the hospital, and I saw him in the passage, on the telephone to Bobby Burns and Nobby Clarke, saying: "I have fallen off my horse and dislocated my neck, and I am holding my head on with my hand, and can you come and sort it out for me, please?"

X-rays confirmed his diagnosis, and Bobby and Nobby came that night and tied his cervical vertebrae together with stainless steel wire. When I next saw him he was in an extraordinary plaster-of-Paris coat, which went down to his hips and up over his head like a modern day hoodie.

He was terribly ill, got pneumonia more than once, lost much more weight, and I could tell that people were thinking he might die. I trusted that his extremely tough personality would not let him die, and anyway, he had a score to settle. A very experienced rider, Tommy Phillips, was on the horse beside him at the last fence, and my father thought Tommy had kicked his foot out of the stirrup on purpose. The horses had collided at the fence, and Tommy fell off and got trodden on by another horse, and lost a kidney. He was in the same hospital. Totally immobile, my father was snarling away, threatening to kill him. I did not worry about that, because I knew he was in no position to do so.

Because he kept getting ill again, he took ages, weeks and weeks, to recover. Then, what seemed like months later I went to see him and we were alone and he said, "Quick darling, quick, you must help me".

"What shall I do?"

"Get my big sponge and put it in the basin full of water, and don't squeeze it, just bring it here."

He put the sponge on his stomach and said, "Now get my nail scissors, and start cutting at the bottom, where I have wetted it."

"Your pyjamas are wet, and so is the bed."

"Just cut."

It was desperately hard work. The curved nail scissors had blades about half an inch long, and the plaster-of-Paris was nearly two inches thick. I wetted and cut and wetted and cut until I had bleeding rings round both my thumbs. The water soaked through the bed, and dribbled white melted plaster-of-Paris onto the linoleum. Finally I had it cut all the way up to his neck and he sat up and said, "Now help me out".

It was still so stiff that he could not get his arms out, and much more wetting was needed before I managed to pull it off him. He put his feet on the floor, and then stumbled off down the corridor, carrying the plaster cast, saying "You stay there. I'm going to go and kill Tommy Phillips."

Horrified, I crept quietly behind him, knowing he could not turn his head to see.

He walked into Sister's office, plonked the soaking cast down on her desk, and said: "There you are. I told you it was itching and you took no notice. Now you'll have to have another one put on. Can you get my stooge to come and see me?"

I had never known a woman stand up to my father before, but Sister, his very own Orthopaedic Theatre Sister and his right hand, stood up and said angrily: "How dare you, Mr Brittain? Go straight back to bed at once."

And he humbly turned, and shuffled back up the corridor towards his soggy bed, saying to me: "What are you doing here?"

"I was going to try and stop you killing Tommy Phillips", I replied.

They put a new plaster on and weeks later, when they finally took it off again, and took out the steel wire, he said to me: "Look, I've got a great idea. They're going to take me off to X-ray in a minute to check they've got it all out. They gave me the wire, here it is. You pull the dressing off the wound on the back of my neck. Gently, it's sore. Lay the wire on the wound and put back the dressing. Now we'll have some fun."

Bobby Burns and Nobby Clarke had stayed the night at our house, after taking out the wire, and were waiting in his room in the hospital when my father came back from X-ray. They were having a drink to celebrate, and about five minutes later a wide-eyed radiologist arrived with the films, still dripping.

I had already been told that I would say nothing, and that my face would not give the game away. The surgeons held the X-rays up against the window for minutes, and then were very quiet.

"Well then. What is it? Lost your tongues have you?"

Reaching behind his neck my father pulled the wire out from under the dressing and held it up, saying: "Gentlemen, was this what you are looking for?"

Bobby and Nobby believed my father to be so extremely ill that he was beyond practical jokes. Their straight and worried faces in an instant creased into wide grins of relief, and loud laughter. My father winked at me.

The dislocated neck had taken months to mend, but he did recover, and started working again, and riding, and hunting with the same old enthusiasm and recklessness. Once he was convinced there was no danger of me trying to become a doctor, he allowed me to watch him operate.

"You'll wear a gown and mask, and these things on your shoes. You'll keep your hands in your pockets, and touch nothing. The most important thing is, you will *say* nothing. If you don't like what you see, or feel sick or faint, don't tell me, bloody well go outside, and be sick there. I don't want to see you, and I definitely don't want to hear you. If I have time while I am operating, I will call you to explain what is going on, and you can come and see. Is all that clear? Because if not I don't want you anywhere near."

Ah, what a challenge. I was as good as gold. The first operation he let me see was the removal of a torn cartilage from a patient's knee.

"Easy one first", he said, "no blood. We put a tourniquet, a rubber strap, see, tightly round his thigh, and then we can see what we are doing, because it doesn't bleed. Mustn't forget it, though." He said that one of his colleagues (one I knew well because he was often staying with us), had operated in the morning, and only remembered the tourniquet when he did his evening rounds. To his horror, it was still there. He undid it, and later, the patient died.

"Why did he die, Daddy?"

"No circulation in his leg for eight hours. Lot of bad blood in it. Let it all go at once, and his kidneys tried to sort it out. But it was too much for them, and they packed it in, and he died."

I could hardly wait for the operation to be over, so that I could see them take the tourniquet off.

Patients always looked so mysterious on the operating table. For one thing, they had a big orange balloon coming out of their mouths, inflating and deflating regularly, almost as if they were a character in a comic, about to give an opinion on something. And for another, the patient was just a heap, lying on the table all covered in green cloths. Only the skin in the place where they were to operate was visible: you had no idea what sort of a person was under there. They started by painting the skin with pink stuff, and always the most shocking part was when my father, with what seemed no effort at all, drew a scalpel down the line of the operation, and the skin opened up and little pin-pricks of blood seeped all along the edges.

Theatre sister seemed to be in telepathic communication with my father. She had a tray of instruments in front of her, and as soon as my father had finished with the scalpel, he held his hand out to her, and she took the scalpel and put the next thing he needed in his hand. He did not even look at it before he used it. She always chose the right thing.

Once, they were putting a bone graft in a woman's back. They cut the graft out of the front of her leg below the knee. Then the young assistant surgeon, with a pair of forceps, lifted the piece of bone to put it in a kidney dish, and dropped it on the floor. There were 30 seconds of silence. I felt terribly sorry for him, on the wrong end of my father's extreme displeasure. They had to cut another from her other leg, with my father snarling "Just bloody remember, Charles, that she only has these two legs". They injected a lot of saline into her, either side of her back, to stop her bleeding too much. Nonetheless blood poured from her, gobs of it dripping to the floor and making a huge congealing puddle for the surgeons to stand in. They stuffed many swabs in either side of her spine to soak it up, but still she bled. Eventually the graft was in, the wound was stitched, and they went to stitch up her two legs. "Charles", my father said, "race you." At this sign of forgiveness Charles relaxed, and together, like magicians, they whipped along either leg, Charles very wisely just losing the race. After they had finished, my father said "Swabs?" to Sister, and she replied "24". They were laid out in lines, ten in a line, on a piece of rubber matting. He counted them, said "Good", and to me, "It is all too easy to leave a swab behind. I left 20 once. Awful".

I said, "Will she die from losing so much blood?"

"So much blood? Go and get a glass of water from the sink, fill it to the brim and bring it here."

I did, and he said "Now pour it on the floor".

"On the floor?"

"Yes, for God's sake, just get on and do it."

I did.

"That's a half pint glass", he said. "You have eight pints of blood in you. Now look at the size of the pool of water, and the pool of blood. Did she lose a lot of blood? She did not."

It is Christmas Day, 1946, at the Norfolk and Norwich. My six foot father, chief orthopaedic surgeon, arrives at ten thirty in the morning, and is surrounded by shrieking nurses, seized, forced struggling into a Father Christmas cloak, has a beard stuck crooked on his face, and is pushed down onto a hospital trolley. Squealing with joy, the nurses (quite drunk on the sherry they have been given as presents by patients, which they have been drinking out of hospital tumblers since just after their early breakfast), run the trolley headlong up and down the male and female orthopaedic wards, my father girthed on with restraints used for violent patients. In another part of the hospital, the Lord Mayor of Norwich, wearing his chain, is having the same treatment. Every patient well enough to be sent home has gone, so only the seriously ill remain. At the top of the men's ward, my father is allowed to get off the trolley, and, still dressed as a rumpled Father Christmas, carves with surgical skill the giant turkey. Nurses add hard roast potatoes, long-cooked grey sprouts, slimy bread sauce and congealing gravy, and take the plates to the patients who are too ill or in too much pain to touch it. A group of carol-singers from the hospital choir sing 'Away in a Manger' very loudly, and during it my father says to me, "We're not going to have any of this. You and I will have ours at home". It is only just noon when we leave.

On the way home, we pick up a couple of cold-looking American airmen walking on the pavement, who were from the nearest air base. They are having 24 hours' leave for Christmas, and have come to Norwich looking for something to do. There is nothing to do in Norwich on Christmas day.

"Come and have Christmas dinner with us," my father invited them. "There really is nothing to do in Norwich, even the pubs won't open today. And there are only two of us: we need some company."

I think we did that every year for about three years, and it was always a happy occasion. They drank chilled champagne in front of a roaring wood fire, and took out photographs of their wives and children from their pocket books, and said how lonely they were, and how nice it was to be in someone's home for Christmas. They said we had a lovely place here, which always delighted my father: he liked the 'Americanness' of using the word 'place'. They told us about Thanksgiving while they ate the turkey and plum pudding and drank red wine, and they were made to listen to the stuttering King's speech on the radio with brandy afterwards. When we took them back into Norwich to be picked up to go back to the base, they were warm, rather drunk and happy, and thanked us for the best Christmas they could possibly have had. For many years afterwards, two of them, from two different Christmases, each sent us a huge bouquet of flowers on Christmas day.

I knew my father was not a mild man, neither cautious nor prudent. He was a wild, exciting man who never dipped his toe in the waters of life to test them, but leapt in up to his neck, swimming furiously. What of course I could not know, until I met them, was that in the medical profession there was a gang of men with these characteristics, who behaved almost as if they were related, like brothers. These were all his colleagues: other orthopaedic surgeons. About twice a year, all his orthopaedic friends came to stay a long weekend at Witton, and I wondered if the place would not explode with their reckless excitement. They used to tell each other silly (and very rude) poems they had learnt as medical students, and one in particular remains with me.

In Corsica so I am told, at least that's where my story begins,
Two brothers were born at one moment, joined together like Siamese twins.
Their parents were certainly cranky, for what did the old buggers do,
But send for Sir Lucius de Franchi, who cut them from one into two.

In spite of this operation, each brother could still feel exactly what was happening to the other.

When Mum wiped the bum of one brother, the other one felt it so keen,
He took down his trousers *instanter*, to see his own bottom was clean.

Of course, as the twins grow up, the poem gets ruder and ruder. I can remember some of the rest of it, which is exceedingly coarse. It must surely have come from at least a generation before these surgeons were students, maybe even longer ago. It ought to be possible to date it from the given fact that when this stuff was written, the price and style of a cheap prostitute was 'a fourpenny touch in the park'. The scatological poetry of today's medical students must be different, and may be constrained by the fact that nowadays half the doctors of medicine are women.

I have looked everywhere for this poem, and could not find it. But now, to my great pleasure, I see it is based on a perfectly serious novella of 1844 by Alexandre Dumas, père, entitled 'The Corsican Brothers'. The conjoined twins Louis and Lucien de Franchi were highly sensitive, and, in spite of being separated and living far apart, instinctively knew what was happening to the other. In the real story, their father is named 'Sir Lucius'.

I remember, after dinner, the surgeons all stood on the landing in their pyjamas, offering each other the latest thing in sleeping pills. Someone said "Try some of these, these are not barbiturates. These are from Switzerland. They are hypnotics". And they all had some, and then presumably they all fell asleep at the same moment.

Once, when I was 14, I had to hire a cabin cruiser for six of them for the day on the Norfolk Broads. The cook made them an elegant picnic lunch, which they were going to eat on the bank somewhere, and they took several crates of champagne along.

Nobby came. As it happened he never drank alcohol, but nonetheless he knew, as all Irishmen do, how to party and was one of the naughtiest; and Bobby Burns came and threw himself into everything, ending up quite paralytic, with apparently no thought for the morrow. Really nice Pete Smith Petersen came, the inventor of the Smith Petersen Pin, or Nail, which was used as another way of holding a hurt hip stiff. He had left Sweden when he was 16, and arriving in the United States with one dollar in his pocket had taken the opportunities that the country offered, and became its greatest orthopaedic surgeon. Reg Watson-Jones came. Years later he was Surgeon to the Queen, and my father claimed that he keenly looked forward to the Trooping of the Colour, the great annual State event when the Queen took the salute riding side-saddle on a big chestnut gelding called, most politically incorrectly, Winston. Probably the only chance Reg had of getting his hands on Her Majesty, my father said, was if Winston took fright and the Queen fell off and broke something.

The day was lovely. I piloted the boat, and from time to time I looked down into the cabin and said "Tell me when you want to stop and eat lunch". They were laughing and chattering down in the cabin like small boys, and they shouted "Keep going, we'll eat it in here". They passed some up to me, and I watched the reeds slip by as we chugged along. Then my father had what seemed to him a good idea. He bet Reg Watson-Jones that he couldn't fire a champagne cork straight out of one of the eight tiny portholes. "If you do it, I pay you a pound. If you fail, you double up and bet the next man he can't do it for two pounds."

There was no point opening a second bottle until they had drunk the first, and the afternoon wore on to the bellows of excitement and popping and banging of ricocheting corks flying round the cabin, while they ducked and swerved and started betting serious money. By the time the sun was setting over the glittering water, and the reeds were golden, they had still not come on deck, let alone onto the bank, and had seen nothing of the Broads. But tears of helpless laughter streamed down their cheeks, and I realised somewhat indignantly, as I brought the boat alongside and moored her, that I was in sole charge of some of the nation's and indeed the world's greatest orthopaedic surgeons. It was down to me to help them climb up the companionway and along the plank to terra firma. And peering down at them, I could see that several of them were incapable of standing. As with two hands I carefully steered them, one by one, along the gangplank, I wondered what they would have done without me.

Chapter 16
Side-saddle

Sir Alfred Munnings painted a shining portrait of Sybil Harker, Master of the Norwich Staghounds, riding side-saddle on her huge horse, surrounded by her giant hounds. She is wearing a black velvet hunt cap, with her black hair in a net, white stock round her throat, navy blue Melton riding habit, and she carries her crop.

I knew her in my early teens as a tall striking woman, with a deep man's voice. She rode powerfully but elegantly, and looked magnificent. They say that on a side-saddle one rides two stone heavier than astride, so a bigger, more powerful horse is necessary. Sybil Harker was a big tall woman, and she had an enormous horse, or so it looked to me, and I thought that no form of address could have suited her better than 'Master'.

I hated the very idea of hunting: it seemed so unkind to chase a frightened animal with slavering dogs. I did not want to enjoy that, and I did not believe I could. But after a summer holiday of Pony Club gymkhanas I found that at Christmas all my friends were hunting. My father cleverly suggested that I might try, and if I really hated it I need not go again. So I weakly gave in, and tried.

I first went out with the Dunston Harriers, a few miles south of Norwich. At the meet the harriers seemed to me delightful: full of enthusiasm and affection, wanting to stand on their hind legs and reach up and lick everyone's face. I could not see them as slavering. Beagles are the smallest of all hounds, and you hunt hares on foot with them, so they must not go faster than a human can run. Harriers are the next size up, half way between beagles and foxhounds. They also hunt hares, but followers are mounted on horses. Hares have territories which they are reluctant to leave, so when hunted they hurtle round the edge

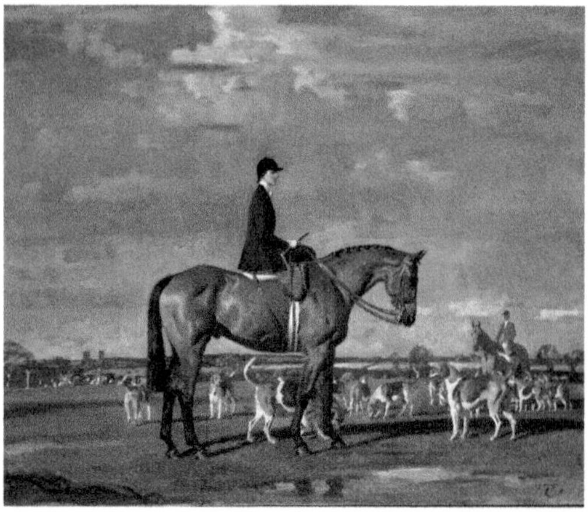

Sybil Harker, Master of the Norwich Staghounds, on her enormous horse, Saxa, with her favourite hound beside her and Tom Thackeray the huntsman in the background. Painted by Sir Alfred Munnings (Photo © Christie's Images / Bridgeman Images).

of their homeland and often return again to the same spot, a bit like the false hare on a greyhound track. My father was extremely scornful of this kind of hunting, and said you might as well just climb a haystack, and watch it all from there.

In those days there were haystacks, plenty of them, because the landscape had not yet been disfigured with big Dutch barns, or rooves on steel stalks. Haystacks were not always in the farmyard, many were in a corner of the field where the hay was made. In a yard, if one burned they all went. They were safer in the field. Once the crop was cut in August, the stubble was just left for the winter, and serious ploughing did not start till after Christmas. Flocks of black and white lapwings rose up and down over the stubbles, wheeling together in dense formation, crying 'Peewit'. Unless the stubble had a layer, a second crop of clover coming up beneath it, you could ride on it, and it was nice and firm. The field gates were often left open, because there was nothing valuable in the ground. So the riding was easy and it was often not necessary to jump.

In the hunting field there were many parents on foot urging on a great many mounted children, tightening the girths of fat ponies, smacking them on the bottom with the flat of their hands to improve their keenness. I never did see a kill, and am not sure we ever made one. There was a great deal of standing around on impatient ponies, and very little action. But the worst was over: I could face the idea of hounds killing a hare, even though I never saw it.

Shortly after we came back to England, Caravan, my father's heavyweight hunter, was brought up from the marshes to Henry Bothway's stables, to get fit for hunting in the autumn.

"Henry has a beautiful pony you might want. Shall we look at her?"

"Oh, mmmh, she's beautiful."

"Put her through her paces, then."

"Daddy, I'm frightened: she's very excitable and nervous. I may not be able to stop her."

"If you want this pony you will make her trot, canter and gallop, yes fast, right round this field. And then you will take her over that jump. Now."

"I can't, I can't, I'm afraid."

"OK. Get in the car. We're going home. Stop snivelling."

"Oh please, will you give me one more chance? Let me try her?"

"Try. I'm watching. Good. Now the gate, come on."

"We did it!"

"Yes you did. And you both looked good doing it. She jumps very big and you rode her perfectly. I'm very proud of you. I'll tell Henry. How about that?"

That's how he got his patients to walk again. They really did not have a chance not to.

I had two ponies now. Beautiful Dinah, liver chestnut with a black mane and tail, a real delight for the eye, she almost always came first as best pony in her class. My father and I often sang:

> Dinah, is there anyone finer,
>
> In the state of Carolina. . .

Her full name, of course, was Dinah Lee.

Her winnings were very useful to me. Although horseboxes were always allowed to take my father's hunters to meets, and I could share his if I was hunting, I could only have one to go to local shows and gymkhanas if I could afford it. If I got Dinah to enough little shows, she won enough money so that we could afford a horsebox occasionally. However, I mostly had to ride there. This often meant setting off the day before, riding all day, and putting my pony up

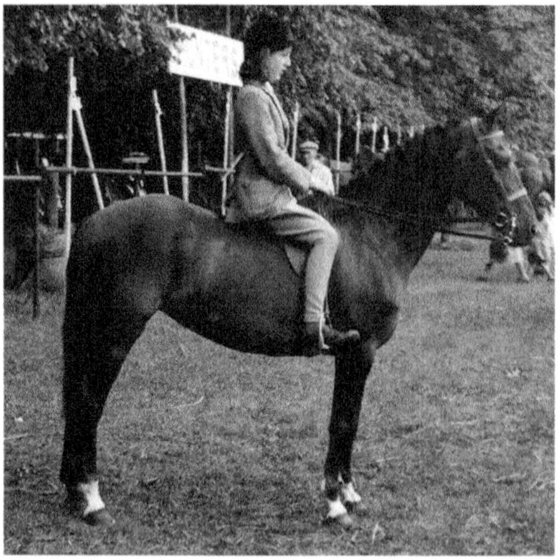

Beautiful Dinah at the Royal Norfolk Show in 1946, about to win a rosette in the Royal Norfolk Show. Photograph by Baron.

with a friend with whom I also stayed. I was quite nervous setting off to go 20 miles on the lonely Norfolk roads, but my father said: "Come on. Let's see a little courage there. Guts, and fortitude, please. Just take a map and get on with it." I learned years later that he was in quite a twitter about it himself, and telephoned all his friends who lived in houses on my way, telling them what time I might pass, and asking them to ring him when they had seen me. It was in fact great kindness to make me do it. I did learn confidence, and some courage.

Dinah was an angel in the show ring, but the cries of hounds or a hunting horn gave her instant hysterics, and I simply could not control her. Failing to stop her with the reins, I once set her at a straw stack in the hunting field. She just charged at it, ending up more than a yard inside it. My face was raw and bleeding from being slammed into the cut straw stalks, and I took her home, never to hunt her again, realising that trying to go hunting on her was stupid, dangerous, and unkind.

I had another, steadfast pony, Danny Boy. He had a head that looked too big for his body. His body was too long. He had rough hair round his heels and a wide shaggy tail clamped to his bottom. He was, sadly, most unshapely. But he was as cunning as a fox, and he loved hunting. When you rode him, you could feel, and see by his ears, how he was thinking.

I graduated to fox hunting. The West Norfolk Foxhounds were the real thing. We moved off at the trot from the meet and then sat silently on our ponies outside a covert, a small bit of woodland, listening to hounds crashing about and occasionally yelping. Sometimes Danny knew, before I did, which way the fox had gone, and was staring, head up and ears pricked, in the right direction. We heard one hound crying, then another, until the whole pack was giving tongue, and music filled the air. Hounds streamed off out of the covert after their fox, heads down, tails up, singing with excitement. The Huntsman and Whips were after them straight away, and then the Master led the rest of the field behind them.

A huge shot of adrenalin fires through you as you start to gallop, you are grabbing breaths against the rushing air, your eyes are streaming in the wind, and you feel your heart wildly thumping. I know that I have never done anything in my life so exciting, so completely thrilling, as hunting. Once away, nothing will stop you. Your mount is tearing across a ploughed field facing an unknown obstacle at the end, which absolutely must be got over, no matter how.

Much of the West Norfolk hunting country was rich land, suitable for growing sugar beet. For this relatively new crop, very important during the war, the ploughshare had to cut a sod ten inches deep. It turned up plenty of earthworms, eagerly grabbed by the following crowd of crying gulls and cawing rooks. Because of the new depth of ploughing, wonderful golden Saxon torques, bracelets, buckles and other jewellery, buried for a thousand years, had been turned up in sugar beet fields. These were the fields in which the prisoners of war were made to work, topping and tailing the crop with bare hands in freezing November. After the sugar beet was dug up, the fields remained heavy sticky clay, and you tried never to ride on them.

Hedges here were often on top of banks, with old oak trees in them. In the autumn, as the vegetation was dying down, a ginger fox against a ginger-brown bank was almost invisible. Once or twice we caught the smokey-urine whiff of one, but we could not have chased it without hounds: we needed their noses.

Sometimes a clever fox ran zig-zagging through a field of kale, grown for cattle fodder. Hounds had difficulty finding their way through, and horses had a horrible time. The kale stalks were thicker than my legs, the plants came up above the pony's back, and enormous drops of water rolled round their waxy leaves, soaking us.

There is nothing to break the wind from the North Pole as it rushes over the sea to Norfolk. Sometimes when it came whistling down, in spite of the warm pony beneath me, I froze. My fingers in string gloves were numb, I could not feel my upper lip, my feet were dead. If my father saw me like this he would say, "Follow me" and, with an unerring sense of direction, lead us to the nearest pub. I was too young to be allowed in, so I held the horses while he bought me ginger wine, himself a double whisky. He told the publican how cold I was, and asked if I might, as a special favour, be let in to sit by the fire. It was mid-afternoon, there were often no other customers, and the publican usually took pity on me, and I slowly warmed up. Before we left, we begged to be given some old newspapers. We helped each other stuff pages of these up our jerseys front and back, and down the back of our jodhpurs for wonderful insulation. Warmed up, I could stay out another couple of hours.

Danny looked small and insignificant, but when I was 14, he brought us in first in the Open West Norfolk Hunter Trials, where we were competing against experienced riders on big horses. Danny, at 13.2 hands high, was about ten inches shorter than the 16 hands of an average horse (a hand is about the width of a human hand, it is measured at four inches). We hopefully walked the course together, and he knew he had to scurry round it full tilt. He did it brilliantly, cutting all the corners that he could, a perfect gentleman at opening the gate, keen as mustard, right as rain. West Norfolk was the territory of the Boos, and to my great satisfaction, we even beat them. When we got home triumphant, my father was out to dinner, so the first he knew of it was our picture on the front page of the *Eastern Daily Press*.

"You might have bloody well tied your hair back, and you are growing out of your jodhpurs," he said. "And surely you could have made a neater job of plaiting his mane."

I had at this age grown 'teeth like tombstones' my father said, and a strong bony nose that my face had not yet caught up with. I was all too well aware that nothing I did could make any difference to those disasters, and tying my hair back was only going to show them up more. And no amount of plaiting would make Danny look pretty. But I knew my father was very proud of us, because he bought the picture from the paper and bored his friends with it. He wanted to know who the other competitors were, was pleased about the Boos, and absolutely delighted that I had beaten Michael McKee, the son of the second orthopaedic surgeon at the Norfolk and Norwich. My father absolutely loathed McKee, and I was constantly told that I must never let Michael or Theodora, his children, win anything on their ponies when I was competing. Theo was not a specially good rider, but she had a pony, 'Stormy Night', more beautiful

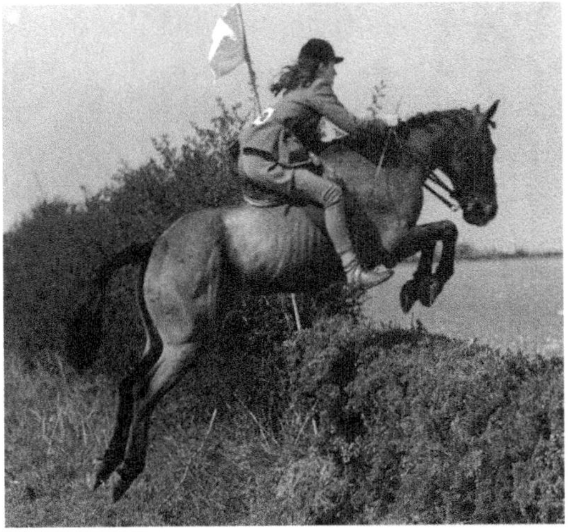

Danny Boy winning the Open West Norfolk Hunter trials, 1947. He is only a pony, 13.2 hands high competing against full size hunters at least a foot taller.

than my Dinah, and the judges often (and often quite rightly I thought) gave her the red rosette. Michael was different. Most boy riders are pretty hopeless at it. They grip with their knees, ride with strength, and seldom use balance. When they are young they have not the strength to do the job properly, and girls who ride by balance, particularly if they have learned bareback, easily beat them. Michael was tall and strong enough to ride very well. I was lucky if I beat him.

My father hunted with the West Norfolk sometimes, but always with the Norwich Staghounds. He said the staghounds were too fast for me, and galloping long distances jumping so many fences could be very exhausting, and he was afraid I might get so tired I would fall off and get hurt. Of course, this was a challenge, and I wanted to go stag hunting, especially as we were not trying to kill the stag.

Foxhounds are twice the size of harriers, but staghounds are even bigger. Straight after the war the Norwich Staghounds could only find five (two and a half couple in hunting parlance) staghounds to hunt with, but as their quarry was there before them, they had not nearly so tricky a job to do as foxhounds, and even so few hounds provided a great hunt. My father of course was properly dressed for the hunting field: black silk top hat, scarlet coat (you have to be invited by the Master to come out in scarlet), and nylon stockings over his socks to help him pull on his boots. These boots took three days to dry out after hunting and had to be polished by the butler with a bone, a flat piece of a cow's tibia. Until I was about 16 I just wore my ordinary riding clothes, but once out with the staghounds I wore a bowler hat and a stock. Some women wore a veil, which sounds silly, and is no longer worn, I think, but it did its duty protecting your face from the great lumps of mud flying up from other horses' hooves. And the stock: a great fuss was made about this stock, and my father insisted on tying it for me. It is a scarf made of tough linen, with no give in it, folded in three lengthways. Beginning at the front, the ends are crossed over the back of your neck, brought round to the front again and tied in a granny knot. It is the only use for a granny knot that I know. It forces one end of the stock up in the air beneath your chin, and you can turn it over and fan it out a bit to cover the knot. You can put a stock pin in it to hold it there. The tightness and stiffness is all important: I went pink in the face, and the vein on my forehead stood out as he tightened the noose. In vain did I gurgle, as if I were Kipling's 'Elephant's Child': 'Let go, you're hurtig be'. To tie the knot your head must hang right back with your chin in the air (it is very hard to tie for yourself), and when I complained "I'm strangling, you're throttling me, ug, ug", he just said "It's got to be really tight: that's all there is to stop you breaking your neck if you come off".

My father's hunter, Caravan, was bought before the war from gypsies: his mother pulled a wagon, his father was a thoroughbred, and he was chunky enough to be up to my father's weight. Typically, he first bought the horse, then learned to ride him. He had bravely spent a fortnight at Cavalry School in Aldershot, then came back with many blisters and sores, and straight away went out hunting. Now we were home Caravan was brought up from his war time retirement in the marshes, put in a livery stable again, and exercised daily until he was fit to hunt. Although the Irish horse, O'Hara, had to be seen out hunting to qualify for racing in point-to-points, he took such mad delight in shaking off his rider and hunting all over the world on his own, that his efforts at hunting were limited to about three days in a season.

People who came from the smart packs in the Midlands to hunt with the Norwich Staghounds were astonished at the toughness required to hunt in flat, watery Norfolk. We said: "If you can't see the ditch, it's the other side," and that meant you had to hammer away, flat out, towards the fence so you had enough speed to clear the ditch, which definitely would be the other side if you could not see it. Landing in the ditch could break your horse's neck, or yours. A 'bullfinch' was a hedge that had not been cut recently, and was growing tall and straggly, 15 or 20 feet high. You hurtled towards it, hoping to see a gap anywhere, and then tucked your head tightly down into that comfortable dent between the horse's neck and shoulder. Eyes tight shut as the horse jumped, the saplings struck your hard hat, and most painfully your knees, which would be bruised the next day. But no matter, you were over it, now where was the next?

Norfolk skies are wide open. They have huge horizons: we galloped with the pale turquoise bowl of the sky above us, the grey-fawn of the dead grass at the field edges and the dark chocolate brown of the plough beneath our hooves. The slanting winter light often made magic of the horses, dark silhouettes against golden back-lighting. Spiders' webs and hawthorn berries hung glazed with frost, black tarmac roads had icy patterns traced all over them.

I had some of the most wonderful days of my life hunting with the Norwich Staghounds. Foxhunters sneered at hunting a carted stag. It was all too predictable, and hounds had little work to do. The deer was caught in its deer park in the morning, brought to the meet in a box that just exactly fitted it, so it stood still and could not struggle. It could see out from slits at its eye level. It looked extremely uneasy, and we were asked not to go close and stare at it. To see it running was beautiful: it always appeared to run much faster than hounds, like the hare and the tortoise. If it ran through an open gateway, it leapt the full height of an imaginary gate as it passed. We often lost sight of it, but hounds seldom lost the scent: there was no hanging about all morning waiting for hounds to find a fox. It was straight off go, and gallop all the way.

We often started at 11 o'clock, and did not finish till four in the afternoon: five hours hunting with very few pauses could be hard on the horses, and they needed to be fit. After hunting, the horses had to be ridden home. Long distances had often been covered, and it was a chore for tired rider and tired horse to go slopping along at a jog for miles and miles. When about a mile from home, the horse, recognising where it was, perked up, and started to go faster and faster. A sweating horse in a cold stable gets ill, and the groom will be angry if you bring in a hot horse. Having been digging it in the ribs to get a move on for miles, suddenly you are shortening your reins and pulling it up to keep it just walking: the thought of the furious groom weighing on you. If there is no groom when you get in, the horse must be looked after first. It will want a long drink of water, mostly from the cold tap but with a kettle of hot added. It must be rubbed down all over with a twist of hay, and all the mud got off it (these days they are often hosed down). Its hooves must be picked out. When it is dry it needs a rug put on it, and deep clean straw for bedding. You must give it a bucket of hot gruel made with linseed, and a meal of crushed oats and chaff, and the rack filled with hay. And not till then can you go indoors, have a hot bath and an omelette, and go to bed.

When the deer was tired out, it would finally seek refuge in water. You could tell it was going for water as the hunt went plunging downhill, and there at the bottom would be a stream, river or lake with the deer bravely swimming in it. I greatly hoped for its safety at this stage, and now an extremely skilled and coordinated job was required of Huntsman and Whippers-in. Hounds wanted to swim after it, and if they could have caught up with it, they might have paddled on top of it and drowned it. So the Whips had to call and beat them off, to make sure they never connected, while someone, usually some very brave member of the hunt, jumped into the water, swam to the deer, and with an arm round its neck and a thumb in its mouth, brought it ashore. Sweaty, muddy and whacked from a ten-mile gallop, it is a brave man who jumps fully clothed into an ice-fringed river to grab a deer. The frightened deer will kick hell out of its rescuer. A hunt enthusiast, a greengrocer who followed every hunt in his van, jumped in once. He put his thumb in the wrong part of the deer's mouth. There is a gap between the incisors and molars, which is where the bit goes in a horse's mouth, and where it is safe to put finger or thumb. He put his too far up and the deer chomped right through his thumb so it was dangling by the skin. My father abandoned his horse to a friend and drove the victim straight to hospital and stitched it on again, which saved it.

I have held horses for men doing the rescue, and once for my father, and I would find myself praying equally for man and deer. Once ashore, hounds are drawn well away from the deer and a collar with a lead each side is buckled onto its neck. A strong man leads it on either side, and usually, because it is now exhausted, it walks unprotesting to the road, where the box is pulled up and it willingly goes into it, seemingly with relief.

A-hunting we will go, a-hunting we will go,
We'll catch a fox and put him in a box,
And then we'll let him go.

I know 'deer' does not rhyme with 'box', but this is a very old jingle, and there is nothing I can do about it.

Within about half an hour the deer's ear is notched to mark it so that it is never to be hunted again, and it is released back into the deer park and rejoins the herd, to live out the rest of its days in peace.

When I was about 16, I still weighed as little as a flea, and I was so used to riding that unless my mount fell I never fell off. So people asked me to qualify their point-to-pointers out stag hunting. They had a young, inexperienced horse, three or four years old, which they hoped to run in the point-to-points that happened around Easter after the hunting season. If it won, it might graduate to proper steeple-chasing, and might even, for instance, if it was that marvellous, end up running in the Grand National. It was so valuable its owner definitely did not want it to fall and injure itself, and it would be less likely to fall with a very lightweight rider. However, to qualify for the point-to-point, it had to be seen by the Master out hunting, properly hunting, up with hounds not straggling at the back of the field, for two hours at a time on three separate days. So, as I was now growing out of my rough little pony Danny, and wondering how I could hunt in future, along came this wonderful opportunity. I was not nearly strong enough to hold a young horse, but I could just about hang onto one rein to turn it in circles in a field, to stop it overrunning hounds. But hunting on such a horse was glorious. A horse like this would fly over fences as if it had wings, and I was flying with it. Oh the delight of watching it point its ears as it saw what was coming, feeling it size up the jump for itself, and leap at it.

No, of course we had no excuse for hunting a terrified and completely harmless animal, which we did not even hope to eat. Hunting a carted stag from a deer park was, not surprisingly, one of the first kinds of hunt to be stopped. Years after I stopped hunting, I kept and dearly loved a tame fox, and I personally would never hunt one again, although I must say I can see no reason to stop people hunting if they want to do it. But I do know that no other thing that I have ever done or wanted to do, neither sailing nor skiing, could begin to be so exhilarating as hunting, and I admit, bravely, that I am glad I did it.

I remember the very first time I went out with the Norwich Staghounds. There was a meet at the house of a friend, and Judy, Sara and I (three close pony-riding friends) were allowed to go, and told that whatever happened, we were to pull up and go home as soon as our ponies were tired.

At the meet, grown-ups ate cheese straws and drank punch while the deer was released and given 20 minutes' 'law', or time to run away, and then the Huntsman moved off with hounds. Even at the meet I felt sick with excitement, and I could never eat or drink. In the echoing clip-clop of the followers, keen, oat-fed, clipped-out horses mad with excitement sidled along the frosty road, striking sparks with their iron shoes, behind the Huntsman and Whips. The horses were so pent up that many defecated, and steam from their dung rose to our nostrils as we trotted along the road. The Huntsman held his hunting crop out dangling the thong and lash, and a sea of hounds trotted around him.

The worst crime you could commit out hunting was to let your horse charge up among hounds, and scatter them. My pony, Danny, was old and wise, and never tried it. But one girl's pony got away with her and galloped up with the hunt servants, snorting and bucking. Gnarled, purple-faced Tom Thackeray, the Huntsman, turned to her and shouted "Take your thucking pony home!" and the poor humiliated child went. Judy, Sara and I all heard it, and were fascinated. We wanted to know, of course, what 'thucking' meant. We would not have dared ask Tom, but we soon discovered that every grown-up we knew would not tell us either.

We gossiped on the telephone daily, endlessly discussing the magic word 'thucking', and telling each other which grown-up in particular had now refused to say what it meant. We had high hopes of Judy's brothers, who were in their late teens, but even they just sniggered. It became for us a magic word that we tried out with many different meanings. I did not ask my father, of course. With him, there were things you could not ask or discuss, like why had he told me that birds would fly in through the bathroom window and nest in his chest, when he knew that was not true? And although I so much wanted to, I could never discuss Pinkie, or even mention her name, or talk about any of the things she and I had done together while he was away. I did not need telling what these no-go things were. I knew. And I knew for absolutely certain that 'thucking' would be one of them.

My father registered that the door of the telephone box was shut and the light off, and I was missing. He picked up a telephone somewhere else in the house and breathed down it like a horse. I could hardly hear Judy for the heavy huffing, so I said: "I'm on the telephone". This enraged him. He shouted "Ring off, I want to speak to you." Then he furiously explained, "You're costing me a fortune in telephone bills, I can't afford it, and if you don't look out, I'll marry Sybil Harker and she'll sort you out."

It seemed quite possible that he would marry Sybil Harker (who quite often came to dinner parties in our house) and that she would marry him: she was unmarried. Apart from his theatre sister, I had never seen a woman able to refuse him anything. After all, it must have been she, the Master, who had done him the honour of inviting him to come out in scarlet. So I supposed that even splendid Sybil Harker might not refuse his hand in marriage. I had no doubt that she would have sorted me out, but on the other hand I could not believe that that majestic woman would have any interest in small matters like telephone bills. This frightening liaison was threatened every time I annoyed him, but it never materialised. When there was no sign of it happening, I decided that he was quite afraid of being sorted out himself. I doubt if he ever asked her, and I know she never did marry. Only her exquisite portrait remains to remind me of her glory days.

Chapter 17
Greek Dancing

Hampden House, in the village of Great Hampden, Buckinghamshire, was the stately home of the Earls of Buckinghamshire, and the 8th Earl rented it out to stage-struck Mrs Robley-Browne, who ran an acting school there. In 1946, at the age of 12, I was sent to this boarding school. I had no idea why this particular school was chosen for me, until a girl in my form, called Minty, or properly The Hon. Araminta Yarde-Buller, told me my father had had an affair with her mother and thought she must have told him about it. This was news to me, but I thought it quite likely.

New girls arrived one day before the others, and there were only two of us in our big dormitory, where we felt lost. The empty beds were jammed together with a very small dressing table between each, and the floor was swirling green linoleum like a shallow sea. The other girl was called Pixie Marlowe. She said to me that first evening, "You're not to worry, but tomorrow morning early, I am going to run away."

I was surprised. It was very cold, but otherwise it seemed so soon that I had not really had time to see if I liked or hated it. I asked her, "Are you unhappy here?"

And Pixie replied, "No, not unhappy, but a bit worried. I have to run away, because it is a family tradition. My father and both my brothers ran away from Eton, and I must run away from here. It's best if I go straight away, before they think I might. I'm only worried that I might not get all the way home, before they find out. They might make a fuss when they notice I've gone, but you won't tell, will you?"

"No," I promised, "I won't."

Pixie vanished after breakfast, without saying goodbye, and the school did not discover until all the girls had arrived in the late afternoon and there was a roll call. Pixie was the only girl I had so far talked to, and I made myself as small as possible in this big crowd. However, when the police came round, my name was called out, and I was made to go into the Brick Parlour alone, to talk to them. The three of them seemed very large, very intimidating in their navy blue uniforms, with their helmets on the table. They asked me if I knew anything about Pixie running away, and I said "No". They asked me if she had seemed at all unhappy, and I said "I don't know". Could I imagine why she had done it? I replied, "No". Did I think she was a little bit upset, a bit mad? "I don't know".

That night I was worried about her, but I had promised to tell nobody, and that was that.

In the morning we had Assembly, the daily meeting of the whole school for prayers and announcements, in the Great Hall, one of the biggest rooms I had ever seen: two floors high, all panelled in oak, and surrounded at first floor level by the Minstrels' Gallery. We were told that Pixie Marlowe, a new girl, had disappeared, but that she had arrived back at her home late last night. She was unhappy, upset and a little bit disturbed, and so would be staying at home to settle down for the next two days. When she came back we were to treat her as normal, as if it had never happened, and not to ask her anything about it.

When she came back I asked her: "Were you really unhappy, upset, and feeling a bit mad?"

"No, of course not" she said. "I told you I had to, and I did it. I got quite cold waiting for buses, because I didn't know when they went, or where they were going. At least I had enough money. I had to make some sort of excuse, or the school might not have had me back."

I told her about my negative answers to the police interrogation, and she said "Thank you", and that was enough for us to become best friends.

I had not been at this school very long before I realised that my darling nursery governess, Dickie, and Miss Ivens of Aylsham, had already taught me everything they were trying to teach us here, so I sat back and enjoyed myself while the others struggled with fractions, or the past imperfect, or whatever. I, meanwhile, mastered the art of carving pencils. The delicate turpentine scent of pencil sharpenings always reminds me of this time. Just after the war, there was no paint to coat pencils with, so they were just plain wood, very soft and easy to carve. I did all sorts of designs: probably the multiple twisted spiral was my favourite. I tried to carve some patterns inspired from the pillars in the nave of Norwich Cathedral. I was only carving in soft pencil cedar: the Normans had carved in hard stone, yet I had to admit they were incomparably better at it than me. At first, about two out of every three pencils got confiscated by a teacher, infuriated by my sitting in her class carving away with my penknife. However, I got good at arranging piles of books in her line of vision, and I always sat at the back of the class. I carved them for all my friends.

We also bred silkworms. A girl brought some eggs in: little grey dots on a piece of brown paper. I begged some from her, waited for them to hatch, and then the fun began. I knew where all the white mulberry trees were in the grounds, and to begin with, 20 tiny caterpillars only ate one leaf every two days. But by the end, I was going out twice a day for leaves for my huge greedy grey pets. They seemed to change their personality when they started to make their cocoons. They forgot their greed, and moved to and fro in a steady, purposeful way, spinning their beautiful cream silk. Then I kept them in a shoe-box with holes in, under my bed, until one day they woke up, ate their way out of their cocoons and pumped themselves up into silkworm moths. Then they mated, messily, and the males died at once, the females as soon as they laid eggs. I gave eggs away, and after some time, everyone had them. We decided to steel our hearts and save the silk. To do this we had to boil the cocoons alive.

There was a wretched 15-year-old Irish girl called Mary, not a pupil at this school, who had been 'adopted' by Mrs Robley-Browne, and had become her slave. She was made to work long hours washing up and cleaning, and we befriended her, and persuaded her to boil our cocoons for us, because she had access to saucepans and stoves. The cocoons bubbled a bit, making no other protest when we did it, but I still found it very painful. They turned the rich golden yellow of the best egg yolks. We put them in the inkwell spaces in our desks, and unravelled them. There were no china inkwells, only the holes where they should have been, because, it was said, they got broken during the war, and could not be replaced. We pulled out a loose end of silk, tied it onto a pencil and twiddled and twiddled the pencil, pulling the silk off the cocoon as it bumped around in the inkwell hole. It seldom broke, being extremely strong. For a long time the teachers had no idea what we were doing. We could do it in our laps, below the desk, while still looking the teacher in the eye, and the faint bumping of the cocoons did not attract their attention. We soon all had pencils, some carved, and all with bands of golden silk around them. They were much in demand.

I sometimes think, if I was very grand, or royal, that I would have a full-length evening dress made out of this glorious golden silk, in its natural colour. I would wear it with a golden crown for the opening of parliament or some very great occasion. Nothing else would come near its brilliant perfection.

So why was this an acting school? The reason, we were told over and over again, was because Mrs Robley-Browne, our large, fat, floppy headmistress, who dyed her hair a most unrealistic red, had been the 'First Person to Introduce Greek Dancing to the New Zealanders'. We found it hard to believe that the New Zealanders had taken to Greek dancing keenly: we did not like it much ourselves. We thought it soppy. This oft stated achievement appeared to be how she had got acting into her head, and she went at it very thoroughly. She had built a gymnasium with a stage at one end. The stage had footlights, spotlights, floodlights, coloured lights, every sort of stage light. It had heavy curtains, with three wings on each side. We had masses of dressing up clothes, Leichner stage make up, and we acted.

We learned classical mime. We learned stage falls. Sideways is easy, forwards is possible: in both cases you protect your head with your arms. But straight backwards is really hard. I still watch with awe if I see it done in the theatre today. You have to fall with your head sticking up a bit. You absolutely must not let the back of your head crack on the floor, but it is all too easy to do. After every lesson several girls had to go to Matron with terrible headaches. Me too, sometimes.

We learned classical ballet. Only really small girls were encouraged in this, because one day some man would have to lift us, and tower over us, even when we were on points. We did not much fancy that.

We learned tap dancing, which was exhilarating. At last I got to wear a pair of the school's tap-dancing shoes. They were bright shiny red leather, with high heels, and we tied them on with red ribbon bows. They were heavy, with metal taps at heels and toes. We were not allowed them until we were competent at some tapping routines, and they were so very desirable that when we were queueing for our bread and dripping at break, the whole school was bobbing about, tapping. Once you had them on, you felt yourself a new and special person. The taps they made were so loud and positive: a mistake so clearly heard, and so humiliating. But getting them to work for you was such a joy: standing in a line in the dark wings of the stage, the music starting, prancing out into the dazzling footlights, clattering and tapping furiously as we moved lightly over the stage. The routines were so familiar that we moved our feet almost automatically. But we had to swing our arms for balance, hold our heads up, and grin into the blackness of the invisible audience beyond the footlights. I was 13 the first time I got them on, and I still remember the excitement of feeling sexy for the first time in my life.

And then we had to do Greek dancing. Step-kromat, step-kromat, we went, rising and falling on our toes, waving our arms about like seaweed. We were supposed to be very graceful, but we were actually very bored, and to show our sympathy with each other at having to waste so much time, we made soft groans on every down-beat. We knew Mrs Robley-Browne was a bit deaf.

We did not enjoy lessons, except art, scripture, biology, and sometimes geometry, so we needed ways to avoid them. We particularly disliked algebra, and French. Miss Gook taught algebra, and was the extreme pencil confiscator. She would peer round the pile of books to see me carving pencils, and say: "Give that here, Alison Brittain. I'm not as green as I'm cabbage-looking, you know." And I am afraid I did think she looked quite like a very cross cabbage.

Mam'selle was almost a man. We liked calling her, among ourselves, "He, She or It". She sat at her desk smoking Gauloises, asking questions in her gruff man's voice about the pluperfect, which did nothing for any of us. We could just about manage stupid poems about foxes and crows, and mice, but grammar was unbearable. We had to go.

Fortunately, we were forever doing school plays of one kind or another. Just about the whole school was always rehearsing something. When we had a lesson we did not like, we arranged for a friend in the next classroom to put up her hand and ask to be excused. Then she came round to our door, knocked, put her head in and said, "All gnomes and elves for the court scene". We snapped our books together and ran out, in the direction of the gym, then slipped out of a door near the practicing rooms, into parts of the grounds never visited by teachers, and just sat on an old fallen tree chatting till the bell rang. It was a win-win situation: we were free, and so was the wretched teacher who no longer had to struggle with reluctant pupils. We of course performed the same kindness for neighbouring classes. We varied the wording sometimes: "Warriors down to theatre for the battle scene", "Courtiers and nobles for act three", "Storming of the Bastille now", "The Queen, please, and all ladies in waiting". We used to try and think of the most outrageous thing we could get away with, and I remember desperately trying to suppress giggles at "The whole herd of elephants now, and the snakes". We would try anything, really, which the teachers might believe, since none of them taught acting.

We did like scripture, because it was taught by the only married woman on the staff. Mrs Lovibond was an absolute darling, full of interest and encouragement. She treated all her pupils as if they were her own dear clever children, and we said to each other that she was a great recommendation for marriage. She was small and dumpy, and when she sat down at her table, she lifted her two enormous breasts with her hands and set them gently down on it. I once asked her what circumcision meant, because I genuinely did not know and it seemed an important distinction in battles between the Israelites and their enemies. She said she simply could not tell me, but I was at liberty to go out into the library and see if I could find out. The Earl's magnificent old Library was in a long corridor, which seemed like one side of a cloister, a floor of black and white marble diamonds, and the busts of Roman senators on marble pillars all down one side. We were not encouraged to use it and almost never went there. That morning I finally thought I was getting close, and came back into class and asked what 'foreskin' meant. The bell went, and I never did find out until I was grown up.

The only other sweet teacher was Miss Motchalov, who taught biology. She had not the faintest idea how to keep order, and her classes were always a riot. Luckily for all of us, her classroom was miles from the main house, way beyond the practising-rooms, so no one could hear us. She was unable to teach us anything above the din we made, but one day she said: "I have put a question box here on my desk, and if any of you want to ask a question, please write it down and put it in here, and I will try to answer it next week."

Oh, poor Miss Motchalov. Every single girl in Form Two put "What is sex like?" on a piece of paper and put it in her box. Next week Miss Motchalov went very pink, and said it was a difficult question for her to answer, because she had never had sex. But she did have a married friend who had, and this friend said it was very nice.

We already knew more about it than she did, actually. There was one girl in the school, in our class and in our dormitory, who had had sex. She had two older brothers at home, and when each of them was about 12 their father had invited them to come to his study, and had told them how sex was done. Burdened with this new exciting knowledge, when they each came out, they said "Felicity come here", and raped her. She said they were trying it out to see if their father was right. We wanted to know if Miss Motchalov was telling the truth. Felicity said she was not. If we wanted to know, it was rough and it hurt, and she had no intention of ever doing it again.

We were supposed to write a letter home every Sunday. I usually failed. What could I possibly write? 'I am carving pencils. We loathe Greek Dancing. Mam'selle is probably a man. We are learning about sex'. I simply could not imagine telling him anything like that, so I did not write a letter. Then one day a telegram came for me. You had to open a telegram in front of matron, who could presumably counsel you if the news was bad. Mine was unsigned. The message read, 'SO SORRY LEARN YOUR ATTACK SCRIVENERS' PALSY'.

Matron was pretty dim and she was not sure what it meant, which was just as well. I said it was quite clear to me, and private, and took it away. That Sunday I wrote to my father saying I was sorry, but I could not think of anything to say in a letter.

We did almost no games. Instead we had to go for walks in twos, forming a crocodile. Pixie and I always walked together. Sometimes, if there was an odd one out, we walked in a three with Minty. Then one day the accompanying teacher shouted at Minty to walk singly at the back, and Minty argued that then she would have no one to talk to. So she continued to walk with us, and then the teacher noticed she had her gym shoes on, not her outdoor ones. With a frenzied bellow she made us all turn round and go back to the house. Minty was sent to the headmistress and disappeared. We were told at assembly the following morning that Araminta had been extremely rude and disobedient, and been found walking in her gym shoes, so she was being punished by having to spend one week in solitary confinement in the sick room. Minty came to school very young. She was only ten. We wondered if her parents knew she had been shut away for a week, and wished to pay for a week's solitary for their daughter, or might have preferred her to do lessons. The sick room was above our bedroom, and Minty sent a dressing gown cord down from her window to ours, with a note attached declaring, 'I'm not allowed books. Can you send me some?'

We thought it was outrageous, and tied books and comics and a few sweets to her cord, and she drew them up and dealt with them under the blankets.

One autumn day Pixie and I were walking down the avenue of plane trees, just losing their leaves, and she asked me: "You're always talking about your father. What about your mother? What happened to her?"

"Oh she's dead, I think," I said. It seemed quite unimportant to me now.

"What do you mean, 'you think'?" said Pixie. "Don't you know if she's dead?"

I stumped along, making a shsh-shsh sound by kicking up the fallen leaves.

"Well she's not around," I said. "I've never seen her, so I suppose she's dead."

"OK," Pixie said. "So she's dead. What did she die of? Where is her grave?"

I thought about that. "Well," I said. "Those are good questions. I've never been told. There is a photograph of her on my father's consulting room desk."

We shsh-shshed the leaves together, arm in arm.

"Ask him", she said, "Ask him. Why haven't you?"

I did not know how to tell her that I knew this was not a practical idea. This, I knew, was absolutely a question I could not ask him.

"You don't know him. He's not the sort of man you could ask that sort of thing."

"Come on. You must. This is your own mother we're talking about. You have a right to know. He knows. Why shouldn't you? When you get home in the holidays, choose your moment and ask him."

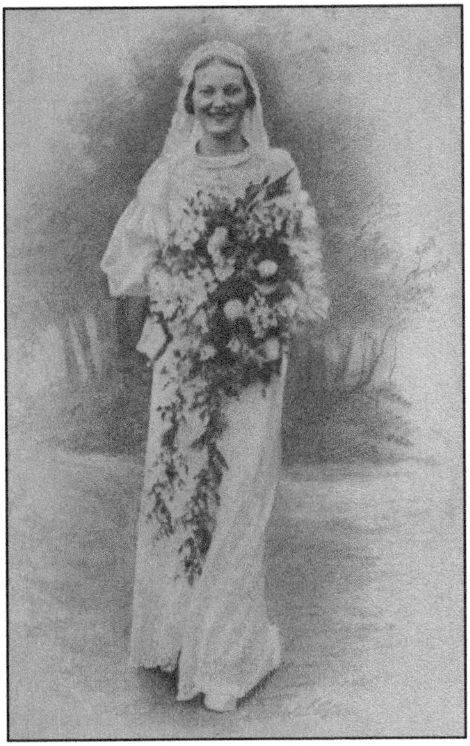

Photograph of Dorothy on Tommy's desk in 153 Newmarket Road, Norwich. Alison believed she was dead.

When I got home in the holidays I took one look at my father and knew I was better off as I was, not knowing. I could never ask him a question like that.

Every Saturday evening the whole school, including the teachers, and Mrs Robley-Browne, assembled in the gym, and one form performed a play to the rest of the school. The seniors performed real plays, often very well. Mrs Robley-Browne expected a high standard, and had no time for those who forgot their words, or could not be heard. The juniors could perform a story: Red Riding Hood, say, or Cinderella, or the plot of any book we all knew. The Second Form, in which I had arrived, turned down my suggestion that we act Black Beauty. I had hoped to be Black Beauty's friend, a horse called Poor Ginger, and get carried about on a cart with my head drooping down and my tongue hanging out. So we decided instead to do a variety show, in which groups of us performed whatever we could. Some tap danced, some said poems they knew, some sang songs. Angela Coburn and I finished the show with one of my father's bath songs. She wore a brown rug safety-pinned round her, with a dressing-gown cord pinned on her bottom. She trotted about, snorting, holding two empty lavatory paper rolls on either side at the top of her frizzy-haired head. Another girl had a red cloth wrapped round a stick, and poked at her quite hard. I sang:

It was at ze bullfight that we met him,
While watching his daring display,
I went for ze chocolate and programmes,

And ze dirty dog stole her away.
When I get Alphonso Spigone the toreador-or, diddle-om-boom boom boom,
With one mighty swipe I will dislocate his bloody jaw-aw,
diddle-om-boom- boom-boom.
He shall die
He shall dieeeeeeeee,
When I get my bunion on his Spanish onion
With one mighty swipe he shall die.

This rendition was wildly applauded by the girls, not so by the staff, who seemed rather shaken.

The first summer term that I was there, in 1946, Mrs Robley-Browne decided we would have a pageant on the lawn outside the house. The best of us had to do Greek dancing, the rest of us did maypole dancing, all in bare feet. In order to get in enough practice, we were roused by the fire alarm at 5 o'clock every morning, when it was just getting light, and those of us detailed off had to bring down the gramophone, records, maypoles and the tops with the ribbons. Maypole dancing looks quite easy, but it is not. There were a dozen of us round each pole, and if one of us hesitated or went the wrong way, we ended up with an ugly knot. We could not easily see to the top of the pole as we danced, so we went on making the mistake worse until Mrs Robley-Browne noticed it. With a bellow of fury and a scraunch on the record, she would stop us, and make us walk it slowly backwards undoing the ribbons until she had discovered the culprit. She was not at her best in the early mornings: she stood there in her dressing gown and great big slippers sucking at her cigarette in its long tortoiseshell holder, and gave the culprit a punishing piece of her mind. She was lucky. She was warmly dressed. But we were not.

At the beginning of term she made all 80 of us together do sinuous Greek dancing in a figure of eight around the gym. Right at the back of the gym, up on stage in a wheelchair, in the gloom against the curtains with the lights off, sat 'The Captain', also known as 'The Doctor'. He was Surgeon Captain Robley Henry John Browne, 84, husband to Mrs Robley-Browne, our headmistress (she had fancied her name by adding, and hyphenating his). I think we were supposed to think that he was paying medical attention to us, but we thought not. We had to perform in only our knickers. She had a great long pointing stick, and as we danced past her, she tapped us with it, shouting "Bra!" or "No bra!" How I longed to be 'Bra'. Only well-developed girls could wear one, and I am sorry that while I was there I never reached this summit.

Later, I discovered there was quite a class thing about nakedness. Hampden had some fairly upper-crust pupils, and none of us turned a hair about undressing for swimming, or prancing about half-naked to see if we needed a bra. In other, less smart schools that I went to, the girls looked very surreptitious changing, and turned their backs and wiggled about under their towels.

Anyway, for fire practice, which was really rehearsals for the pageant, those with permission wore bras and knickers: those without wore knickers only — nothing else. This was both humiliating, and terribly cold on the wet grass at early dawn.

The day before the pageant, we tried on our costumes. They were shaming: floppy sort of tunics with jagged hems and no waists. On the day of the actual pageant, we were up at five as usual, and we had to bring every single chair in the school out to the lawn and set them up in rows. The Duke and Duchess of Gloucester sat on two front ones, with cushions on the seats. We had no idea why they came, and felt sorry for them. We had not been told how the pageant was to start. To our amazement, the show opened with the arrival of Mrs Robley-Browne herself, wearing a strange laced-up riding costume that made her bulges resemble the segments of a caterpillar, and with her dyed red hair scraped back, which was supposed to make her look like Queen Elizabeth I. There was a most beautiful portrait of the young Queen Elizabeth I hanging in the Main Hall (a present from that Queen to the then Duke of Buckinghamshire, Griffith Hampden, after a regal visit to Hampden, painted about 1563) and certainly Mrs Robley-Browne bore no resemblance. We were astonished as she solemnly rode, from stage right to stage left (in other words, across the lawn from one yew hedge to the other, the whole length of the house) on a richly caparisoned and extremely stout chestnut mare, with a groom leading her. She looked fat and frightened, and not how we imagined good Queen Bess.

One of the dormitories, in one of the oldest parts of the house, King John's Tower, which had a spiral staircase leading up to it, was called The Tapestry Room. I do not remember seeing any tapestry there, but the room was completely panelled in old, very dark oak. It was a gloomy room, and I was glad not to be put there to sleep. One night, a few days after the pageant, it caught fire. It was now light at 4 o'clock in the morning. The fire alarm bell went, and we tumbled out of bed, put our knickers on, grabbed the maypoles and the rest of the gear, and presented ourselves on the big lawn, thinking 'Not more pageant, surely?' We could see big blue curls of smoke coming out beneath the gutters, and realised that it was a real fire. So we lined up in twos neatly on the gravel path in front of the house, just under the fire in the Tapestry room, which was where we were supposed to go in a proper fire practice for a roll call. But no one came to take the register, and the fire got stronger, and we watched the red flames behind the windows blacken the glass. There was a loud crack, and another, and the glass burst open, shards falling around us. Flames roared out of the windows, and we ran back over the lawn. Then five or six fire engines came charging onto the lawn, ringing bells. In only a few minutes the firemen did severe and terrible damage to the house, thrusting their hose nozzles up through the beautiful rococo plasterwork ceilings and putting so much water up there that the loveliest ceiling crashed to the ground. Then Miss Gook came out and asked us what on earth we thought we were doing, standing around half naked gawping at the fire. We were to go indoors immediately and put on some clothes. Refugees from fires are not usually sent back into the burning building, but I guess Miss Gook could see that 80 nymphets in their underclothes on the dewy lawn were making the firemens' day.

Chapter 18
The Great Lover

My father was a great lover. On a journey on the way to King's Lynn to hold a clinic, he once told me, with considerable glee, "I have slept with Judy's mummy, and Sara's mummy, and Bridget's mummy: all of them."

I could not imagine why anyone would want to sleep with him, to me he seemed so old and hairy (he was 43), so I asked "Did they want to?"

"Yes," he said. "They did."

"And did Uncle Geoffrey, Uncle John and Uncle Peter want you to?" I asked. These were not my real uncles of course, but most of the women to whom my father had made love became my aunts, and so their husbands were my uncles.

"They didn't know", he said. "I hope. And you don't tell them."

"I won't", I replied, and I never did.

I did get chapter and verse out of him. Judy's mummy acted in Shakespeare plays at the Maddermarket in Norwich. The Maddermarket Theatre, converted in the 1920s, was the first re-creation of an old Shakespearean theatre with an apron stage that stuck out into the audience, a tiny version of The Globe in London. One night Judy's mummy came to our house instead of going to a rehearsal.

Sara's mummy slept in a different room because Uncle John snored loudly, and my father and his horse Caravan spent a night there after hunting.

Bridget's mummy was very upset because Uncle Peter had invited Claire, referred to by my father as the 'hotel tart' from Shepheard's Hotel in Cairo, where both men had been stationed in the war, to come and live with him in Norwich when the war was finished. Claire was French. Bridget, Sara, Judy and I were fascinated by her completely plucked eyebrows that were replaced with lines drawn in purple indelible pencil. Bridget's mummy had not been warned of her expected arrival, and it had all gone very badly, and Uncle Peter had had to rent a flat in Norwich for her and had gone to visit her there, so my father was able to comfort Bridget's mummy.

Secretaries, nurses, even hospital sisters fell like ninepins, and private patients fought the secretary to have the last appointment in the afternoon in his consulting rooms, because after that he might ask them out for a drink, or I suppose, more. People said he looked like a film star, though I could not see it, but he could certainly be very charming.

One evening during the Christmas holidays, six months after the pageant, my father took his live-in secretary out to the cinema. I did not call her aunt, but she was one, I knew.

I was 13 years old, alone in the house, and not sleepy. I wandered about a bit, going from room to room, looking for something to do. I played the piano downstairs for a while, and eventually I ended up in the secretary's office. I loved playing with her typewriter, and stapler, and paper punch, and she was not there to stop me. I glanced at the box files, and noticed that there were two with the same name as ours: 'Mrs E. Brittain', and 'Mrs D. Brittain'. So who were these? I decided to take the files back to my bedroom so that I could read them in private, and if need be I could slip them back in the morning.

Mrs E. Brittain, it turned out, was my grandmother. There were a few short letters from her, always starting, as he would have wanted, "My dear Tommy". No mention of Herbert Alfred. How annoying it must be to give your baby boy two good names, that seem to you, his mother, both fashionable and of the right class, and find them rejected in favour of what sounds all too like Tom, Dick or Harry.

There were some carbon copies, typed, from my father back to Granny. There was a copy of her will, and lists of things that my father had inherited. It was boring legal stuff.

Mrs D. Brittain, on the other hand, was extremely interesting to me. She was Dorothy, and that was my mother's name. It seemed to be mostly bills. Monthly bills from St Andrew's Hospital in Northampton for 25 guineas a week, all paid. What was he paying for? Perhaps my mother spent many months dying in that hospital, and he had to pay for that. Pinkie had said she was extremely ill when I was born: that was why I was christened late, in Heydon. And there were some letters from her sister Alice saying that Dorothy would like to have the sewing machine if that could be spared. She must have been getting better if she wanted the sewing machine: perhaps she got a bit better before she died? And Dorothy 'would like a pair of slippers, size 4'. Ill again, was she, needing the slippers? At 13, I already took size 6 shoes: my poor dead mother must have been tiny, I thought.

Was there anything to tell me how she had died and of what? Where she was buried? I flipped the pages to and fro. Mostly bills. And then, at the very back of the file, on blue writing paper with our old address on it, were about eight pages in my father's handwriting. As with nearly all doctors, his handwriting was scarcely legible, usually, but this was him as a younger man, and very clear. The date was 1933, the year they were married in January: the year I was born in December.

It said, in very medical terms, that three days after I was born my mother could not sleep, and went mad, and had to be put in a mental hospital. St Andrew's Hospital in Northampton was a mental hospital, and that was where the bills were from. I looked at the most recent one. It was dated a fortnight before. Two weeks ago. How could I believe that? I felt sick, and I could hear my heart beating. That jolly well meant that at least until a fortnight ago, she was still alive, she was locked up in a mental hospital and still mad. Was she quite completely mad? Oh please, make it not be true that she was there alive in Northampton, and I had never seen her and no one had ever told me. But it was true. It could not be anything but. You can change some things, but not a truth like this. I should have been told this, I thought, I should have. Why not? I am afraid I was simply not prepared for such news, and I did a very strange thing with it.

I put the files carefully back, and managed to convince myself for the rest of the holidays that I had never read them. Somehow, it seemed that if I had not read them, it was not true. Discussing this with my father seemed beyond all possibility now.

The Christmas holidays were over, and we were back at school. In our acting school, we did not only act: we sang. In my thin treble voice I sang, as clearly as I could:

> The blacksmith I hear
> With clash and with clamour
> Resoundeth his hammer
> His mighty arm swinging
> His mighty strokes ringing
> Like bells, loud and clear.

As it happened, I had arms and legs like knitting needles. Nothing could less have resembled a mighty blacksmith than me. But my singing this got me into the school choir. Pixie and I were the only ones in the bottom form to get in. We were quite proud of ourselves. Now we could sing exciting shivery pieces like Schubert's 'Earl King's Daughter', and we sang lovely sad anthems in church. We were so unimportant that we stood in the back row of stalls in the choir and were taught to sing 'fear' as 'feeeer', and 'God' with a clear 'd' at the end, and not 'Oh littol town of Bethlehem' but 'Oh littl town. . .'. We often spent hours singing in an ice-cold church, with breath coming out of our mouths like steam, but we loved it. And of course it got us out of a lot more lessons.

The church where we sang was, of course, Great Hampden Church, in the grounds of Hampden House. We walked past it every day. We were told at school that it was where lovely 'Gray's Elegy' was written: 'Elegy Written in a Country Churchyard' by Thomas Gray, 1742.

> The curfew tolls the knell of parting day,
>   The lowing herd wind slowly o'er the lea,
> The ploughman homeward plods his weary way,
>   And leaves the world to darkness and to me.

Pixie said, at the beginning of that term: "Oh, not another holiday and you haven't asked your father what happened to your mother? What's wrong with you? Why are you so frightened of him?"

"I didn't need to ask him. I've found out. I do know now."

"Well, come on, what happened to her?"

"She's mad," I said.

"There you are," said Pixie. "I knew it was a mystery but I never guessed that. How exciting. Like Mrs Rochester, only she didn't set fire to the house."

I felt rather proud to have an exciting mystery about me.

"Not very nice for her, though," Pixie said. "How did you find out? Have you seen her? What is she like?"

I told her how I had found out, and said: "I don't know what she's like. She's got very small feet."

"And?" said Pixie, "And? What else?"

"I don't know anything else," I said. "That's all I know."

But now that I had let the cat out of the bag, it would not get back in. I lay in bed at night in our dark dormitory with seven other girls in it, and tried to think clearly about my newly discovered mother. Why had nobody told me? Why did not anybody think I had a right to know? Why did they think that telling lies about Father Christmas was right because it was such fun for them, even if horrifying for me? Why had Dickie actually lied to me? And Pinkie must have known. And so must all my Dublin aunts. That must have been what Happy meant when she told me she knew a secret about my mother. All these people who I loved and trusted had known, and not told me. What stopped them? And my father, my beloved father, so insistent on the truth, who told me everything he knew, who even told me which of my friends' mothers he had slept with: how had he failed to tell me this?

Because I had never suspected madness, or given the subject much thought, I had never realised the horror with which madness was regarded. A severe psychotic illness in the 1930s was regarded as terribly shaming. I worked out, eventually, that there could be only one explanation. It must be that they all knew that it ran in families and it was going to happen to me too, that I was going to go mad like my mother, and that it would be unkind to tell me in advance. That explanation was not much help. When was I going to go mad? Now? Later? When I had a child? How long had I got? How could I find out? Who on earth could I ask who would tell me?

I found it hard to sleep for worry, and wandered limply round the school failing to turn up anywhere at the right time, or do any prep, which got me into lots of trouble. Pixie said: "You're not taking this very well, you know. You are behaving very oddly. I think you'd be better to tell someone. Get it off your chest. Perhaps better tell Mrs Robley-Browne."

That was an absolutely abominable idea, but I did not like being told I was behaving very oddly. I was sleeping badly too. Was I going mad now, so soon? Where could I turn for help?

Perhaps to relieve my terror, and find some substitute for the fear that visited me every night, I fell in love. I had a 'crack', as it was called, or a crush in other schools, on a girl in the fifth form. Fiona Campbell Walter was the daughter of an admiral. She had auburn hair, honey coloured skin and greeny-grey eyes. I thought she was stunning. Later on, so did the whole world. When she left school, she became Britain's top model for years on end, and was often referred to in the gossip columns as the most beautiful woman on earth. She married a German baron, who was said to be the richest man in the world, but sadly, that must have been unhappy, because it ended in divorce.

Having a school crack on someone is surely the purest love of all. I had absolutely no wish to touch her, or have her touch me. It never occurred to me to want to kiss her. I knew about sex, of course, but it did not seem to me that being in love with Fiona could have anything to do with that: I never thought about it in that way. I did not even want her to talk to me, which she would not have deigned to do anyway. I did greatly hope to be able to rescue her, but rescue from what exactly I had difficulty imagining. Very occasionally, through intermediaries, I managed to be allowed to clean her shoes, or darn her stockings. Of course she had no idea I did it, or she would not have let me. Having some junior with a crack on you is boring and embarrassing, and you give them as little encouragement as possible.

But I did put a lot of effort into what all small girls with a crack on an older one did: they tried to stand in front of them in Assembly, so they could hear them sing. Assembly was held every morning in the Great Hall in front of the wonderful portrait of Queen Elizabeth I.

I had been told that Fiona said, with some expression, "Ah men!" at the end of hymns, and I did so want to hear it, because I thought it was so witty. This required enormous guile. We went into Assembly in height order. You had somehow to discover the exact height of your loved one, and of the nine girls just shorter than her, and make yourself the tenth one. We measured each other endlessly with the stick in the gym when the games mistress was not there. We peeped into her book before she gave it to Matron after measuring us. Knowing the height that we had to be meant adjusting it by crouching slightly, or by putting rubbers in the heels of our socks. We congratulated each other with many grins and winks when one of us found ourselves in exactly the right position.

One morning in Assembly when I was in the perfect position, and Fiona had clearly said "Ah, men!", in a thoroughly satisfactory way, Pixie was somewhere in the row in front of me. We all turned right and marched out row by row, but Pixie held her ground. You only did this if you wanted to talk to the headmistress, which was extremely rare. So I said, out of the corner of my mouth: "What do you want to talk to her about?"

And she said: "You and your mother. Either you do it, or I will."

"No!" I shouted, "No!"

"Stop shouting in Assembly," yelled Mrs Robley-Browne. "Which of you wants to see me?"

Pixie glared at me. "I do," I said, with a knot in my stomach.

I went into the cigarette smoke filled so-called 'Nest', her study, with Mrs Robley-Browne, and she said "Well, my dear?" She had a false plummy accent, so she actually said "Well moi dear?" We all imitated her at this. I was alas quite right not to want to talk to her about my mother.

She said: "Speak up, we haven't got all day you know."

I blurted out, "Do you know about my mother?"

And she replied, "Yes, my dear, and what do you know?"

"She's mad."

"And how did you find that out?"

When I told her, she said "You wicked, wicked, wicked little girl, reading your father's private papers. I shall ring him up at once and tell him. He will be very angry with you."

I fell on my knees and wept. I clung round her fat calves that strained her lisle stockings, hating the way she smelled of smoke, begging her not to. I said it would be much better to talk to him at home: that I couldn't bear him to come down to the school and be angry with me and then go away again. I needed to be at home with him for that. Promise, promise to wait: I would tell him in the holidays, which were not far away now. In the end she promised. But I went away concerned that my father, when I finally told him what I knew and how, was going to be in a terrific rage with me for reading his private papers.

Easter came early that year. We were still at school for the Easter service in church. I had a thin, clear voice like a choirboy's, and it was my turn to sing solo the introduction to the anthem in church. I think it was 'O God(d) how manifold(d) how manifold(d) are thy works. . .' from Psalm 104. The organ played the first few bars, and the choir stood up. I took a deep breath. I was in the front row now. I looked down the nave as I was trained to do, and there in the front pew beside Mrs Robley-Browne, less than four hours since she had promised she would not tell him, sat my father.

I opened my mouth to sing, and nothing came out. The organ went back to the beginning and I tried again, but I was utterly dumb. The third time the choir came in and sang it for me. So much for my first solo.

My father caught me up coming out of church. We went for a walk together, and I said I was sorry for reading his papers. He said he was extremely sorry that I should have found out about my mother like this: he had wanted to tell me himself. He was sad, not angry.

So I asked, "If you wanted to tell me, why didn't you? Or why didn't anybody: Dickie, or Pinkie, or the Irish Aunts, or even Mrs Robley-Browne? They all knew, even awful old Mrs Robley-Browne knew: you told her, but not me." He said that he had wanted to tell me himself, and would not allow anyone else to tell me. I had seemed too young when he went away to the war, and when he came back he decided to tell me when I was old enough to understand.

"I do understand," I said.

"I know you do if you've read all that," he said. "But is there anything else you want to know about her?"

I did not know where to begin. We walked on in silence. How could I ask him what I most desperately wanted to know? I needed to know that my mother was different, special, in some way much, much better than all the other 'aunts', better indeed than my friends' mothers.

"All right," I said. I was crying. "I want to know if you loved her?"

"Of course I did, you Chucklehead," he said. "I *married* her."

I realised that my father felt degrees of love. Affection for my friends' mothers was overwhelmed by the strong emotion he still felt for his wife. There was a catch in his voice and tears in his eyes and I suddenly realised how much it hurt him. I had been selfishly thinking only of the effect this awful news had on me.

Only now did I realise the anguish he had been through. It was so terrible for him that he simply could not bring himself to discuss his agony with me, and that, I think, was why he failed to tell me for so long.

There seemed no point continuing this painful conversation, and it only ever came up again in odd phrases, like: "Your mother used to sing, too." Or "Her family thought it was all my fault, you know." He never brought the subject up, and answered questions as briefly as he could. If I learned anything else about her it was much later, after he was dead, from my real Aunts: my namesakes, Alice and Betty.

As we were saying goodbye in the drive, my father caught sight of Fiona, standing like the goddess of spring among the daffodils on the lawn. "Oooooooh," he said. "Well, lookee there. Now, then, she really is quite something." Conflicting emotions churned up inside me, and I wanted to hit him.

Chapter 19
Murder at Chequers

My father was a great lover, but he was also a great hater. The things he hated mattered enormously to him. I knew them all well, and stepped carefully around them, even if some of them did not seem very hateful to me.

He hated people who drove Jaguar cars; really viciously hated them, and would have liked to see them run over and squashed flat, he said. He hated *The Observer* newspaper. It was ordered every Sunday, along with all the other Sunday newspapers, including left wing ones like the *Sunday Herald*, *The People*, and *Reynolds News*. They were brought up to him in bed, and he sorted out *The Observer*, scrambled out, screwed it up, page by page, and burned it on the big wood fire in his bedroom, cursing it for being the 'pink 'un'. He never read it, but he seemed to feel much better with its ashes smothering the fire. Of course it was not pink, like the local racing edition of the *Eastern Daily Press*, that was always referred to as the 'pink 'un', and it took me a long time to realise that it was being cursed and burnt for its political views, not the colour of its newsprint.

My father's greatest hatred was for Socialists, and pink was their colour. They were the enemy. He went to the election meetings of all local Labour candidates and shouted at them and interrupted and made such a nuisance of himself that he had to be dragged out by the party heavies or the police. He felt certain that this was an important democratic duty, and the very least they deserved.

He was Surgeon to the Course at all the Norfolk point-to-points. After the last race, cars queued up to get out of the field, sometimes two or three rows of them, churning up the mud. A policeman stood at the gate, allowing, say, ten cars from any row to go before he stopped them, and let another line go.

If he held his hand up and stopped our Rolls, my father would wind down his window, purple-faced with rage, and yell "Bloody Socialist!" at the astonished policeman, who very probably had voted Conservative all his life.

When I was 18, at my finishing school, the House of Citizenship, we held a mock election. In 1950, there was a real general election going on in the country at the time. It appeared that having a mock election would teach us useful citizenship skills about the difference between the party candidate, the agent, the party secretary, understanding 'one man one vote' (except for the University vote, which had only recently been stopped), how to make public speeches and posters and all the different ways of persuading people to vote for your party. I believe that probably the parents of almost every girl in that school voted Conservative, out of habit and tribal solidarity. We knew that Winston was wonderful, and had won the war for us almost single-handed, but apart from that our knowledge of politics was superficial. In the school we voted for who should be what, and to my surprise I was elected the secretary of the Communist Party. I had a forthright, tough, anti-apartheid thinking, motor-bike riding South African candidate, and she had a quiet determined agent. Since we realised we knew so little about politics and what was important in this election in particular, each party secretary telephoned their party's real headquarters, and asked if they would kindly send us any literature they had.

The poor Conservative was asked if she had not the faintest idea that there was an election going on, and told they could not possibly help her. Labour Party headquarters were very nice, said they were very busy, but if they could they would send something. They never could, it seems, because nothing ever came. The Liberals were charming, said they would send as much as they had when it came in, and did indeed send dribs and drabs of publicity stuff as they got it from the printers. My Communists were completely different.

"Wonderful," they replied. "Absolutely."

They spoke with very nice accents. They sent us, immediately, 500 copies each of the Red Flag and the Internationale including the music, books and pamphlets by Marx and Engels, and a term's subscription for six copies a day of the *Daily Worker*. I left copies of the *Daily Worker* lying about everywhere. I learned to play the Red Flag on the piano, and we had singalongs: we found this attracted the interest of quite a few potential supporters, and all of us enjoyed the bloodthirsty words: 'The people's flag is deepest red, It's stained with blood of martyrs dead. . .'

All I had known about communism before then was that Russians did it, and brainwashed people, and they were bad. I remembered that I had learned at Hampden House that I should never forget Yalta, Potsdam and Teheran, places where there had been meetings of British, American and Russian leaders, and it was there that we had gone wrong with the communists. That was the limit of my knowledge of this subject.

I read the *Daily Worker*, Marx and Engels with enormous interest. Engels had spent some time in England considering the working classes. After a week or two, I felt that the ideals of communism were absolutely right, and that other parties' beliefs were at best watered down versions of the truth. Communist ideals seemed to me to have the same ring of goodness about them as the best precepts in the bible. They were not that dissimilar to those 'Do as you would be done by' and 'Love thy neighbour as thyself' directions that Pinkie had said were the golden rules of Christianity. Everyone giving as much as they could, and getting as much as they needed, seemed so fair. Everyone being equal, and all working for the state, greatly appealed to me. I said so, with passion, to everyone in my bedroom, everyone I sat next to in classes. I was busy explaining the virtues of communism to a heavyweight blonde Finnish girl I was sitting next to at dinner and was extremely surprised when she stood up and brought a chair down on my head. I did not know, unfortunately, that Finland had suffered terribly at Russian hands during the war. I was told I must apologise to her, and said "Certainly not, I am the secretary of the Communist Party, this is what I believe, and I believe in freedom of speech and my right to say what I like to anyone." She never spoke to me again.

My candidate gave excellent speeches, coached wisely by her agent to speak of a worldwide movement bringing fairness and equal chances for all, and to prevent her getting too carried away and recommending things like striking and rioting, and supporting the working class struggle. Towards election day, we really put the pressure on. We stayed up all night drinking black Nescafe made with hot water from the bedroom tap, making posters. Each was decorated with a red flag, and they declared sensible things like 'WE ARE ALL EQUAL

– VOTE COMMUNIST', or 'WE SHALL ALL WORK FOR EACH OTHER – VOTE COMMUNIST', or 'WORKERS OF THE WORLD UNITE – VOTE COMMUNIST', 'WE MUST RISE TO RULE – VOTE COMMUNIST'. We tried, 'We shall grind down the bourgeoisie', but it did not seem to make much sense, so we left it. We went into every lavatory in the school (it was an absolutely vast house, about a quarter of a mile long, and there must have been near a hundred lavatories) armed with a red ball point pen (red ball point pens were rare and special then). Lavatory paper then was not soft and furry: it was hard and shiny, smelled slightly of creosote and had 'IZAL' written in the corner of each piece. I still have friends in unspoilt Norfolk whose downstairs gentlemen's lavatory has not only photographs nearly a yard wide of the pupils at Eton College in about 1945, sporting the owner as a very small dot in the third row, but it is also provided with Izal lavatory paper. To use it, you took a double sheet and rubbed it vigorously between your hands to soften it. We unrolled all the rolls, and wrote in red, on every tenth piece, 'If nothing else works, try Communism' and rolled them all up again. It was widely noticed and remarked on, and we felt we were hitting home. At 5 o'clock on election morning, we hung our posters everywhere: over the banisters, over the pictures, above the fireplaces, completely covering every notice board.

At breakfast, there was no breakfast. We all had to go out to the kitchens and fetch our own cornflakes and milk. The 20 or so underpaid teenage Irish maids who slaved away for us, cleaning, cooking, and serving at table, had gone. They were Catholics, rose early to work, had seen the posters and walked out, on strike. They knew communism was wicked. They had to be rounded up and taken in a coach down to the town to see their priest, who made an enormous effort to convince them that this was a mock election, and to send them all back by lunch time.

We were told we should vote, not as we might in a real general election, but for the party which seemed to us to have made the most effort, and which we personally would like to see running the country. We all thought it would be a landslide for Conservatives, and were mightily surprised when the results were counted. The Liberals won, and the Communists came less than ten votes behind them. A long way down came Conservative, and eventually Labour, which sadly totally lost.

I felt sure there was hope for the world yet, and took all the literature home at the end of term. The day after I got back I said to my father: "Daddy, I know you are a true blue Conservative, but I wonder how much you have thought about the other parties?"

"What are you saying?"

"I never thought for a moment I would become a Communist, but when I was the secretary of the Communist party in our mock elections I read a lot of stuff about Communism."

"You shouldn't have bothered."

"Well, I've brought it all home."

"Brought it home, in this house? How dare you?"

"I thought it might interest you."

I was still in my 'freedom of speech and saying what I thought' phase.

"I'd like to talk to you about it. Maybe you don't know what it is all about. Maybe if you do. . ."

"Of course I bloody do. Do you take me for an idiot?"

"Well I think there are a lot of good and true things about Communism."

I handed him all the copies of the *Daily Worker*, Marx and Engels, omitting the Red Flag because it did not seem to me to be his kind of song: not really in the same style as the Daring Bullfighter or the Drunken Sailor.

I have never seen him so apoplectic. He became red then purple with rage, tossing the copies of the *Daily Worker* all over the room like confetti. He yelled: "Christ alive! Jesus bloody wept! I am bloody paying bloody good money for you to learn this utter bloody bunkum! Bloody BUNKUM!" And I was made to clear up all my deviant literature and take it out to the garden and burn it on the bonfire, while he stood over me. After that, whenever I met him walking round the house, he sang loudly, to the Tannenbaum tune of the Red Flag:

> The working class can kiss my ass,
>
> I've got the foreman's job at last.

Some days later he took me into the library, searched around, found the two books he was looking for, and presented me with George Orwell's 'Animal Farm' and his most recent, '1984'.

"You read those," he said. "They're about communism. And when you have, I'll talk to you about it."

I do not remember us talking about it, but I certainly did read them and I do remember how queasy they made me feel. It seemed that, having spent a whole term thinking about almost nothing except communism, there was a lot more to it than I had thought. I found it very worrying that some animals were more equal than others. It seemed that communism could go too far, and turn out to have power over you, rather than you have power over it. I was not sure how that happened but I could see it was a great danger that wanted watching. I rather lost my great enthusiasm for it, but I certainly was not going to tell that to my father.

Years before that, when I was 13, back at Hampden House, one day the choir was told that the Prime Minister's daughter was getting married, and that her father would like our choir to sing at her wedding. Only it was not to be all of us: I think only 16 were wanted. Our school grounds lay right next to those of Chequers, the Prime Minister's country house, and he had visited Great Hampden church and heard us sing. Pixie and I knew we were surely too small and useless to be among the chosen 16, but we also had another problem. Pixie's father was the highest paid journalist in Britain; he wrote a political column for the *Daily Express*, the most Conservative paper of the day. When my father heard this he wanted me to invite Pixie to come and stay with us in the holidays at once: her father was a hero after his own heart.

But the Prime Minister of the day, whose daughter was getting married, was a Socialist, Mr Attlee. He had cruelly usurped the God-like Winston Churchill, and after the election my father often moaned that he wondered why anybody bothered to stay in England now.

Pixie said, "My God, the ogre himself: Heavens how exciting!"

"Even if we were chosen, my father wouldn't let me sing for him, I'm sure," I said.

"Mine would not be best pleased either," said Pixie. "But if we don't tell them, they'll never know."

"We are not very likely to be chosen, anyway" I replied.

"But we must see him," Pixie said. "If he is so awful, it will be very exciting."

"All right then" I said, "We'd better get chosen."

So we sang our hearts out in practicing rooms, and distant parts of the grounds.

Could we get that high 'G'? What about the 'A' above it? We needed three octaves, and three octaves easy, no hoarseness or squeaking. By about half-term, we got them. We had strong voices down in our boots, and clear voices floating up to heaven. We did get chosen.

At the wedding, Pixie and I were in the front two seats in the choir stalls. We were so close we could have reached out and poked Mr Attlee as he gave his daughter away. But he seemed small and quiet and rather harmless really.

The singing went well. The anthem, while they signed the register, was long and lovely, and the soloists got it all right. The blessing was devastating: it always was, to me. 'The Lord bless thee and keep thee. The Lord make his face to shine upon thee and be gracious unto thee. The Lord lift up his countenance upon thee and give thee peace.'

My father said that once, when he was a houseman at St Bartholomew's Hospital in London, he had come back from a pub-crawl late at night, and there was a parcel for him. He opened it, and it was a bible from his mother. He wished she would leave him alone. On the inside cover there was a text written in her hand. Numbers 6, 24. 'Oh Jesus,' he thought, 'I know. It'll be 'Keep to the straight and narrow path', or something like that'. But it was instead that lovely blessing, and he forgave her.

I still sing it, sometimes, in the bath, and I wish I could find again the music to which we sang it: I would love to hear it again.

Afterwards we had been told that we were invited to Chequers for the reception, and that we should mind our manners, and stand at the back, and not speak until we were spoken to. No one spoke to us, but we ate the most delicious canapés, and had a glass of champagne each. So we talked among ourselves.

Suddenly, I caught sight of Aneurin Bevan, the Minister for Health. He was the monster who had started the National Health Service, and he, I knew, was the ultimate enemy. My father used to go on lecture tours in America to warn them of the horrors of the National Health Service.

"Look there," I said to Pixie. "Do you know who that is?"

"Of course," said Pixie. "It's Aneurin Bevan: he'd be bound to be here."

"But do you know what my father wants to do to him? He wants to put him on a bacon slicing machine, and slice him from the toes up, and have the slices fried, and make him eat them."

"Good God!" Said Pixie. "I'm afraid your father isn't quite right in the head, either."

And we eyed up our victim, imagined his fate, and fell into helpless giggles.

The afternoon wore on. The bride and groom left, in showers of confetti. Guests went home, and servants cleared away the food and glasses. The coach that had brought us failed to come and get us. It had to be telephoned. Apparently it was busy, and would come later.

So the ogre himself, Mr Attlee, suggested to us that the choir might like to play games until it came. Did we know how to play murder? Indeed we did. We were pretty amazed at this turn. He said we could play it in the hall and on the stairs. The stairs at Chequers go round in a square. They have lovely oak-panelled walls so you cannot see around the next corner. The banisters are great thick ropes like dressing gown cord, but much more beautiful. Mr Attlee obviously really enjoyed playing murder. He threw himself into it. He was seriously good at it. He even allowed himself to be murdered, once.

I never did tell my father about singing at the Prime Minister's daughter's wedding. And playing murder with Mr Attlee. It would not have done him any good. And I thought that if he could decide not to tell me details about my mother, I could decide not to tell him about murdering the Prime Minister.

Chapter 20
Making a Book

My father drove down from Norwich and took me out from school, when that was allowed. All the other girls were taken to the cinema to see 'Snow White and the Seven Dwarves', and on their return boasted of having eaten fantastic quantities of ice cream. Not me. I spent my days out at the races. I knew the lie of the track at all the home counties race courses: Lingfield, Goodwood, Ally Pally and the rest. We used to sail from school in the magnificent Rolls to a large house in a cul-de-sac in Mayfair, to pick up Vsev (pronounced Sev) and Maimie, our racing companions. Vsev was my father's wine merchant, but he was also one of the last of the Romanovs, Prince Vsevolod of Russia, and I suppose if Russia had ever had another Tsar, he might have been it. Lovely Maimie was the daughter of an earl. She was brought up in Madresfield, the great house that had been the model for Evelyn Waugh's Brideshead. At Madresfield, Elgar's father tuned the pianos, and it is thought that the thirteenth of Elgar's Enigma Variations, the Romanza, may have been written for Maimie. She and Vsev were tremendous fun: very grand, very clever, and she was a smiling blonde beauty. They laughed all the way to the races. But before we set off Vsev and my father stood in the drawing room drinking what seemed to me a great many whiskies and soda. Vsev smoked lovely smelling Russian cigarettes which he got out of a case made of three kinds of Russian gold: white, gold and pink. The cigarettes were khaki coloured, with long hollow cardboard tubes for mouthpieces: much more tube than tobacco. I do not like the smell of cigarettes normally, but these were delicious.

I went up to Maimie's bedroom to help her dress. All I had to do was sit on her bed and watch, while I fed what Maimie said was the smallest dog in the world (and I have never seen a smaller) on Ovaltine tablets. The dog lived on her bed. I thought it was a Pekinese, but she said no, it was a sleeve dog: so small you took it about in the long hanging sleeve of a kimono. She asked if I thought it looked like a lion. I said, "No, not a bit", which was the wrong answer.

When she had done her face and hair, and was ready to dress, we opened a few bottles of scent, and tried them. When we found one we liked, Maimie poured the entire bottle over herself. She went about in a great cloud of scent. I actually think that if I were taken, blind and deaf, into a room where Maimie and Vsev were, even today, I would immediately recognise them, as a dog does his master, by their smells.

Alas, I was not up to Maimie's style. I wore school uniform, of course. This was a grey pudding basin hat with a grey ribbon round it, a grey tweed coat with a tweed belt pulled too tight, the buckle crooked and the long end dangling loose, brown lisle stockings that wrinkled on my pinstick legs, and brown lace-up shoes. When we got to the course they all went to drink more whisky and soda, and I was given my father's race card and a five pound note, one of those crisp white ones with black copper plate writing on it, rather like an invitation, and told to go and look in all the bars for the Pie Kid. I had to give him the fiver and invite him to mark my father's race card. The bars were all dark, smoky and smelly, and it took time to adjust my eyes to see if the Pie Kid was in there. If he was, he was up on a stool by the bar. He was small and thin, and wore a shiny brown pin-striped suit and a greasy trilby hat, even in the bar. Spotting him from the door, I had to make an absolute dash for him, in order to get to him with my father's money before the barman shooed me out. School girls were not allowed in bars in those days. After a time he knew me, and said "All right Pet", thus protecting me from the barman. He opened the race card, removed the fiver, and put a tremulous cross by the name of one horse in each race. While he did that I studied his astonishing nose, which was like a huge purple sponge. I thanked him, took the card and fled back to my father in the stand.

I was utterly passionate about horses. Thoroughbreds were the most beautiful things I had ever seen. As long as they were in the paddock, I was there leaning over the rails, choosing a winner, and drinking in the excitement, the tension like a taut wire, before the start of a race. Unhappily, I had few funds for speculation: only what I had won in Pony Club gymkhanas in the holidays. Worse still, school girls were not allowed to bet with bookies. My father, if I could find him, would allow me to bet with him, so long as he approved of the bet, using the bookies' odds, but only for two bob at a time. Bookies are not allowed in the Members' Enclosure, so they lean over the rails. I would run up and down trying to find the best odds before betting. My father allowed and encouraged this. However, if he did not like the horse I fancied, he refused to take my bet, and once or twice, when it won, we had a hell of a row. I said he owed me my winnings; but he, doubly humiliated now that I should have guessed the winner, and he had not even tried an each-way bet on it, said I could hardly expect winnings when the fact of the matter was that I had not placed a bet.

My job during the race was to position myself exactly opposite the two winning posts with them in line. I shared this position, on the other side of the track, with the bookies' runners. We were waiting for a dead heat. Twice, it happened. The first time it really was hardly a dead heat. The crowd was sure they knew what horse had won, and they were right. There was no point betting on it. But the second time it was very close. I saw a chestnut nose flash by just ahead of a brown one. So when my father came running down from the stand, pink-faced with excitement, asking "What won? What won?" I said, "The chestnut, number two, by a nose." He replied "You'd bloody well better be right", and went off to place a huge bet on it. Maybe, in these electronic days, you can no longer bet on a dead heat: I do not know. But then you could, because an automatic blurry photograph had been taken, and everyone had to wait while this was developed. I went and stood by the place where the photograph was to be pinned up.

"Please God," I said under my breath, "*Please God*, if you really do love me, make it be number two by a nose. *Number Two*."

We waited in anguish. What seemed like days later a grey man with a wet grey photograph arrived, opened the glass frame and pinned it up with four drawing pins. We could not see till he had finished, and shut the frame. Then it was as clear as day: Number Two, by a good nose. Wonderful relief. I only remembered to thank God much later.

Unlike my father, I never ended a day's racing much richer or poorer, due to the measly bets he allowed. If he had won he was elated. If he was seriously down on the day, he drank a lot more whisky, got very red in the face, and snarled, "Where do all the bookies go for Christmas?"

To which question I always answered correctly, "Barbados". I had no idea what or where Barbados was but I imagined it as some kind of bookie paradise, and wished I too could spend Christmas there.

When I got back to school, later than I should have been, usually, I was walking on air, in a state of ultimate bliss. Matron and the head girl and anyone else who wanted to could tick me off for being late, but I didn't care. I had had a day entirely to my liking, of beauty and excitement. I would have liked to go to the races every day of my life, and had decided that as soon as I got out of this much disliked school, I would become a bookie. At that time I had not noticed that there were no female bookies, but I doubt if it would have affected my decision.

The girls who had returned to school from their day out, and who had half decent parents (among whom alas my father was not counted), had been given small tins of Nestle's sweetened condensed milk, which they had brought into school up their knicker legs. After dark that night in the dormitories we had 'LickySticky', a heavenly and longed for event. The owner made two holes in the top of her tin, and we all stood in a line, palms upwards and touching, while she poured a thin greenish white trickle of sugary condensed milk up and down the line, leaving a gorgeous smear on the palm of each upheld hand. We can buy any food we want these days, but nothing I now eat can produce half the anticipation, the desperate mouth-watering, of watching that line of goo and waiting till you could put your hand to your face and lick it off. Because we were deprived of sugar, that sugar shot gave us happiness and pleasure near delirium; nowadays I suppose probably only a crack cocaine addict may get such a rush.

Other girls at school had photographs of their mothers and fathers (could they not remember them?) and their horrible home counties houses on their bedside lockers: I only had ponies and horses.

I took a great interest in breeding. I kept my father's out of date copies of *Raceform* and *Chaseform* under my pillow, and read them by torchlight under the blankets after lights out. We were supposed to own up to crimes like that, and for talking, but I could never see why, and I never did. I knew the names of the winners of the St Leger since the start of the race in 1776, and was pretty good on the Derby too.

One Easter, when I was 14, the Grand National was run towards the end of term. I knew the jumps were stunning, but apart from the sports pages of the newspapers and *The Illustrated London News*, I had little information.

However, the year was 1948, the War was over but there was still food rationing. We were allowed to bring a term's worth of sweets, which were stored with Matron, and she handed them out on Wednesdays and Saturdays. We were allowed four on Wednesday and four on Saturday. Half a Mars Bar was four, two sticks of a KitKat was four, and you could have four squares of chocolate, or four Liquorice Allsorts and so on. In other words, they were absolute currency: as if they had been pieces of gold. So, ignorant but hopeful, I decided to make a book on the Grand National in sweets. I accepted bets from girls in almost every form in the school over several weeks. I changed the odds quite often, depending on how many bets I had taken on that horse, and what the out of date *Chaseform* said about its previous performance and its ancestry. I kept the bets in a box in my games clothes locker. We all hated games, and seldom played them, so the lockers were little used. All punters were sworn to secrecy, and as far as I knew, they were trustworthy.

I had one of the first so-called 'portable' radios. It was made of cream coloured plastic, with a curvy front and an enormous battery. It came up to my knees, and it required an almighty effort to carry it anywhere. Games of netball or lacrosse only happened rarely (hockey was thought quite disgusting and emphatically not played: something to do with the risk of getting our front teeth knocked out, I remember), so when there were no games we were supposed to go for walks all afternoon. This suited us fine, and with massive effort we hauled the radio up into a live oak tree in the Pleasaunce. Our school was a mixture of an old Elizabethan manor house, with a Georgian front on it. We used to refer to the 8th Earl, its owner, as Bertie Bucks, and he came to read the lesson in church once or twice a year. He was not married. We used to sit there in our grey tweed cloaks with yellow insides to the hoods, ogling him. The whole school was trying to imagine what it would be like to be married to him. And in the crocodile walking back to the house, the whole school loudly agreed that it would be absolutely awful. Definitely. Sadly, I can only remember this bit about him, but not at all what he actually looked like, nor exactly why we did not want to marry him. So I have looked him up.

He was 'Known affectionately to his friends and family as 'Bertie Bucks'', so we were right there. Perhaps some of our parents knew him.

'In his youth he was regarded as a very handsome and dashing young man, much sought after by his female contemporaries who thought him adorable'.

I very clearly remember that we did not think him anywhere near adorable. Was it just the generation gap that made him seem so impossible for us? He was, at the time, about 40.

'He was marred by the whiff of a scandal in his youth but the press did not publish the story and the full details of the 'scandal', allegedly involving a young woman'.

Exciting. I fear we might have thought better of him, not worse, for this scandal.

'He died a chronic alcoholic on 2nd January 1963 at King Edward VII Hospital, aged 56, unmarried and without legitimate heirs to inherit his titles'.

'Without legitimate heirs' makes it sound as if there were illegitimate heirs, which we would certainly have thought exciting. But 'a chronic alcoholic', was he? Ah, maybe we somehow picked that up as he read the lesson? I certainly do not remember him seeming drunk, but we were not wrong in our judgement, it would have been disastrous to be married to him.

Hampden House had once been the home of the Parliamentary rebel, John Hampden, and he had been arrested in the Brick Parlour. Luckily I did not know about that when the police talked to me in the same room after Pixie's escape, or I might have been more unnerved. All the wrought iron door locks in the Great Hall had been personally made by Oliver Cromwell, we were told. They were lovely; he was talented, even if he was terrible. There were tall yew hedges against which we learned to do handstands, a lawn big enough for two or three lacrosse pitches, a ha-ha, an avenue two miles long ending in two pepper-pot lodges which had been made for a visit by Queen Elizabeth I, and a Pleasaunce, an enormous medieval shrubbery in which, because of war time neglect, the shrubs had grown into tall crowded trees and the paths were overgrown and many completely obliterated. The ground sloped steeply downhill, and I carefully never mentioned to my father that if I had climbed a tree at the top, I might have been able to see Mr Attlee walking around in the grounds of Chequers. I never did see him, actually, though I climbed most of the trees, but I could have. I now know that our school was in a house of outstanding beauty, but at that stage of my life, it did not impinge on me at all.

So we sat on the branches of the dark tree, about a dozen of us, me shaking with excitement, to listen to the Grand National, and see how we had done. Lots of horses fell, including the favourite, at Becher's Brook (hooray!). The winner was Sheila's Cottage, and though I had given pretty long odds, hardly anyone had bet on it. I suddenly realised that I was richer than I had ever been in my life. I had taken about eight pounds of sweets, and I owed very few of them to anyone, and mostly in each-way bets, so the winnings were small. My friends and I were going to eat and eat and eat sweets that evening after lights out. We would have sweets coming out of our ears. Triumphant, I walked back up to the house, swinging the portable radio as though it weighed nothing.

In the doorway in the centre of the long façade of the house stood the head girl. She did have a remarkably beautiful singing voice:

> Trees where you sit,
> Shall crowd into-oo a shade,
> Trees where you sit,
> Shall crow-ow-owd into-oo a shade,

This is what she used to sing to us, as if she were a man dottily in love. But she had nasty hairy legs, and a nasty tough temperament.

"Alison Brittain come here", she bellowed. I wandered towards her. "Matron wants to see you," she said.

"Matron can jolly well wait," I replied.

"Oh no she can't," she said, "Matron has been to your locker and she wants to ask you some questions."

A spider with ice-cold feet crawled up the back of my neck. 'How dare she?' I thought, 'How dare she?' It was none of her business to go poking about in my private locker: had she stolen my winnings? I could explain exactly how I came by them, perfectly honestly. Angrily, I stormed off to find Matron.

"Go to the sickroom," Matron said, "Your father has been telephoned."

"Those are all my sweets," I said, "you mustn't confiscate them. I earned them. I made a book on the Grand National. And I won. Look, here's the book." I showed her the neat exercise book in which all the bets were recorded, which lay on top of the huge box of sweets. She was tight-lipped.

"Do you think I stole them?" I asked. She said nothing.

"I did not. And I need them back now, because I have people to pay out. And why has my father been telephoned?"

"Get up to the sickroom right now," said Matron. "Your father is coming to take you away."

I sat on a bed in the sickroom, astonished. I was locked in, and not spoken to or fed. Late that afternoon I saw the Rolls arrive. I was taken down to the headmistress's 'Nest', her horrible dark smelly study. My father stood with his back to the fire, not looking at me. Mrs Robley-Browne was in total drama-queen mode. All of her wobbled. She was acting 'shaking with rage'. I was nothing but a nuisance in this school. They had done their best to cope with me, but I was incorrigible. I disobeyed the rules. I was never in the right place at the right time. I talked after lights out. I had a bad effect on other girls. All of which they could have put up with until they discovered this ultimate wickedness: betting. Betting on horses. Involving other girls, corrupting them too and teaching them vices. I must go at once: not another night would I spend under her roof. "Take her away," she said, tearfully.

My things had been packed for me, and were in the hall. But not, alas, the sweets. Just as I thought, Matron had stolen them.

My father, grim-faced, said nothing as we got in the car, and nothing for an hour or two on the journey. I was half delighted to be going home to my ponies, and half completely at a loss to know what I had done wrong. Was he too very angry? Was betting a vice? Did it corrupt you? How? No one had told me that before.

As we went through Newmarket, and I was admiring the strings of racehorses out for exercise, my father turned to me and asked: "So what odds were you giving on the favourite?"

I told him how much and said, "But it didn't matter because it fell." He put both hands to his face (still driving), then looked at me and said "Jesus Christ, you were lucky!"

Years and years later, I was standing in the cosmetic department of Harrods, thinking how unfair it was that I should have spots, and wondering if there was any potion there that would cure them, when a voice cried out "Potty? Potty, it's got to be you". I used to be in trouble at school for deliberately disobeying the orders of staff. If I thought orders were stupid, I did not do what I was told. I would run with knitting if I wanted to, whatever was said. Friends thought I was inviting punishment for this, that I was living dangerously, so they called me 'Potty'. "Potty" this voice called out, "I was at school with you, don't you remember? I'm Jane Baker."

A vision of glory stood in front of me. Tall, thin and elegant, in a pale grey coat and skirt, and a dream of a hat with a feather, stood what had once been insignificant little Jane Baker of the second form. These days she was a model, she said, and she looked it every inch.

"And as a matter of fact, Potty, she said with a radiant smile, I've been looking for you. You owe me half a Mars Bar."

Chapter 21
Crimes and Punishment

I left Hampden House in disgrace in 1948 and was sent to Tortington Park later that year. I was 14 years old.

Dear Daddy,

This is a very funny school. All the girls say 'pardon' and 'serviette'.

Miss Le Sage's best friend, Miss Callahan, sits beside her at high table crocheting doilies. There are 400 of us here, and she has made two sets of them, in beige cotton thread, to cover our place mats. She is now on her third lot. They live together. Before supper, while our soup is getting cold, we have to stand up and say a prayer. Miss Callahan crochets while she prays. At first it sounded like you, because it begins: 'Oh my God,' But then it goes on:

I present myself before Thee,

At the end of another day,

To offer Thee anew,

The homage of my heart

And it goes on and on and on and I don't know it but they say I will learn it in the end. But the thing is, it is a Catholic prayer, because Miss Le Sage and Miss Callahan are Catholics.

I thought you didn't like 'pardon' or 'serviette' or 'doily', and you particularly didn't like Catholics. Did you know about all this? Did you mean to send me to this school?

Love from

Alison

He replied tersely, saying he was glad I had noticed, and beggars cannot be choosers. What I do know is that he thought the letter highly amusing, and showed it to all his friends.

Is it not odd that there were some words that I must not say? Not 'pardon', 'serviette' or 'doily'. It is a ridiculous way of distinguishing class, and far from admirable. If you find someone who does not say these things, what does it tell you about them? Will you know, just hearing them speak, that they are kind, gentle, clever, fun to have about, that they do not cheat, beat, or hate you? No. I fear that all you will find out is that they were brought up to avoid the same words that you must avoid. You join a club of people who do not say this or that. If they do say these words, you have no reason to believe that these are horrible people and you would not want your daughter to marry one of them. And as for Catholics, I had never seen my father show the slightest interest in any religion. I think perhaps in Dublin, Protestants took themselves to be better than Catholics. That certainly does not mean they were better but that is how they thought in those days. It took me a long time to realise how stupid all this is.

We had to write letters to our parents on Sundays. But if he was going to read my letters out to his friends as a joke, I wasn't going to write them. After that I preferred the punishment for not doing so. This was going to Catholic Mass, as well as Sung Eucharist. It was much easier than being afraid he would laugh at what I wrote. Anyway, I quite liked the 'bells and smells', and Mass was shorter and nothing like as bone-achingly dull as Eucharist.

This 'funny' school was in the former dower house of the Dukes of Norfolk, at Arundel. The stationmaster on the platform when we arrived shouted, to rhyme with 'trundle', "Ar*und*el, Ar*und*el, Ar*und*el". The school houses were called after the family names of the Dukes of Norfolk: Howard, Maltravers, Fitzalan and Mowbray, but they were entirely imaginary, as the girls were simply divided into four equal clumps and allotted a 'house' name. We all lived together. The school motto was 'Guard Thy Speech', which my father strongly approved of, and often quoted. The motto of my house, Howard, was 'Do It Now' which would today be an appropriate slogan for the front of a T-shirt.

There were many enjoyable things about the school. The best teacher for most of the time that I was there, an Irishwoman called Miss Neilan, taught Science with enthusiasm and brio. She encouraged us each to ask questions, and all the others to try answering them. If your guess was right she was delighted, you never forgot the answer, and we all learned to think. Her pet was my best friend Carol, the only girl in the school at that time ever to get into university, and that at 16, to Oxford, to read Chemistry. Carol had the freedom of the laboratory: she had been given the key to it, and we used to go there most nights. None of the staff lived near the dormitories, nor along the corridor to the lab, and although Matron sometimes came on the warpath, she was listening for talking, and we only whispered, so we were safe.

We collected sugar lumps from girls who did without them with their cocoa at break, and margarine from the lunch and supper tables. We kept a record of who had given us what, and then made fudge for them in large quantities in beakers over Bunsen burners at night. The smell was glorious, and we took a percentage as our reward.

The drains of the lab sinks were filled with thick cylinders of pierced lead, and we discovered that if you heated them up in a crucible they melted, and then we poured them into big jars of water, and they set in the most beautiful, flowing, raindrop shapes, like magma from volcanoes, we thought. We did it to all the lead cylinders, and it was not noticed until one of the drains got blocked with glass from broken test tubes, and even then, when boring new steel drains were fitted, no one could quite decide what had happened to the old ones.

We were very fond of silver nitrate. All science enthusiasts took a crystal, dipped it in water, and rubbed it on the ball of one thumb. You were left with a striking oval patch of black skin, glinting silver in certain lights. We held up our hands to show each other as we passed. No one ever asked how we got them.

Then we read that if you could heat a solution of silver nitrate to a high enough temperature, it would go 'blick', and you would be left with only the silver. Night after night we put three Bunsen burners together, tried blowing them hotter through a straw, but all we got was silvery bubbles stuck to the bottom of the crucible, never what we so hoped for, pure liquid silver. We used up the entire jar of silver nitrate crystals, and when Miss Neilan noticed she was furious, and we were sorry. What we had never thought about, of course, is that silver nitrate is very expensive.

We tried making explosives, with gunpowder we made ourselves in the lab, but it was a failure because we put the stuff in a pipe and lit it, and though a jet of flame like a comet's tail shot out of the end of the pipe, we could never get the really loud bang and proper explosion we wanted.

A friend complained that there was a horrid girl in her dormitory who stole her pillow, and threw her teddy bear all round the room for other girls to tug at and bash. I got a reel of magnesium ribbon for her, and a box of matches, and told her to lay it under the bed of the bully after lights out, leading a fuse wire from it to her own bed. I said: "If you light your end, a bright light will run along the fuse and when it gets to the reel under that bully's bed it will go up so brilliantly that you will have the shock of your lives, and your bully will be cowed forever."

It achieved the right result, but unfortunately the ribbon burned a track through the carpet leading from my friend's bed to a big burned hole beneath her enemy's, and there was trouble, though no one knew exactly what had happened.

We learned fencing: great fun cantering to and fro with one hand in the air behind you for balance, and with the other going poke, poke, poke with the foil, at your enemy. And Miss Le Sage taught us what she called History of Art. All I really remember is long lectures on Corot (she was a great admirer) and hour after hour of sitting on hard benches looking at black and white photographs of the Winged Victory of Samothrace (I never realised until I saw the marble base of her in the flesh, so to speak, on the Aegean island of Samothraki, that she was the prow of a marble boat). We also gazed at Praxiteles' The Scraper, and learned that he was scraping the sweat off his arm after playing games. After games we ourselves tried scraping our arms with the backs of combs, but we got no result.

We were taught scripture by the frightful, prim Mrs Taylor. She would get us reading the Old Testament round the class, and said: "All right, Penelope, you read from verse 1 to verse 6, then Janice read from verse 9 to the end." We then concentrated on verses 7 and 8, knowing that these would be the ones about how he took the virgin, and went in unto her and knew her, and she bore him a son. One day we decided just for fun to ignore the instructions, and whoever it was would just go on reading straight through, including the forbidden verses.

Mrs Taylor absolutely shrieked, "Stop it, stop it, stop it at once. No more." Mrs Taylor decided that I had organised this (I think it was probably a community effort) and so I had to be sent to the Headmistress, Miss Bevan (Miss Le Sage was the Principal and Founder, Miss Bevan the Head) for a punishment. I was always getting punishments. But I also sometimes got awards, and that was not thought good, either.

We had to write essays once a week on sickening subjects, like 'Honour Thy Father and Mother', or 'Honesty is the Best Policy', and for some reason I was very good at these: they tripped sweetly off my pen. Poor Miss Le Sage was plainly choking as she presented me with the term's Best Essay Writer Prize, a copy of Wuthering Heights, which I still have.

And talking of books, there was a school library, where we had to do prep. It was surrounded by locked glass-fronted cases full of books, and if you wanted to read one, you had to go and ask Miss Le Sage.

"Please, Miss Le Sage, I would like to read a book in the Library."

"What is it called, dear?"

"Murder in the Cathedral."

"Who is it by?"

"T. S. Eliot."

"What is it about?"

"I don't know."

"Why do you want to read it then?"

"I like the title."

"That's not good enough, is it? I can't let you have it if you don't know what it is about, and you don't know why you want to read it."

I never tried that one again, but I did think that if I ever had to run a school (which Heaven forbid), I would probably keep the library shelves open, and perhaps lock the laboratory.

And then, like a summer's day, a new teacher came to teach us English. Miss Cox did not just like her subject, she was absolutely passionate about it, and was supremely able to pass her excitement on to us. I read aloud in class Cleopatra to her Anthony, and she stopped it for Enobarbus' speech on Cleopatra's arrival.

> The barge she sat in, like a burnish'd throne,
> Burn'd on the water, the poop was beaten gold. . .

How did Shakespeare know how hot it was in Egypt, and how the sun's heat would be reflected off the gold? She said we could learn it by heart if we liked, and we did.

Miss Cox helped us to discover that if you relaxed a bit and went with the flow, Chaucer made sense. Having read the tale of the 'verray parfit gentil knight' we voraciously read many of the others to ourselves, and begged, in the next lesson, to be allowed to read The Miller's Tale aloud.

"It's hilarious, isn't it?" she said. "But those of you who have read it will perfectly understand why we cannot read it aloud in class. Those of you who haven't read it: borrow a copy."

And then we came to sprung rhythm, and Gerard Manley Hopkins' 'Glory be to God for dappled things', and poor unselved 'Binsey Poplars' which, as she read the poems aloud, lit up the classroom and fired our brains with pleasure. We tried and tried; they were really hard to read aloud, but well worth the effort. I am happy that today I live within half a mile of the lovely, felled and re-grown, Binsey poplars. We had our noses in Shakespeare or Chaucer at every opportunity. And we took to Browning: we went mad for 'My Last Duchess', and were delighted when Porphyria's lover strangles her with her hair, and says "And all night long we have not stirred, and yet God has not said a word".

At night we often sat in twos or threes leaning against the radiators in the long corridors wrapped in our eiderdowns, discussing (in whispers) where you might try to cut off a pound of flesh, or how our current stuttering king seemed to have none of the boldness, weakness or wickedness of Henry V or Richards II and III.

Not all the water in the rough rude sea,
Can wash the balm from an anointed king;

Did George VI believe in the divine right of kings, we wondered?

We loved Miss Cox, but we were not in love with her. Many of us were, however, in love (only in the sense of having a crush) with the 20-year-old Games Mistress, and to my great good fortune I had succeeded in taking a rather nice photograph of her, with my box Brownie, in her bathing suit on the edge of the pool. I could not have cared less about her, but many girls asked me to get and give them copies of her photograph. I sent the negative off to Will R. Rose, the photographer in the High Street, Oxford, who always sent back by return of post, and ordered ten copies which I easily sold for half a crown each. Then one girl, madly in love, asked me to get a half-life-sized print with the Games Mistress cut out and stuck on a piece of board, with a stand behind it so it could be stood up in her room. She paid me three times what it cost. I had not thought of the consequences. All parcels had to be opened in front of Matron, to see you were not secreting forbidden goods into the school (sweets, perhaps, or weapons; what on earth did they fear)? Of course this photograph came as a parcel. Matron was astonished, and made off with it, and I never saw it again. Nothing else happened, and I was never questioned, so I do not know what she did with it. I told the girl, and gave her the negative, and said "You can get one in the holidays, can't you?"

I was very bad at prep. Or perhaps I should say, at not doing prep. But I enjoyed the challenge of exams, and managed to get quite a bit of revision done in a short time. I once got a term average (for prep) of 18 per cent, and an exam average of 96 per cent. The staff resented it.

Several days before School Certificate exams I had Castlereagh's foreign policy written on the fingers of my left hand, and Canning's on my right, and the History mistress saw it, and claimed that even by cheating like that I would not pass and I would end up in Borstal. I had no intention of cheating, and had scrubbed the foreign policies completely off both hands at least a day before the exam. I felt lucky to find a nice question to compare and contrast Canning's and Castlereagh's foreign policies. I passed. I even got a credit.

Unfortunately for them, and for me, I infuriated the staff. I committed crimes and needed punishment a great deal of the time, much more than most other girls. Talking on the stairs was a crime. And all the usual crimes, like talking after lights out, going out in indoor shoes, passing notes in class, feeding scraps to the stray cats outside the kitchens needed punishment. Punishments in this school were the very opposite of poetry.

Any member of staff or senior girl who had it in for you could shout at you "House Point", and you had to accept it. Miss Bevan could give you several at a time. In Assembly, where the school was gathered together on Saturday mornings, it was announced that the girls who had let down their House by acquiring points would now stand up and admit it. One Assembly I had to announce the exceptional disgrace that I had 36.

For one house point you had to spend an hour of Saturday afternoon being punished. So for 36 house points I was obviously going to spend all my Saturdays until the end of term on punishments. We had to queue up in alphabetical order, and go into the gym and do Civil Service tots. These were addition sums, seven figures wide and seven deep, if I remember, that came in a short wide booklet, and were intended for the Civil Service to judge hopeful entrants and distinguish the corn from the chaff. No doubt about it, I was chaff at tots. But then the headmistress said that we could either sit there for an hour of each punishment, or we could get out sooner, indeed as soon as we had got the answers to four tots right. That seemed easy. I immediately wrote away for the answer book, which the teacher in charge of us had in front of her. The address was in the back of our books, and I ordered one. I got a stuffy letter back from the Civil Service. I had failed to give details of the position I held in the school, or of the degrees I had been awarded. I had to think of another way.

We could choose to do tots from anywhere we liked in the book. I went down the line waiting to go in, saying: "I want you all to do different tots, and if you get them right, give me the answers."

I arranged for the first girl to do the first four tots, and the second girl to do tots five to eight, and so on. Within three weeks we had all the answers, and after that punishments were not so grim. As I did punishments every week I was able to share the answers with all my fellow victims. We sat as far away from the teacher as possible, right down the other end of the gym, and listened very quietly to horse-racing or tennis on the wireless, and after about half an hour was up we presented our (correct) answers. Everyone, including the wretched staff member on duty, thought this was much better. Much better, that is, until someone split on me and they discovered how we were doing it. Miss Bevan challenged me, and I owned up. I was told to be truly sorry for my fraudulent, dishonest behaviour; a severe letter was written to my father and in the holidays he asked me to tell him what I had done. I explained, and he said "Oh for God's sake, do be careful." But he seemed quite satisfied.

The senior girls had two-bed dormitories, and unless you shared with a friend, you often went to see a friend in her bedroom, with your pillow and eiderdown. You sat at either end of the bed, and chatted, or even side-by-side with the eider-downs drawn up to your neck. We discussed whether our parents were alcoholics, since we knew they mostly needed a drink at about 6 o'clock. We thought they probably were. We did a survey among the so-called Study Circle (today's sixth form), asking everyone if they had both parents happily married and living together at home. Of the 32 of us, only four replied 'Yes'. So then we discussed how we were the dumped daughters of disastrous divorces, and whatever was wrong with our parents that they could not stay married?

Two close friends, always called 'London' and 'Birmingham' after a running game we played, were found sitting in bed together one night by Matron. A horrible thing then happened. We were told in Assembly the next morning that these two were a disgrace to the school (though we were not told why) and were being sent away. London's mother came that day, but Birmingham's parents lived abroad and it took them two days to fetch her. Why on earth their parents failed to ask the school for proof of what was suspected, I do not know. I do know now that London and Birmingham were just friends, and definitely not lesbians. In the meantime, we were told that Birmingham was so wicked none of us could speak to her. She must be kept in silence. Birmingham had a tear-stained face, and looked terrible. During an art lesson she sidled up to my easel and painted quickly on it 'WHAT HAVE I DONE?' I had to write, 'I'M SORRY, I HAVE NO IDEA'.

I do not think any girls in the school knew what a lesbian was: I certainly did not. I can only suppose that after they got home and told their parents what they had NOT done, none of them wanted to have anything further to do with the school. Maybe their parents wanted to sue the school, to clear their daughters' names, but how could they prove anything? What exactly did Miss Le Sage and Miss Callahan think they were up to, and how did they manage to insinuate it, the horrible old toads?

After writing this, I looked up Tortington Park School, long since closed, on the internet. One old girl had organized a website, and old girls were sending in letters about what they remembered of the school. Niki Bartman wrote: '*Last night I dreamed of Tortington Park and of Miss Cox who used to teach us English but who left unexpectedly suddenly in 1957 - allegedly to do a psychology course at London University. I didn't particularly like English (and went on to do science with Miss Cobley in the Study Circle) but Miss Cox was the best teacher I have ever had. . . and I should love to be able to tell her that now that we are all grown up.*

When I finally finished with formal education Miss Cobley took me out to tea at the Dorchester Hotel and got me to join her London club. In the course of a very smart afternoon, she told me that Miss Cox had been 'invited to leave' Tortington following an indiscretion with our French mistress (as I understood it, it was Mrs Taylor, the First Form mistress and scripture teacher, who told on them).'

Oh, Heavens, were those aged Irish lesbians, Miss Le Sage and Miss Callahan, jealous of the most wonderful teacher the school had ever had? What disgusting hypocrites.

'*Since then*', Nikki goes on, '*I have often thought about Miss Cox and very much wanted to tell her how wonderful she was. She made English come alive for all of us. She was the best teacher in the school. We loved her but were too little and ignorant to know how to tell her. I hope she will one day read this message, but don't know how to include it on your website and so must ask you to please do so for me*'.

Then came the beginning of the end. My friend Carol had to work hard for Oxford entrance, and it was decided that she could no longer spare the time to be Head of Howard House. Since this was only to be for half a term, Miss Le Sage decided that the girls of Howard House could vote for who they wanted to be Head. To my consternation and horror, they voted for me. The last thing in the world I wanted was to be set in authority over anyone. But luckily I thought I was saved by Miss Le Sage who announced at lunchtime that the girls of Howard

House had been very silly, that I was obviously unsuitable to be Head, and they should vote again, and this time think what they were doing. In a defiant and frolicsome mood, they voted for me again.

Miss Le Sage sent for me. I said she was absolutely right, I was the wrong person for the job, and recommended the girl I had voted for. I said I greatly feared I would be no good at it, and that would be tough for the girls of Howard House. They were just being naughty, voting for me. Please, for goodness' sake, let me off this hook. Miss Le Sage said I had to do it, it was my last chance.

She was right. It was ghastly. I was completely unsuitable. I was supposed to prevent the girls in my house getting points, but how? In the very last days of term, when the whole school was excited about going home and people were chattering at night in normal voices, and flashing torches round the room, I saw Matron on her rounds. The next room she would come to had five girls from Howard and only one from another house in it. I had to warn them, or they would all be given house points. My room was on the ground floor, so I jumped out of the window, gathered a handful of stones off the path and flung them at the upper window. One girl finally opened it to see what was going on, when Matron came into the room. She came to the window, saw me and reported me to Miss Bevan, then dealt out house points to all the girls.

Miss Bevan said that Matron had informed her that I was dancing on the frosty lawn in a long white nightdress at 10 o'clock at night throwing stones at windows. Was that true?

I replied "Yes", because, apart from the dancing bit, it was true.

And so my father was told he could come and fetch me a day early, and the school did not want me back next term. I felt terrible about getting the sack from school again, especially as I had not intended any wickedness: quite the reverse. I am sorry that the best things about the school, the science mistress Miss Neilan and the English mistress Miss Cox, went unrecognised. Looking back, I now know that I was lucky to be taught by them, and that there was nothing bad, as my father seemed to fear, about it being a Catholic school.

I left Tortington Park in disgrace when I was 16. I did worry about a few traits: why did I keep getting the sack? Why did I fail to obey authority? Why could I not do as I was told? I think if I had had a mother or a mother-figure at home to soften my father's rule, to explain why I was being asked to do this or that, perhaps to give praise if I did what was wanted, maybe I would not have been such a stroppy little pig. If I was told not to run with knitting, not to talk on the stairs, not to feed the hungry stray cats outside the kitchen, I wondered how that had been decided. When my nice knitting was confiscated, or I was not allowed to speak or be spoken to for 24 hours, or I was searched leaving the dining room, I simply decided that the women put in authority over us were unpleasant and despicable, and even if I did not say so, they knew I thought that. And I got the sack.

For years I did not know I had a mother, and when I did know I was not allowed to talk about it. I found it really hard to accept that I had not been told all that there was to know, and that people thought that was a kindness to me. I did not really trust anyone completely, and felt I must deal with everything from first principles. As Pixie had so clearly seen and said, I was not handling things very well.

I just knew that being sacked would upset my father. All he said was, "Oh my God, what am I going to do with you now?"

Chapter 22
Love and Marriage

I had three sorts of aunts. My Irish aunts were my father's sisters: Mabel, Doris, Phyllis and Ann. My English aunts were my mother's sisters, Alice and Betty, who I did not meet until I was 28. And then I had more aunts, both English and Irish, who were mostly not my blood relations but my father's girlfriends, who I always had to call Aunt 'So-and-so' even though they were not really aunts. I had at least six of them, probably more if I think about it, but I need not name them now.

My Irish aunts, Mabel and Ann in particular, described to me my father growing up as their brother. They said he learned very young to make the world go his way. Their mother and father sent him, alone of his siblings, to public school in England, and he wanted to go and liked it. He refused to learn anything to do with the family laundry because he said he hated and despised it and did not want to take over the business from his father. He told me about that when I was a teenager. 'Taking in other people's dirty washing' he called it. In a difficult interview with his father he had apparently said it was fine by him if his younger brother Eric learned the laundry business. He told me that, challenged by his father, he announced "I'll be. . . I'll be a doctor," on the spur of the moment. He remembered that his father was disappointed, and said he would

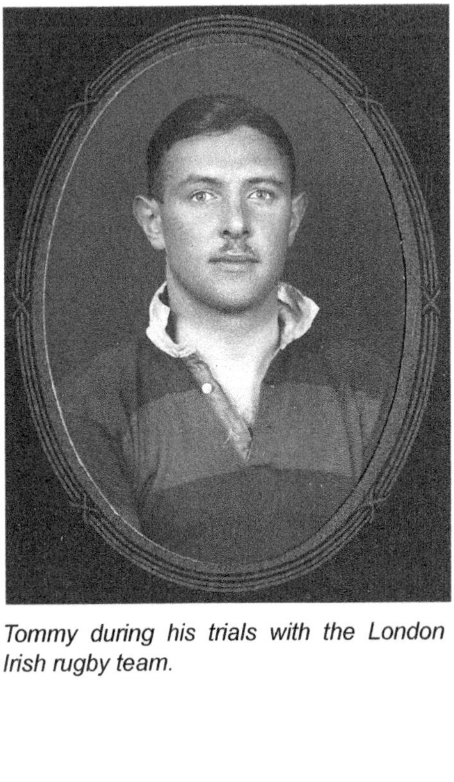

Tommy during his trials with the London Irish rugby team.

pay for his training, but he must understand that after he qualified he would be on his own. His brother Eric would inherit the Swastika laundry. This upset his father, of course, but it suited mine. He passed his medical exams and left Dublin for London where he thought there were greater opportunities. He boasted to me that he was trialled playing rugby for the London Irish, drank all other medics under the table, and passed his Fellowship first time. He said he enjoyed all his house jobs (and happily told me that he had been caught in an airing cupboard making love to a nurse in Portsmouth General Hospital: and had had to move on quickly).

Nearly all that I know about my father and mother meeting and falling in love, and marrying, and having me, I only learned decades after it happened. I was married, and had children myself, before I finally met my mother's relations. That was long after my father was dead. It was even after his brother and sisters were dead.

Of course I was not born then so all I know I gleaned from others. I can only tell it as I heard it. Occasionally, I have to fill in gaps: although I was not there I know what happened because I asked, or I was told.

When my parents first met, my father was just qualified, aged about 28, and my mother was a young girl of 22, living at home.

My English aunts, my mother's sisters, Alice and Betty, told me my father was doing a house job in Ipswich (in about 1932) when he was invited to Hyntle Place for the weekend by the hospital's chief dental surgeon. Alice and Betty described their father, Jackie, the dentist, as a very jolly little man, only five feet tall, wearing cork wedges in his shoes in a brave attempt to raise himself up, and joking and laughing all the time. He said that his wife insisted that he bring home three eligible young dentists or doctors every weekend to meet his three beautiful daughters Dorothy, Alice and Betty. My father keenly accepted the invitation. Hyntle Place was a 16th century brick-built house (once the dower house for the nearby hall), much older, with far more character and with more elegance than any house he had ever lived in. It had very low ceiling beams everywhere. If he was not careful he used to bang his head on quite a few of them. The very short dentist and his petite daughters roared with laughter every time he did it, though they were also very consoling. The dentist's wife,

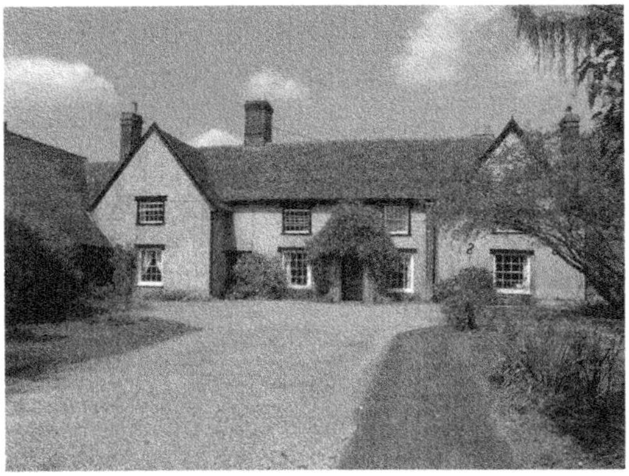

Hyntle Place, the Payne-James' home in Suffolk, where Dorothy first met Tommy.

Bella, was a good organiser, the bedrooms were gracious, delicious meals were produced, the tennis court was ready. The daughters hugely looked forward to the fun of the weekend, they wanted it to be really exciting, and they were full of life and go. They were small, and like their father they had no need to duck under the beams. They were ready to play games, practical jokes, charades, act, sing, everything. My father found the weekend exhausting, hilarious fun. He hoped he would be asked again, and he was, often. After several visits he had got so used to the house that he instinctively ducked under every beam.

He discovered that this family, unlike his, enjoyed being a little outrageous. The daughters referred to their father Jackie, in front of him, as the 'Little Bugger', and indeed he was never called anything else. Jackie was a Methodist, as was John Wesley Brittain, my father's father, which probably seemed a good omen. Dignified John was head and shoulders taller than Jackie, and indeed, it was impossible to imagine anybody calling him by any sort of nickname, let alone one like that. The girls told my father, naughtily, that their father got their mother pregnant when he and she were both 19, and she was the daughter of his landlady. "So he had to marry her you see" they said, pointing, "and that was Dorothy". In my father's own family, if such a thing had ever been true, which seems impossible, it would never, ever have been spoken about.

The girls, with their delicate skin and hair the colour of ripe corn, were all lovely, but everyone in her family agreed that the oldest sister Dorothy was the most talented, liveliest and loveliest of all. As well as her clear-skinned fair-haired round-faced beauty, she played the violin brilliantly, and had an astounding, clear, true singing voice. Her singing teacher, from London, was excited by her lovely singing, and said he believed that when trained her voice might be really outstanding, even the best in the country. Aunt Betty told me Dorothy 'threw herself at Tommy'. It was not long before my father knew she was the girl for him.

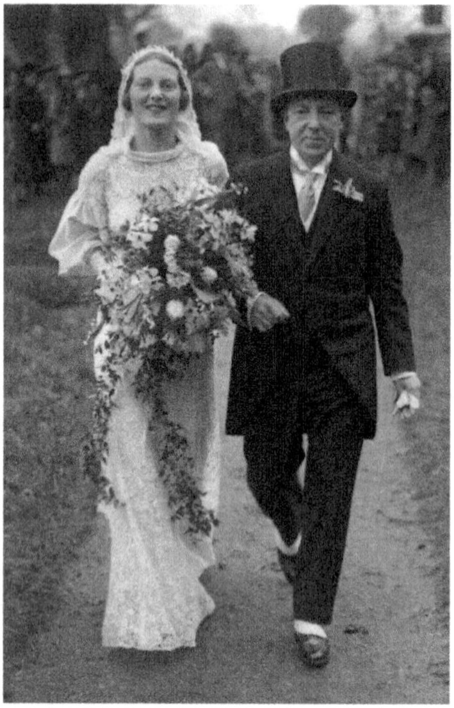

Dorothy walking with her father Jackie (the 'Little Bugger') to St Nicholas church, Hintlesham, for her wedding. 18th March 1933. They are Alison's mother and grandfather: Dorothy and Jackie Payne-James.

One of the first things my mother told me, when I finally met her, was how she remembered being terribly excited when Tommy took her out in his thrilling new sports car, and asked her to marry him, and she said yes. She said that then life became extremely exciting and delicious. He brought her over to Dublin to meet the family and she took to them at once. Used to sisterhood, she quickly became friends with his three youngest sisters, they were all fond of each other and they did everything together. She was so pleased when Doris asked her to be a bridesmaid, with Phyllis and Ann, at her wedding later that year. I think the resulting photographs seem today absolutely grotesque. They wore fashionable Tam-o-Shanter hats like dinner plates on the sides of their heads and were weighed down with bouquets the size of 6-month-old babies, made of gigantic dahlias. Dorothy was told by my father at the wedding that, pretty as his sisters were, no bridesmaid compared with her.

A year later on 18th March, 1933, the Little Bugger walked proudly up the aisle of St Nicholas, Hintlesham, with Dorothy, to give her away, and my father was walking on air down the aisle again with her on his arm. He did not know two people could be so happy. Both of them were head over heels in love. All his family came over from Dublin, and his brother Eric was best man. This time the bridesmaids were my father's two sisters, Phyllis and Ann, and my mother's two sisters, Alice and Betty. Even my father's dog, Stephen the Sealyham, was there in the photographs. It was a splendid family wedding, in the church a short walk from the house. As for the newly-weds, my mother announced, 30 years later, that neither of them would ever forget their honeymoon: the brilliant sunshine and sparkling light of Spain in springtime etched pictures in their memories of snow covered mountains, green valley slopes covered in wild irises, an army of orange trees lining the streets of Seville. He was so pleased to find red wine cheaper than water. He seemed absolutely delighted with Dorothy – so happy, so pretty in all her new clothes, so proud of signing the hotel register 'Dorothy Brittain'.

The honeymoon occupied the interval between leaving Ipswich and going to his new job, orthopaedic surgeon (quite a new speciality at the time, but one he thought he would enjoy) at the Norfolk and Norwich Hospital. He was proud of his new wife, his new job, and their new house in Newmarket Road, Norwich, to which Dorothy now turned her attention. Both of them were thrilled with all the changes she had inspired: she had a real flair for fashion. Aunt Betty told me he loved teasing her, jumping out at her from behind a bush when she was hanging up the washing, seeing her so startled and shocked, and then enjoying the kissing and cuddling to help her recover. My Aunt Ann told me that in the evenings Dorothy, with enormous pleasure, used to sing to him, and he accompanied her soaring soprano on the piano. Dorothy remembers they spent days out on the Broads in friends' boats, making love in the cramped cabin as she sailed among the reeds and windmills under huge skies. To complete their delight, my mother told me that she was 'up the spout' (a phrase I have never heard before or since but it may very well have been a phrase of the day, like 'ripping' and 'topping') on her honeymoon in Spain, and was looking forward to having a baby in only 10 months from the wedding.

I know my mother spent much of the pregnancy perfecting the nursery, knitting a fine shawl for me, and matinee jackets and endless bootees with little satin ribbons threaded through them to be tied in bows. She embroidered a sampler that said:

Thank you for the world so sweet
Thank you for the food we eat
Thank you for the birds that sing
Thank you God for everything.

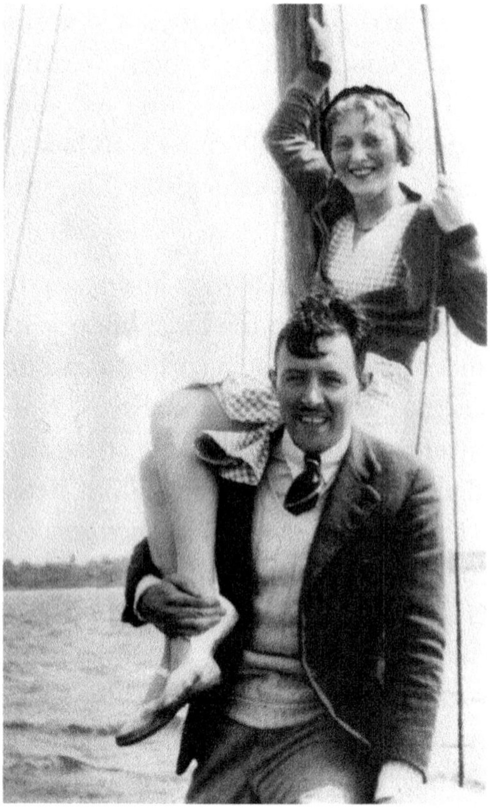

Tommy and Dorothy on the Norfolk Broads in the late Summer of 1933. Dorothy is 6 months pregnant with Alison.

This hung above my cot, where it stayed for years.

This surely was the happiest year of my parents' life. So far as I know, Dorothy's pregnancy was easy, the birth was not hard. It was four days to Christmas, my father was cracking open the champagne. And then it all went unbelievably wrong.

A great silence descended. I only know what happened next from reading my father's notes, in the file in his secretary's room. That was a very long time ago, and they must have been destroyed when my father died: certainly I only read about it once.

For the first few nights after the baby was born, my mother could not sleep. She was terribly excited. Then she became exhausted, and wept. Suddenly, the things she said did not make sense. She said she did not want the baby.

My father could not believe what had happened. Dorothy should have been delighted with her baby. Could this be postnatal depression? He knew that quite a lot of mothers get it, but that they usually recover. He wanted to be reminded about what caused it and what made it better. He asked his colleagues.

They told him it is quite common, something to do with the sudden drop in pregnancy hormones after birth. There seems to be no known reason why one woman gets it and others do not. It may be related to stress, but anyway, after a while they do get better: sometimes in days, or in weeks, or in months. The best treatment is to relieve all stress. Maybe Dorothy should stay in the nearby nursing home, where she could be kept very quiet, and be properly looked after. The monthly nurse could take care of the baby at home. My father visited the nursing home morning and evening, on his way to and from work (she was half way between both home and the hospital). He kept telling her how much he loved her, and waited and hoped for her recovery.

Every day, when no recovery happened, he felt worse. Every hopeful day might be the day she showed a little sign of being better, but it did not happen. My father knew that he would have to get on and do the shaming thing: he would have to tell her family, and his, and in the end, all their friends, his colleagues, the wedding guests, everyone they knew. He had telephoned in triumph and told her mother "It's a girl", and they are arranging to come and see them. Only a day or two later he had to say "No, not just yet, she's a bit upset".

Chapter 23
Suicide or Murder?

When my mother told my father that she did not like her baby she was quite sure about it, and said she knew she must get rid of me, and apparently she tried to do so, quite savagely. She seemed suspicious of everything, and terribly distressed. She heard voices she did not know telling her to do things she did not want to do. She particularly hated my poor father, her husband: she did not want to see him. It was obvious to everyone that my father had a disastrous effect on her.

In only two or three days it seemed worse than postnatal depression. My father really hoped she did not have puerperal psychosis, sometimes called puerperal, or milk, fever – nowadays more usually called postpartum psychosis. His colleagues came to see her again. They agreed on the diagnosis. They said puerperal psychosis was rare, but unfortunately in this state she might even feel driven to kill herself, so for her own safety she would need to be committed to a mental hospital. That must be arranged immediately. This illness was thought to be related to other psychiatric illnesses, and it often ran in families. They asked did he know if anyone in her family had a history of depression, or schizophrenia, had any of them committed suicide, for instance? They suggested he ask them, because it could help in the diagnosis.

So he had to ask them, of course, because the outlook and treatment for the two diseases was different. For postnatal depression, the suggested treatment was to relieve stress. The baby should be taken away, the curtains drawn, the mother left alone and kept quiet, with nothing asked of her. It was thought this would give her the best chance to recover in her own good time. But for puerperal psychosis, which manifested itself in delusional thought, hallucinations and hearing 'voices', it was considered dangerous to leave the patient alone in a darkened room. Someone must stay with her, talk to her, keep her alert, gently point out to her the inconsistencies in her thoughts, not allow her to slip quietly away into a world of permanent madness. That person could not be her husband, because he seemed to upset her most of all.

So he did ask her family, and all hell was let loose.

They said: "How dare you ask questions like that? What do you think you are doing? No, of course there is no madness in the family. What do you mean, suicides? You are going to blame it on her family, are you? As if you thought they had sold you a pup? When you know perfectly well it's your fault entirely. If she is unhappy, you have made her so. If she is mad, you have driven her there. Less than a year ago, she was the happiest woman in the world, with everything to live for. Since she married you she has changed beyond all recognition, and so that has to be something you did to her, doesn't it? You changed her, damaged her, broke her to pieces."

They know more than you think, because, they say, "As a matter of fact, poor Dorothy telephoned home just before the birth, in dreadful distress, saying 'Help me, help me!' because she said she had found you with Thompson, the monthly nurse, in the spare bedroom, having sex".

My father was telling me about asking her family long after I knew that my mother went mad, and I had left my various schools. He was trying to explain to me how it happened. I asked, "And were you, Daddy?"

"No, Darling," he said. "We had been married for less than a year, and I was in love with her."

If I had to bet on my father's answer (and I love betting, but I do also like to win) I would say that he was telling the truth there.

I understand that it is possible, of course, for someone to be 'driven mad' by the circumstances, environment and people surrounding them. But in the case of puerperal psychosis madness seems to come out of a blue sky: a sudden, frightening, horrible change in everything a patient understands and believes. No one or nothing does it to them: it is thought that the big change in hormones after birth may be one thing that can cause it, it just happens.

And, as it happened, when I talked to them many years later in their 90s,

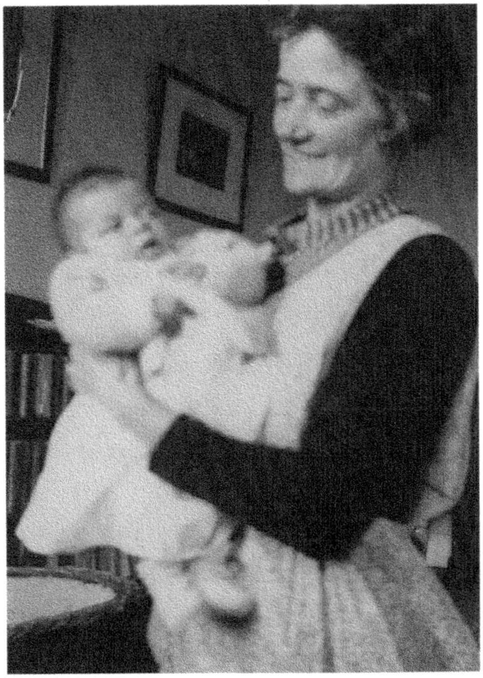

Thompson, the Monthly Nurse, who came to look after Dorothy before the birth, and baby Alison after Dorothy went into hospital.

one of my mother's sisters, Alice, told the story of Dorothy's cries for help. The other sister, Betty, went out of her way to mention it and emphatically deny it.

I asked my father, "But you're a doctor, did you not see before you married her, or at least in the months before I was born, that something was wrong? Were there no signs that you could tell, that she was going to go mad?"

"Yes, I suppose there were, but I did not recognise them. It is easier to see now, looking back. I told you her family said she telephoned shortly before you were born, very upset, and said I was having an affair with a nurse. I couldn't believe it. If it's true she telephoned them, I'm afraid that must have been the beginning of her madness coming on."

"So," I asked, "is there madness in her family?" "No, no special mention of madness. But I did find out they lied to me. Someone who knew the family intimately told me that there was indeed a suicide in the background. It was your mother's grandfather, Thomas James, her father's father, a builder who found himself in financial difficulties."

This member of the family who told my father of the relative's suicide was Angela, the wife of my mother's youngest brother, Ian. Ian was born a long time after the three girls, and Angela was a lot younger than the three sisters. She worked as a nurse at the Norfolk and Norwich Hospital, where my father worked. Years after he died, she told me how hugely popular he was in the hospital; everyone knew of his highly attractive personality and wanted to spend time with him.

Without my asking anything about it, my aunt Betty, aged 92 or 93 at the time, told me about her grandfather who had promised the three sisters that

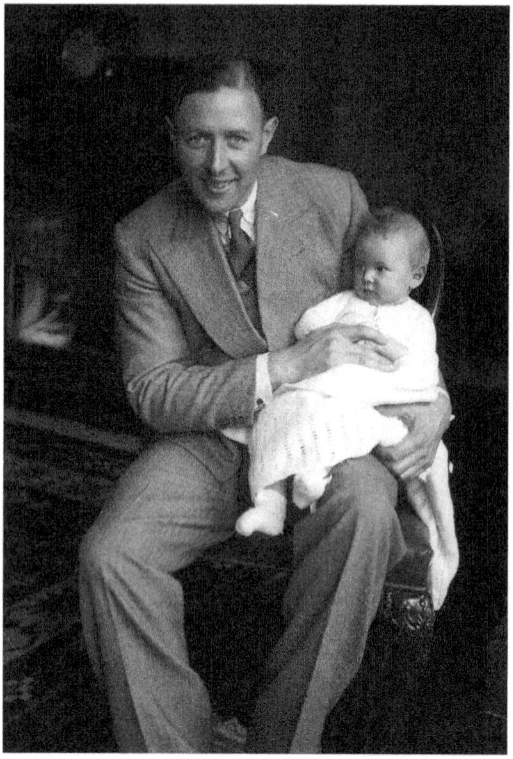

Tommy with Alison on his knee, 1934. Waiting for Dorothy to recover.

he would take them to the theatre, to see The Student Prince. They were all so much looking forward to it, and Betty remembered being bitterly disappointed that day that they could not go. The reason was that the day before the performance their uncle was found hanged in his workshop.

"I was told he hanged himself", my father said. "I had explained why we needed to know, that it might be a way of helping her, but they were too proud to admit it. It probably wasn't all that important, really. He had reason to be depressed. It was not madness out of a blue sky. But her parents lied to me. They denied it. After that I wanted nothing to do with them."

My Aunt Alice told me, years after my mother had died, about her Cornish grandmother Bessie Curnow who, in giving birth to her only child, cracked her pelvis and became a lifelong invalid. Bessie's Cornish miner husband John James later moved to Ipswich and became a builder, for years successful, then cheated by his partner in business who stole the money. James was diagnosed with terminal diabetes, and extremely depressed about this and his sick wife, he hanged himself in his workshop. Alice says: "He drank a bit too". Bessie and John James' small son Jackie was only 5 feet tall, full grown, and weighed 6 stone 12 lbs. Jackie, always known as 'The Little Bugger' in the family, married first Bella Ingles and they had three daughters (the eldest was my mother Dorothy) and a son. After Bella died and Jackie was 59, he married Mildred, always referred to in the family as 'The Black Slug'. They had no children, but when he died Mildred had him cremated and kept his ashes in a serpentine (Cornish stone) vase so huge he could have stood up in it.

My mother's sister, Alice, told me that my father was most unpopular with Bella, the girls' mother. Bella did not want him to marry her daughter. So much so that to indicate her dislike of this alliance, she chose to wear black velvet for the wedding. Marriage in the teeth of her mother's opposition may have caused dangerous stress levels for Dorothy, but in this she was determined. No arguing, she insisted, Tommy was the man for her.

Betty said that they were so wildly in love, both of them, that they decided that her mother's opposition was to do with it being her first daughter getting married: she would come round. They seemed sure they would be wonderfully happy, felt they were made for each other, that Bella would see that in the end, and be happy about it too. And now there was a baby coming; everyone would be delighted, for sure.

My aunt Alice, next in line to Dorothy, said Bella thought my father was a drunk. They knew he was fond of a drink: it relaxed everyone and livened things up. The sisters thought it was just that he was an Irishman: everyone drank more in Ireland. Actually he liked everybody to have a drink, and he brought it with him if he thought there would not be enough. Alice told me that his future mother-in-law found empty Madeira bottles in the wardrobes of seven bedrooms in her house after one of his visits. And Betty said Bella was not amused to see him using the case he had brought for a skeleton that he was supposed to be studying, for storing empty bottles. Everyone else thought it a scream.

My father knew, because he was told by the girls, that his laughing father-in-law, the Little Bugger, came home after work every evening for his supper, and after supper, every day of his life, walked through the village to the pub and drank eight pints of beer: quite a lot for a little man. His wife controlled the money but he saved half crowns for his drinks in dental 'lily cups' for spitting into, or in the turn-ups of his trousers. It may well have been the loneliness of his mother-in-law's evenings that encouraged her strong antipathy to alcohol and those with a taste for it.

So Bella, his mother-in-law, wore black velvet for her daughter's wedding, and Dorothy insisted that black is flattering and slimming and who would not go for that? It was mid-March, and the velvet was warm: Dorothy wore white lace and her mother wore black velvet. But apparently the younger sisters believed that their mother wore black velvet to show her horror and dislike of Dorothy's marriage to my father. Alice told the family, and told me all those years later, that Bella said to her, as they were going indoors after the wedding, "This will end in suicide or murder". My father remembered he was not told that until after Dorothy got ill.

In the mental hospital Dorothy was sent to, she tried to commit suicide. Then her family asked, "Can we have her back? We want our own specialist to see her. Bring her to us, leave her here, she knows us, we'll love her and take care of her, and get her better".

Horrified by her family's accusations, my father decided that it was worth a try at anything to get her better. Maybe it would work. So Dorothy went home to stay with her family. But then he was told that on the second day after she came home Dorothy found her mother in the garden, knocked her over into the rockery, and attacked her with a stone and a fist. Bella was so badly hurt and shaken that she could not get up, and Penelope the cook had to split them up and help her to her feet. In a weird sort of way, Dorothy knew her enemies. Her mother was against this marriage: her mother got the fist. Dorothy had to go back to hospital the next day.

After that visit, there was never any more communication between my father and his wife's family. He told them they need not offer to care for the baby. It was his baby, and he was keeping her. They were not going to take her away: that bit of Dorothy was his. But he felt desperate. He was not used to things in his life going wrong. My father found he could not think straight.

He once broke his silence and told me that at that time his thoughts tormented him, going round and coming back to the same place. He worried, he looked for hope anywhere, he could not sleep. Drink did not help, it only gave him a knocking head, and wakeful nights. I guess, even though he did not say so, that he must have had a miserable sense of loss, of grief and exhaustion, blackness behind the eyes: he will have found it was a real struggle to go the hospital and see patients, let alone operate. And I can imagine how painful it was for him to find an answer for everyone who asked him, "How is she, how is she?" What could he say? He will have wanted a clear head. He needed to calm down. Surely he ought to sleep, knit up the ravelled sleeve of care: he would have done anything for sleep. Maybe, at least, he hoped he could deal with that. He could write himself a prescription for some sleeping pills, for barbiturates, Nembutal.

As he lay in bed, he took two little yellow capsules, with water, started to read, and almost at once fell asleep. The terrible, revolving thoughts were at bay. He will have woken feeling better able to face the day.

I know now that in those days there were no tranquillisers to help shush my mother's torment. There were no tranquillisers to dull the sharpness of my father's pain. Barbiturates are sedative, they settle you down. These sleeping pills will have helped him to lead a normal life, to go to the hospital, to operate. He asked his sister Ann to come over from Dublin to find a proper Nanny for the baby, now called, at Dorothy's request, Alison Betty after her two angry sisters, Alice and Betty.

My father could do no more than wait, for however long it took, for Dorothy to recover in her own good time.

Chapter 24
Blood from a Stone

What is puerperal psychosis? A vivid description of it, written in 1810 by Thomas Dedman, a male midwife, is full of sympathy and deep understanding of how it affected his patients.

> No object, however beautiful or interesting, gives pleasure to their eye, no music charms their ear, no taste their appetite, no sleep refreshes their wearied limbs or wretched imaginations; nor can they be comforted by the conversation or kindest attention of their friends. With the loss of every sentiment which might at present make life tolerable, they are destitute of hope which might render the future desirable.

I was told by my Aunt Betty, long after my mother died, that their younger brother Ian, who was training to be a doctor, visited my mother in hospital and took her out for a drive. Dorothy suddenly reached out and grabbed the hand-brake, pulling it up so sharply she nearly caused a serious accident. Shaken, Ian drove her straight back to hospital.

Betty said that she also tried to get through to her sister, and took her for a ride on the top floor of a double decker bus, but without warning Dorothy suddenly ran down the stairs and threw herself off the platform while the bus was moving. And back to hospital again.

Alice's daughter, Sally, showed me an old grainy film of Dorothy in hospital with her sister Betty and her father, visiting her. Dorothy holds earrings up to her father's ears, seems quite jokey and appears normal: the others are smiling. I do not know which hospital that was.

After she jumped off the bus, although she was visited in hospital, she never came out again for 28 years.

In its effects, my mother's puerperal psychosis closely resembled schizophrenia. My father would have heard about the one experimental treatment for schizophrenia, being performed in Austria in the early 1930s, called Insulin Shock Therapy. The medical papers describing it gave great hope that for the first time, instead of just keeping patients safe from themselves and from harming others, a real cure for schizophrenia might have been found. The treatment in those days was said to be unpleasant, hard to get, and very expensive. It was given without anaesthesia, and was so dangerous that a few patients died. But it did seem that some patients recovered, though many relapsed. No wonder he felt he needed to discuss whether to get this shock therapy for Dorothy, with someone whose judgement he trusted. Some time before the war started, before he met Pinkie, he decided to go and see his sister Ann and talk to her about it. I doubt if Aunt Ann had any idea what would happen to Dorothy, and I expect my father would have greatly toned it down when he told her.

Aunt Ann told me he described it as: "Not a certain cure. Some patients don't respond, a few do seem to recover completely, and the majority recover briefly and then relapse. But it is now being done in this country, the doctor who is doing it has worked in Austria with the man who invented it, and I cannot see how in all human kindness I cannot try to get this treatment for her, if there is any chance at all that she could be cured."

"So what shall I do?" he asked. "Shall I try to get it? It is still very new, and it can be dangerous. Patients may go too deeply into a coma from which they cannot recover. Nobody knows how it works exactly. But properly administered, it ought to be pretty safe. I might be able to get it for her. Shall I try? Should I?"

Aunt Ann replied, "Why are you asking this question?"

"What do you mean?"

"You have no choice, have you? She is your wife. You know what you must do."

She said to me that she thought that Insulin Shock Therapy was indeed given to Dorothy in about 1938, and that because it was very expensive three young men, Harold Cassell, John Barratt and Duncan Begbie, became lodgers in our house in Newmarket Road, Norwich, to help with the expense.

I would like to know where this treatment was done. I wrote to all the hospitals in Norfolk and Suffolk to see if I could find out. But trying to discover something that happened 75 years ago is not easy. I received a letter in 2008:

'Unfortunately it is not the policy of Norfolk & Waveney Mental Health NHS Foundation Trust to automatically release personal clinical information from Health Records for family tree/family interest purposes. The Trust has a duty to protect confidential information even following death'. After appealing to the Patient Advice and Liaison Services, Norfolk & Waveney finally agreed to tell me they did not have her.

I asked St Andrew's Healthcare, Northampton, the hospital where my mother was when my father died. They stated, 'We cannot tell you any more about your mother than you already know. Our records are very limited. Because we have a policy of not disclosing any information about our patients around this period of time, sadly I am unable to fill in the gaps for you. I am sorry that I cannot give you further information, but records were created in those days not to be disclosed. . .' Helped by Michael Gotelee, solicitor son-in-law of my mother's sister Alice, I gave them a legal push.

'I am afraid we cannot give you a great deal more information as we only hold one brief handwritten input form which states that Mrs Dorothy Brittain was admitted on 12th January 1939, that she was aged 29 years on admission and the diagnosis was Paranoid Schizophrenia' (that is how they described her original diagnosis of puerpual psychosis).

'You mentioned in your first letter that your father arranged for your mother to have insulin treatment. As this is a valuable research method, all instances of insulin treatment are recorded. There is no such record in your mother's case so we can only assume that she did not receive insulin treatment at St Andrew's'.

I asked St Andrew's where Dorothy came from, when she arrived there, five years after she first went mad, in January 1939.

St Andrew's Healthcare, 11th February 2008: 'I have checked your mother's brief record and would advise you that no details have been entered in the 'Referred from' section. However, against the heading 'Admission Source' the name 'Moorcroft' has been recorded. This may refer to Moorcroft House, Hillingdon, Middlesex, which I understand was a mental institution until the late 1940s'.

West London Mental Health NHS Trust is where Moorcroft House was. When I asked them they told me on the telephone that they have had fires that have damaged many of their records. And what is more, they only give out details of patient records after the patient has been dead 100 years. I think they ought to know that by 2069 I will be 136 years old, but this appears to be the point. Eventually they kindly do a big search and have found nothing.

Moorcroft House has become the home of an insurance company, who state in their promotion brochure: 'However, we should warn anyone visiting the premises that Moorcroft was a psychiatric institution for many years. As a result we appear to have a resident ghost, who has been seen as a shadowy figure going up the stairs'. How amusing they find it, having a lunatic ghost. Why is being mad so funny?

Moorcroft House was a private mental institution. But Moorcroft is also the hospital where the doctor in charge was once the great and famous Dr Maudsley, he of the Maudsley Hospital, now attached to the Institute of Psychiatry. So I asked the Institute of Psychiatry. The Institute of Psychiatry knows nothing.

Nearly another year goes by and I am canoeing down the Wye with a large party of friends, and I am sharing my canoe this afternoon with a hysterically excited young springer spaniel, muddy all over, who stands staring out on each edge of the canoe in turn tipping it this way and that, and rushes to and fro climbing over me as if I were a sack of potatoes, a dog whose enthusiasm for life is so attractive I would love to own it. Paddling the boat with me is the dog's owner, a psychiatrist.

"Try the archives of the Royal College of Psychiatrists," he says. "They'll know."

I discovered that the Royal College of Psychiatrists' Archives are only available for people with psychiatric qualifications. All I actually want to know is: did my mother have insulin shock therapy? Did they do this therapy, for instance, at Moorcroft House? Because if they did, maybe that is where she got it, just before she went to Northampton.

A week later, it is a cold dull day in June, and I ought to be gardening really, but I am not encouraged by the dry hard earth and the wind. Fortunately, this is my lucky day. I take our old dog for a walk along the river bank, so he can pretend to hunt rabbits, and I can give myself time to think how to persuade the Royal College to tell me what I want to know, even though I have no psychiatric qualifications.

Three young great crested grebes are watching their parents dive, and rushing to them to beg noisily for the fish in their bills each time they surface. Watching them, I marvel that few parents, of any species, have any idea of what they are letting themselves in for when they have babies.

When we get home, the old dog and I have exercised bodies and calm and orderly minds, and I am now ready to telephone the people who 'will know'.

Luckily for me, the archivist is on holiday, and it is her junior who asks how he can help me. He has not asked me if I am a psychiatrist. Maybe he could find out if insulin shock therapy was performed at Moorcroft House? Oh, no, unfortunately for me Moorcroft House was a private mental institution, and there are no records from them. But he will have another little look if I like, he has thought of something else: can I hold on? I can.

"Are you there? I've got something here that might be good. Chap called Freudenberg, have you heard of him?"

Of course I have not. I am not a psychiatrist. If I say 'Yes' he might ask me some questions I really cannot answer. So I say 'No'.

"Well, I've found a paper by him here. It's titled 'Ten Years' Experience of Insulin Shock Therapy in Schizophrenia'."

"I'd like to read that."

"Well, yes, you would, because when he wrote it, he was the resident physician at Moorcroft House, Hillingdon."

I thank him very much indeed. Oh the excellent, kind, helpful and clever junior archivist. He has told me at last the very thing I want to know. They did do insulin shock therapy at Moorcroft House Hospital, and records suggest that my mother went there. So there is every likelihood that she did get insulin therapy. But so very sadly for her she was not cured.

I have a reader's ticket for the Bodleian, Oxford University's wonderful library. I haven't been there for ages, but I must go and get that paper. What was insulin shock therapy?

Chapter 25
Insulin Shock

Unless the book or paper you want is on the open shelves in the Radcliffe Science Library (part of the Bodleian), which in my experience it just about never is, it takes a day for the good librarians to find it underground in the stacks and bring it up for you. A day after the telephone call to the Royal College, two or three papers on insulin therapy, including Dr Freudenberg's, were waiting for me.

As I started to read these papers, I began to feel sick. Until this moment, I had been on the trail, nose down, tail up, hunting an intriguing scent. But now, I came face to face with the fox, bristling and snarling at me, suddenly all too real. What I read seemed horrible. I wondered how anyone could put their wife whom they loved through this? My medical father must have known perfectly well what he was asking them to do to her, and I think it would have been an appalling dilemma for him, trying to decide if he should.

Thinking about the agony in which he must have made his decision, I could not sit there in the warm hum of the underground reading room and take in these words. They were terrible. I had to take photocopies and bring them home and force myself to read them, a few pages at a time, a few pages a day.

I certainly did not know anything about insulin shock therapy until Aunt Ann told me my father asked her if he should get it for Dorothy. Ann told me the rent paid by the three men who had come to live in our house in Norwich was to help pay for my mother's treatment. I have no other record that she did get this treatment, except for this conversation, and the fact that I know that at this date she had not yet gone to St Andrew's, the hospital that told me she definitely did not have insulin treatment there. So if she did have it, it was during the five years between my birth and her arriving there in 1939. If she was given insulin treatment, she most likely got it at Moorcroft House, Hillingdon.

In the hierarchy of treatments, insulin shock therapy was the last resort. The aim was to get the patient into a coma and bring him or her out of it every weekday for at least six weeks, more often, six months. A doctor and a nurse needed to be in constant attendance throughout the treatment.

As I read about it, I imagined what it must have been like for my little mother, the woman my husband Anthony later described as my 'chirpy bird with a broken wing'.

She would have been woken early in the morning, before breakfast, at 6 a.m., dressed in a short-sleeved shirt and long drawers that could be easily washed after they were soiled, and that would keep her decent if she writhed and struggled. The nurse would pull up the side rails on her bed. My mother would have known what was going to happen to her: she must have been wracked with fear. The nurse wheeled in a trolley with a monstrous array of equipment and drugs on it for helping the patient to recover, in case the coma went too deep (it included a mouth gag for use in the event of a fit: a dog's small rubber bone was said to be useful).

To a modern doctor now all this stuff will seem very old-fashioned, although then it appears to have been thought essential. It was said that it also proved to psychiatrists that now they had a proper 'medical' treatment to perform, instead of just 'talking therapies', and that helped them to hold their heads high in the hierarchy of the medical profession.

The nurse would have given the patient an injection of insulin, in either the shoulder or buttock, which were used in rotation. The doctor would have decided on the dosage the day before.

After somewhere between three and five hours of 'treatment', including about 30 to 60 minutes of coma at the end, according to the doctor's prescription, the patient would have been suddenly brought back to consciousness with a large dose of sugar, or glucose. 'The means of nasal interruption are placed on a small portable tray. The nasal tubes selected should be stiff and of fine bore, and should be discarded when they get soft from repeated boiling. The container of warm sugared tea (six and a half ounces of sugar to the pint) is also on this tray'.

If the coma remained deep or other signs of danger were present, the time to interruption might need to have been shortened.

I wondered how did they ever contrive insulin shock therapy? Looking back through the earliest papers, here is Dr Manfred Sakel, a young psychiatrist working in a private addiction sanatorium in Berlin in 1927. One of his patients was a famous actress addicted to morphine. She was also a diabetic. Administering insulin to control her diabetes, Dr Sakel accidentally gave her an overdose. The shock put her into a mild insulin coma. Both the doctor and his patient were surprised to find, when she regained consciousness, that she no longer craved opium.

When Dr Sakel wrote up his findings he was jeered at and mocked by the medical profession, who could not accept such cures that appeared to have no reason to them. So he returned to his alma mater, the University Clinic in Vienna, where he was put in charge of psychotic patients. Still believing in the curative power of insulin, he tried these schizophrenics on his 'Insulin Shock Therapy' too. In many cases he believed he got very good results.

Hospitals were full of schizophrenics: like my mother, they were agitated, withdrawn, hallucinating, hearing voices, suspicious, feeling threatened and sometimes terrified. There was nothing that could be done for them. Here at last was hope. Here was a 'treatment'. No one knew the mechanism by which it effected a 'cure', if indeed it did do so.

What could go wrong? Epileptic fits, respiratory problems, dehydration, heart failure, very occasionally death.

To be effective it was thought necessary to produce a coma five or six days a week for up to six months. Apart from the above dangers, the worst thing was the way it worked, and the long-term effect. Insulin drives sugar from the blood and stores it in the liver, and this starves the brain of glucose. Starving the brain of glucose causes brain damage. Repeated comas cause repeated brain damage.

A dark shadow fell over me as I read Dr Freudenberg's paper. He states that 'Patients with a hereditary taint often do well with insulin'. He means that schizophrenia can be inherited, it does run in families. How lucky that my mother's 'taint' seems not to have been passed to me, nor my children, although I am greatly reassured to be told that it will be so dilute by the time we get to my grandchildren, all now in their 20s, that they will be at no more risk than any normal person.

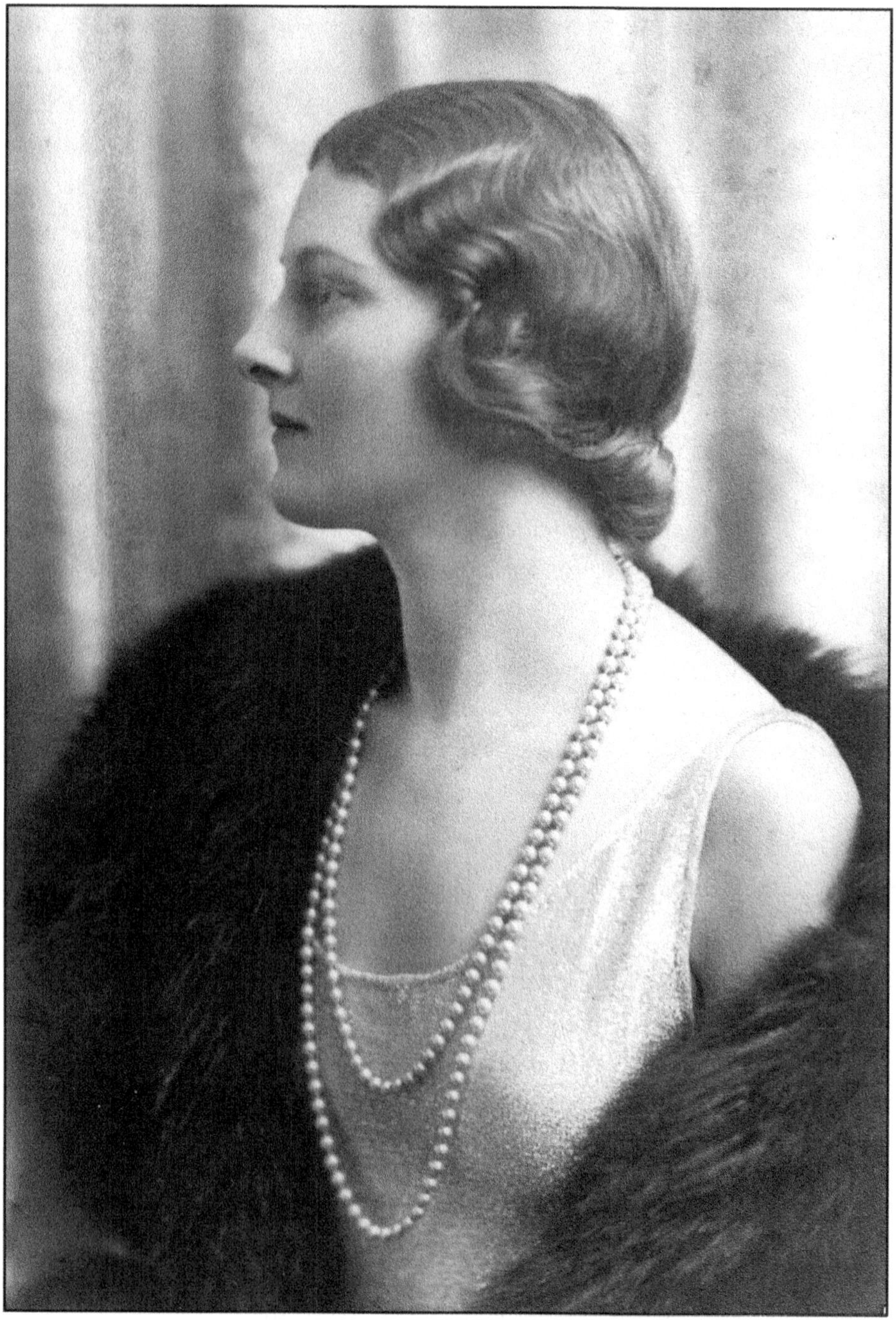

Dorothy as she was when she first met Tommy, in her late teens, circa 1930. Her family agreed that Dorothy was the most talented, liveliest and loveliest of the three sisters.

Dr Freudenberg wrote: 'The production of comas is essential for good results. They should be of sufficient depth, must be clearly defined, and a certain number of them should be administered. The insulin dose should be increased if comas are too light. A total of about 50 comas should be aimed at. . . our own experience shows that the quality of the results is definitely better when more than 30 comas have been given'.

Dr Freudenberg's paper says that in his private hospital he only treated 112 patients in 10 years. In some of the larger hospitals, special wards containing up to 22 beds were set aside for the treatment.

He also recommended electroconvulsive therapy, writing: 'It has also been our practice to use ECT in combination with insulin. . . Many workers combine insulin therapy with convulsants. Most agree that convulsive treatment in schizophrenia increases the number of remissions, and also improves their quality'. Describing the treatment he states, 'If no results appeared with insulin alone after 20 comas, convulsions were added'.

If my Aunt Ann was right, and my mother was given insulin therapy, it does seem likely that she will have received both insulin and convulsion therapy. Electroconvulsive therapy can cause serious memory loss, and brain damage. My father may not have told his sister (my Aunt Ann), but he will have been perfectly well aware of the way this treatment caused brain damage, and no doubt dreaded it.

It was found that as they emerged from a coma, patients became more accessible and open to psychotherapy, their confusions and delusions gone, and they related more readily and warmly to the staff. Although these good results mostly did not last, it was thought that each time the treatment was done the patients stayed well a little longer, and it was hoped that in the end they would completely recover.

But all this huge effort at 'medical treatment' came to nothing. After ten years of giving it, Dr Freudenberg still believed in it, and claimed many recoveries due to it. But he gave a lecture at the end of 1946, after the war was over, and there were questioners in the room where he spoke who plainly did not believe insulin therapy did any good. It was no longer given in England by 1950 (although occasionally in Manchester during the next ten years and there were still reports of it in Russia and China). In the end a randomised trial was undertaken, and the results showed that insulin shock therapy was no more effective than doing nothing. All that cruel effort: for nothing.

Joanna Moncrief, Senior Lecturer at University College London, writes in 2002: 'Insulin coma therapy was always regarded as a specific treatment for schizophrenia. It had a very high mortality rate. It may have had a tranquilising effect on patients by inducing brain damage through the prolonged deprivation of the brain cells of glucose. It was also a very dramatic procedure, with patients being put into this long coma, and then re-awoken quite suddenly by the injection of glucose. A Senior House Officer in Psychiatry in the 1950s suggested that its effect was actually a placebo effect, and a result of the drama of the whole procedure. A randomised trial was then conducted from which it was concluded that insulin coma therapy was not effective. It did not work'.

So, if insulin coma therapy really did not cure, how could Dr Freudenberg have continued giving it for ten years? He writes lucidly, and shows great concern for his patients. It is known that he was admired by his patients and is remembered as a humane doctor, a kind and concerned person. How did he, and all the others who worked for him, believe in the treatment?

Prolonged comas are described as 'the psychiatric equivalent of cardiac arrest, and during them the insulin ward acted like an emergency unit, where the primary motive was keeping the patient alive. Especially tight bonds formed among staff members, as a by-product of the cooperation and collective risk-taking demanded by the treatment. There was a camaraderie and optimism that set the ward apart from the rest of the hospital'. When patients recovered from their coma at the same time 'there was an opportunity for group therapy. They sat and talked together about their experiences, especially that of 'struggling to come back to life, really, from death's door in the coma''. In such a small hospital I am afraid that my mother probably came round all alone, and may have had no chance to sit and discuss her experiences with another patient.

Even though we now know it did not work for patients, the aftermath of insulin therapy must have seemed like a miracle: 'Insulin coma therapy was an effective therapeutic intervention in the minds of the physicians who had experienced their patients' tremendous recoveries'.

This must have been hugely rewarding for the doctors and nurses: 'From an aloof, withdrawn and suspicious individual, the schizophrenic is momentarily transformed into a warm, friendly, responsive and lucid person whose symptoms are either absent or greatly diminished in intensity'.

It seems most likely that my mother will have received a full course of treatment: both insulin and convulsions. And sadly, she did not recover.

In 1946 Dr Freudenberg declared, 'It is generally agreed now that the response to treatment is largely dependent on the duration of illness. There is a decrease in the quality and quantity of improvement as soon as the duration of illness exceeds one year. Amongst the cases with a duration of illness under one year 80.1 per cent were able to leave. Of patients ill from one to three years 53.6 per cent were fit to return to the community. Where the illness had lasted more than three years only 28.6 per cent could be discharged'. My mother became ill in 1933, was certified insane a week later, and did not arrive at St Andrews Hospital until 1939. It is possible that she had been ill for about five years before her treatment started, and the longer it took between illness and treatment the less likely recovery would be. Perhaps Dr Freudenberg already knew this in 1936, and if so it was good of him to accept my mother as a patient: one less likely to recover than most. As the course was coming to an end and she had not recovered, I think my father and Dr Freudenberg would have had to acknowledge the failure and discuss if there was any other help she could be given. Was there nothing else that could be done?

Chapter 26
The Ice Pick

Perhaps it was then that Dr Freudenberg might have described something else: he has written that 'a considerable number of schizophrenics benefit from its use'. Maybe then he might have mentioned prefrontal leucotomy.

I wondered why my mother left Moorcroft House in Hillingdon and went to St Andrew's Hospital in Northampton. I have never been told why.

Both my mother and Aunt Ann told me that she only came home for just that one night. If she had seemed better, if she came home, and if then she relapsed within hours and became very aggressive, a medical friend suggests that the normal thing, when that failed, would have been to take her back to Moorcroft. Dr Freudenberg would have wanted her back for another try. He believed then that if his patients relapsed he could give them a few more comas and convulsions, and sometimes that settled them.

So why did my father not take her back to Moorcroft House? My mother had one night at home, and it went somehow wrong. She attacked Aunt Ann, believing she was my father's girlfriend, and the next day she was taken to St Andrew's. I guess that is the reason for the 'incomplete' admission form. The box 'Referred from' was not filled in. It appears that Dr Freudenberg did not refer her to St Andrews.

Prefrontal leucotomy (or lobotomy in the United States) was a new treatment recommended in 1938, in particular for aggressive paranoid schizophrenics. Taking just a few minutes to perform, under only a local anaesthetic, it was much quicker and cheaper than insulin coma therapy. It made patients easier to manage. It was also believed useful for treating 'backaches, headaches, youthful defiance, moodiness and homosexuality'. Sometimes after insulin treatment had failed, it was thought that prefrontal leucotomy might be helpful. It was surgical interruption of nerve tracts to and from the frontal lobes to the rest of the brain. It was hoped that by this destruction, the nerves would grow again, this time more normally, giving patients a chance to recover. It was devised by Dr Egas Moniz, who received the Nobel Prize for the procedure in 1949. The chief practitioner of this procedure in the States was Dr Walter Freeman. At first the approach to the brain was made through holes drilled in the top of the skull, but Dr Freeman had an improved method. Taking a common tool for breaking ice that he had found in his kitchen, he inserted it, under local anaesthetic, through the upper eye socket. With a sharp blow from a mallet, this ice pick would perforate skin, subcutaneous tissue, bone and meninges in a single plunge. Dr Freeman would then swing it to sever the frontal lobe. Then he did the same through the other eye socket. This would take no more than a few minutes, with no need to admit the patient to hospital.

RME Sabbatini writes 'The procedure was so ghastly, however, that even seasoned and veteran neurosurgeons and psychiatrists would not stand the sight of it, and sometimes fainted at the 'production line' of lobotomies assembled by Freeman'. Looking at that beautiful picture of my young mother in her pearls, it is hard to imagine someone picking up the sterilized ice pick, gritting their teeth and saying "Let's get on with it".

Although Moniz received his Nobel Prize in 1949, a year later people were finding fault with the procedure. Perhaps the most famous case was that of Rosemary Kennedy, sister of President John and Attorney General Robert, whose father complained about the 23-year-old's 'moodiness'. Apparently it was felt in the family that she showed too much sexual precocity. Dr Freeman himself performed the lobotomy. Rosemary was reduced to an infantile mentality, her verbal skills became an unintelligible babble and she was incontinent. Afterwards, the family did not say how this state had been caused. Her father used to describe her condition as 'the result of mental retardation'.

A close Norfolk friend of mine told me the sad story of her uncle and aunt. When her uncle was diagnosed with schizophrenia after the war her kind unmarried aunt (his sister) looked after him. He became increasingly violent. Believing he was a danger to his sister, the family agreed he should have a leucotomy. After the surgery, although he was no longer aggressive, he became so simple, and lived so only in the present, that Mary Anne told me his sister had to tell him each time separately when to go to the lavatory, when to defecate, when to wipe his bottom, when to pull up his trousers and when to come out.

It was usual after the operation for patients to be dull, apathetic, listless, lethargic, placid, childlike, docile, passive, preoccupied and dependent. They seemed confused, showed disinclination to feed without persuasion or assistance, and they were incontinent.

Dr Freudenberg may have discussed this possible treatment with my father. And surely my father would have wanted to know details: how likely was it that this would cure Dorothy, and if it did not, might this treatment harm her more than just doing nothing and having her kindly cared for from now on?

Dr Freudenberg's records inform that 18 patients who had shown no response to insulin had been treated with leucotomy. Of these, two recovered, and two were discharged as 'social recoveries' (a lesser form of recovery). The rest remained in hospital, five of them 'very much easier to handle'. That would be a 2 in 18 chance of recovery, with 16 out of 18 in a poorer state than if nothing had been done.

These results would not have encouraged my father to entertain the idea of prefrontal leucotomy for his Dorothy. Those are awful odds for making a bet on a horse, let alone on your wife. He may have believed that it was still possible somehow, for her to recover. My father knew some brain damage will have already occurred. Given those results he could only have decided that the least he could do would be to prevent any more damage. He could not allow her brain to be destroyed so greatly, just for the sake of easy management to take away forever her faint chance of getting better. She had had her treatment. It did not work. He must find somewhere where she could be looked after for the rest of her life. St Andrew's Hospital, Northampton, is a private mental hospital where well-known and well-off people were confined. When my mother was there, so too were Gladys Spencer-Churchill, Duchess of Marlborough; James Joyce's daughter Lucia Anna, a professional dancer, briefly lover of Samuel Beckett, diagnosed with schizophrenia by Carl Gustav Jung; and the Hon. Violet Gibson an Anglo-Irish aristocrat famous for having shot at Mussolini (she missed). It may have seemed the best my father could do for his wife. Once there, and certified mad, there was very little likelihood that a patient would come out.

And so, knowing my father, and knowing his forthright and impetuous character, I would guess that the next thing he did is to jump in the car, drive terrifyingly fast to Hillingdon, and take his wife away. He would have known as he drove her home, that as the only possible treatment had not worked, she would have to be transferred to another mental hospital. That night was a confirmation of her mental state: she attacked Aunt Ann.

Dorothy went to St Andrew's the next day. My father must have arranged it. The consultant in charge of St Andrew's, with whom he had fixed it, filled in her admission form by hand, and incompletely, partly because consultants can take short cuts, and partly because Dr Freudenberg evidently played no part in sending her there.

This hypothetical reconstruction of events that I have made seems to fit my father's intemperate character, my mother's terrible illness, and Dr Freudenberg's best efforts to save her. By rushing off and grabbing her and arranging for her to go to St Andrew's, he actually gave my mother eight years of wonderful freedom at the end of her life. He never knew it, of course, he was long dead by then, but I bless him for refusing a leucotomy.

At what cost was that to him? He lost his chance of a happy marriage with Pinkie. His resulting misery led to his disregarding the danger of taking too many uppers and downers, and to a disastrous second marriage.

Chapter 27
The Looking Glass

Once my mother had been committed to a mental hospital, my father threw himself into surgery. He was appointed the first orthopaedic surgeon in Norfolk, and was said to be one of the most dexterous and accomplished operators in his field. He was always delighted with his registrar Richard Howard saying he was 'an excellent carpenter'.

'Tommy Brittain had a terrifyingly attractive personality', wrote Richard, my father's registrar and later his junior colleague. The first time they met, in 1940, my father was 36 and Richard was probably 26: 'He asked me, then a very junior house officer, to play squash with him. Naturally I felt highly honoured, but at the same time imagined that I should win as youth was on my side. How wrong I was. He won easily because I could not keep up the pace'. This was typical: my father made sure he was a winner, not a loser.

Soon after he got his first job at the Norfolk and Norwich Hospital he and his old friend Nobby Clarke went to a lecture in France given by the famous surgeon Jacques Calvé. Calvé spoke of one of the 'impossible' operations on Girdlestone's list on my father's bathroom mirror: how to repair the neck of a femur in a hip joint, if it was broken, or riddled with tuberculosis. 'The man who can fuse the hip on the adductor side will make a great contribution', Calvé stated. This was the operation my father invented for which he received national and international fame. He was greatly encouraged by his friend John Charnley who thought it a very useful operation, although it was eventually superseded by the artificial hip joint. We have so succeeded in conquering tuberculosis now, and in improving replacement hip joints, that although the operation still has its occasional uses, it is today very little performed, although then it was most useful and important.

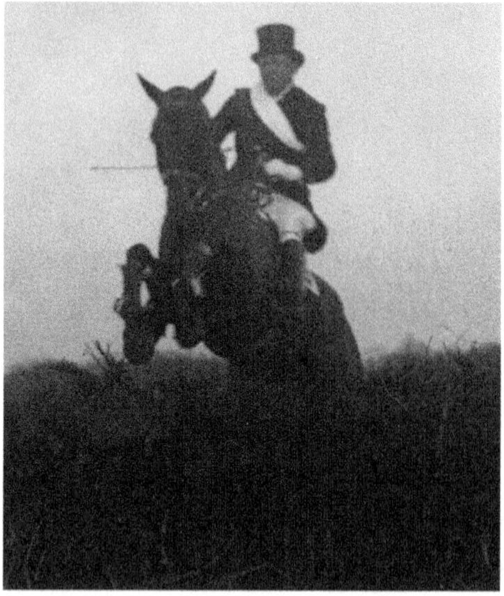

Tommy riding Caravan in the West Norfolk Hunter Trials.

When my mother developed puerperal psychosis, my father would of course have hoped desperately that some treatment would be found that could cure her illness. To begin with, sad and sorry, he waited for her recovery. He organised his life so that he could wait for her.

After a couple of years he took a skiing holiday on his own in Kitzbuhel, Austria, and, typically, left the nursery slopes for the pistes in a few days although he had never skied before. He also decided to go hunting, bought a horse and learnt to ride it. Extremely tough and determined, when that season started, he went out with hounds, and never lagged at the back of the field. He really loved hunting. Hunting was not sexy, and nor was going skiing on his own to Kitzbuhel. For five years he remained hopeful about my mother's eventual recovery. Though he had to have a Nanny for me, all the rest of the staff he employed were male: butler, chef, footman, boots and gardener. His father (my Irish grandfather) told his youngest daughter Ann that she now had a job to do, and she was to come over and run her brother's house for him. She helped to hire Nannies, choose staff, and keep him company. She told me all this, years later, and said he went out very little, and at home played the piano a lot.

I think my father showed great courage and fortitude in waiting for my mother's recovery so long, and in fighting to get her insulin coma treatment when he knew there was only a small chance that it would cure her, because she had been ill for so long. She had been in a mental hospital for at least four years by the time she started the treatment.

One weekend (and I do not remember it, I was probably too young, and kept out of the way), my father brought Dorothy home. It was decided that all excitement must be avoided: they must not sleep together, but she could stay in the room next door. Aunt Ann was staying in the small guest room. During the night my mother got out of bed, then wandered round the house, and found Aunt Ann asleep. She wrenched the heavy looking glass above the fireplace off the wall, woke Ann, and as she sat up, cracked it down on her head. Fortunately she did not do Ann serious harm, but, of course, she was taken off to hospital the next day.

Aunt Ann described it to me years later. "The room had velvet curtains and a kidney shaped dressing table. We were all nervous about the baby (well, little girl actually: you were just about six) with Dorothy at home, but the governess slept with you, in a different part of the house, and understood about your mother's illness. I woke up, hearing a noise, turned on the bedside light and sat up. There was Dorothy running towards me, a huge dark rectangle held above her head. It came whanging down on me. I was hurt, stunned, seeing stars everywhere. I fell back, unable to speak. Then I cried out for Tommy, and nearly got hit again."

As a result of this attack it was obvious that Dorothy must be quickly moved to somewhere that could care for her and keep her safe.

I know that my father decided to send her to what was then thought to be the best mental hospital in England: St Andrew's, in Northampton. She had to stay in a High Observation Unit to keep her safe. It was expensive: St Andrew's Hospital told me in 2010 that then it would have cost today's equivalent of £4,000 a week, payment in advance, to stay in a High Observation Unit there. He would have known or been told of nice buildings, of 100 acres of lovely grounds, with a golf course where patients could play, and its own farm where patients could work if they wanted to; the staff were called 'Companions'. It must have been the best place he could have found for her, and it was probably a faint pleasure to think he could do anything for her at all. The fact that it was very expensive probably confirmed him in the thought that she would be well looked after there although, in fact, at least on some occasions, she was not.

My mother loved him until he died. In December 1943 my father writes to Aunt Ann from Italy: 'I hear quite often from Dorothy – very affectionately, but no change'. How terrible and sad that ten years after my mother went into hospital, she is just as much in love with him as ever she was, and just as insane. I know that he continued to pay for her to stay in St Andrew's long after they were divorced, and he had married again; no matter how high his debts were, he paid her hospital fees until the day he died.

My mother's physical attack on Ann will have ensured that something had to be done quickly. But there may have been another, practical matter that my father wanted to be sure about.

In those early days incurable madness was no grounds for divorce. But three and a half years after my mother first went mad, in 1937, AP Herbert's Matrimonial Causes Act was passed. It allowed for a 'no fault' divorce, and included grounds that the patient had been 'incurably of unsound mind and had been in continuous care and treatment for a period of at least five years' before the petition was presented. That five years must have been almost up. I understood that my father's divorce, under this Act, could be allowed in early 1939.

After that attack it was obvious that my mother must be sent into another mental hospital straight away. She had proved she had not recovered, might not ever recover, and was a danger to others. My father will have been aware of the new humane law allowing divorce after five years between spouses, one of whom was incurably insane. If he considered it at that moment, he will have supposed that by making this move to St Andrew's he would not risk losing his chance, if he ever wanted to, of one day divorcing and remarrying. If, between leaving one hospital and arriving at the other, Dorothy was in his continuous care (my father was a senior medic after all) and since she was insane throughout, he presumably could not see why that should affect a divorce when the five years were up. He must have decided that it would be a good idea, from this point of view, that she was treated formally and medically, and to ensure propriety, she should stay in the spare room. It was cruel for Dorothy, but for my father it may have felt like the only professionally responsible thing to do.

I wrote away for the divorce certificate. There were many difficulties with this request: the certificate could not be found. It took a year before finally I was sent a copy, and it had written on it by hand, 'Reason for Divorce: Respondent was incurably of unsound mind and has been continuously under care and treatment for a period of at least five years immediately preceding the presentation of the petition'.

The date of the divorce is 8th November 1944. Oh, now, look at that. Nineteen-forty-four. My father had to wait ten years not five.

Chapter 28
". . . and not Otherwise"

Dorothy was under continuous care and treatment from 1934 to 1944. Surely that one night at home when she was between mental hospitals could not have made a difference? Sane, witty, polymath Member of Parliament, AP Herbert, had promoted an Act of Parliament that was intended to grant relief for husbands or wives married to those who were diagnosed as insane: to allow them to divorce when there was no hope left, and to make another life for themselves.

I have never been into the Law Library (another part of the Bodleian) except just this once, and it was nearly the end of the summer term and the library was packed with would-be lawyers, mugging up for finals. This was not the right time to be asking help from the librarian, but she saw me from her desk, and smiled, and asked if I wanted help. So I asked about the Act, and could I see it, and I blurted out, in a whisper, exactly what it was I wanted to know. How long did you have to be 'incurable' for? She brought me the Act. She had found a reader's card left in the photocopying machine, and made me a free copy so I could take it home and think about it. It was the most glorious day, green grass, huge white candelabra dancing on the horse chestnuts, playing fields full of buttercups, scabious and daisies, wood pigeons cooing, and I felt truly sorry for the lawyers.

Then the Librarian asked me, "Would you like some of the case-law, which shows how some parts of the Act took effect?" For seven pence, she made me a copy. I had no idea how useful it would be.

Here is a case entitled 'Frank v. Frank – Husband and Wife – Divorce – Insanity – Matrimonial Causes Act 1937', in which the incurably insane wife was moved, under escort, from one hospital to another, arriving the same day and being admitted under an emergency certificate, followed by a sheriff's order the next day. She was still under care and treatment at the hearing of the suit. There was no doubt that she had been insane all that time, and as she had been so for over five years, her husband requested a divorce. Petition dismissed. The technical ground was just three words: '. . . and not otherwise'.

Comments on Section 3 of the Act dictate, 'A person of unsound mind shall be deemed under care and treatment in certain specified circumstances, 'and not otherwise'. . . The safeguards. . . laid down. . . in order to ensure that detention on the ground of lunacy shall only take place in proper cases, are strict, and unless they are strictly observed, the detention of an alleged lunatic is illegal. I cannot doubt that there are many cases of lunatics where, owing to some failure to put the proper machinery strictly into operation, a spouse will be deprived of the benefit of the Matrimonial Causes Act and will be unable, on what very often must be a highly technical ground, to obtain relief'.

Although the judges were cross about it, they decided they had to make their judgement, to quote one, 'on the letter of the law', and in this case they refused divorce. One of them hoped that this part of the law would be changed one day.

Even if Dorothy stayed at home just for one night, during which she was in the care of her medically qualified husband, and even if all the doctors agreed that she had always been, and remained, 'incurably of unsound mind', she would now be out of what the courts considered to be 'continuous care and treatment', she would now be 'otherwise', and the clock must start again.

My poor mother went insane at Christmas 1933 and did not reach St Andrew's until five years later, in January 1939, and the war started in the autumn. She went there about nine months before my father met Pinkie.

Later that year, in the autumn, Pinkie Bulwer, an extraordinarily beautiful young woman, with hazel-green eyes, brown hair, and the softest skin, was sent to see my father. She had broken her collar-bone falling off her horse. He told me "You must never fall in love with a patient: very bad form". But he and Pinkie got engaged a year later, in spring 1940, and he gave her a magnificent engagement ring. Pinkie would have known about my mother: my father would have told her, of course, and anyway, my presence would have needed explanation. And then war came, and he volunteered to fight because he thought he should. He could have had a 'reserved occupation' and stayed in Norwich being an orthopaedic surgeon for the rest of the war, and continued to live with me, and with Pinkie after they married. But at that time he believed decent men fought for their country.

I wanted to know why they did not marry before he went away to the war, as Harold and Ione had done. I went back to Norfolk, to Bolwick, to try to find out. There I found delightful Mark Wathen, Uncle Walter's cousin, who had inherited Bolwick from him. He was charming, hospitable, and in his 90s. I told him my story and asked what he knew. He explained that his family and Pinkie's were related, and living only six miles apart, spent much of their childhood together. "Diana, my sister, who lives in Tasmania now, was especially fond of Pinkie: they went to school at Runton and did a great deal together. Diana's husband was posted to the Middle East, and so she went, with her son George, to live at Bolwick and help look after both it and Uncle Walter. Pinkie was a constant visitor, and eventually came to live there with you". He said he empathised with me and would write and ask his sister Diana what she knew.

So Diana, Mark's sister, was still alive, and living in Tasmania. And Diana was living there at Bolwick with Pinkie and me at the time Pinkie left my father. They were best friends since their childhood. If anyone knew Pinkie's feelings at that time, she did. What would Diana say? After some months I got a letter from Mark declaring, 'I ought to have sent you a line about Diana and Pinkie. Diana wasn't very forthcoming about this. I think all those girls were closeted together at Bolwick, against a background of war and uncertainty, and they just lived from day-to-day in a sort of vague hope for the future'.

Mark continued: 'Diana didn't seem to know whether your father and Pinkie were actually engaged'.

I was sure they were engaged. I had lived with Pinkie at Cawston, Heydon and Bolwick for nearly five years. We lived together, Pinkie, me, Gretchen and Mickey Mouse. Pinkie wore my father's emerald engagement ring. There was the whole page acknowledgement 'To R. D. B.' (Rosemary Dering Bulwer, 'Pinkie') in my father's book 'Architectural Principles of Arthrodesis'. We lived and shared our lives at Bolwick with Diana. And Diana did not seem to know if my father and Pinkie were actually engaged.

Indeed, she was right. Some time then my father must have discovered that he could not yet be divorced, and in that case they could not say publicly that they were engaged. He must have had to tell Pinkie, by letter from Italy, the reason why: that it was to do with the special treatment he had provided to Dorothy. It would mean when the fact of their lack of engagement was known, that Pinkie would not have a right to look after me as a refugee, that some other arrangement for me must be made, and that eventually Pinkie must join up. That was an unbelievably awful letter to have to write, and Pinkie will have been shocked and dismayed on getting it. Three of those extra years had already gone by: there were only two more years to wait, but two more years without seeing each other, even, was a desperately long time to ask for. And no one knew when the war would end, nor whether we would win or lose.

Years later I learned from Mary Anne in Heydon, talking about Bolwick in the war, that Diana had come to stay with Uncle Walter because her husband had been called up, and she wanted the company of her friends Rosemary and Pinkie with her Uncle Walter there at Bolwick. Mary Anne told me that Diana and her husband broke up, and never got together again after the war. I can see how that may have affected Pinkie's decision to leave my father. Diana might have said, "Look, this means you are not even engaged. I'm leaving my husband. Tommy has let you down. You should leave him."

And so Pinkie put away her engagement ring, continued to love and look after me, and the war dragged on and on. She went, from Bolwick, with Diana and Rosemary to dances with airmen on bases: airmen whose aeroplanes they were watching, standing out on the lawn in the early summer dawn, counting them home, coming in on a wing and a prayer. Airmen who the very next night might be shot down and killed.

Pinkie must have been distraught. This was a terribly upsetting and unhappy time in her life. I can feel her anguish and understand her agony. I learned with pleasure, years later, that she remained friends with John Barratt and his wife Baba long after the war ended, and that Duncan Begbie did so too. It would not be surprising if, on hearing Pinkie's sad story, Duncan and his wife kindly asked her out and heard her story with sympathy. Duncan had remained in Norfolk with a reserved occupation: he was a grain merchant, and responsible for ensuring food supplies during the war. I am afraid that by asking her out, he would have earned my father's fury. There goes 'Not fighting in the war', and I fear that 'and other things' might have included that kind invitation from the Begbies. If that was my father's reason for black-balling Duncan in the Norfolk Club it does him no credit.

No wonder my poor father took barbiturates to blot out his thoughts. He really did not want to be reminded of five years of anguish hoping my mother might recover, and five more years of waiting, during which he lost Pinkie. He had done nothing to deserve that awful bad luck.

Chapter 29
"Forget It"

Six years later, in 1949, my father married again. The signs for this were not good. In spite of the madder music and stronger wine of his new lifestyle, a sense of gloom began to hang over our house. Now it was not just the telephone bill that exercised him, but the urgent need for economy drives.

My father paid dire visits to his accountant, after which he simply went to bed till the following morning, and then said nothing to me or to anyone for about a week. I could go out to the cinema with friends and come home to find the house in darkness. Pressing the light switch did not produce light. My father had gone round removing all the light bulbs, to save on electricity bills. He downsized to Bentleys, which he said were better than the Rolls Royce anyway, because they went faster. He bought a new one every year, "because doctors are not allowed to advertise, but if people see me in a new Bentley, they think I am earning a lot, and therefore am a good doctor, so they come to me. Anyway, I am a good doctor".

He always parked it right in front of the front door of the Norfolk and Norwich Hospital, and saw it as more important to advertise thus than to pay for an electric light bulb.

When at last divorced, he decided to marry Sonia (long 'o' as in 'snow'), the youngest of the three Barclay sisters. She was 25 years old, 20 years younger than my father, and only ten years older than me. He always seemed larger than life, hugely attractive, highly amusing, and by Norfolk standards, at 45, a glamorous catch. But he was actually in no state to ask anyone to marry him. He was by now, though he would not have recognised it himself, addicted to barbiturates and amphetamines. However, he was an optimist: he hoped for the best.

The pastime that Sonia most liked doing was acting, and she sometimes got walk-on parts in amateur productions of Shakespeare plays at the Maddermarket theatre. At least two of my father's other girl friends acted there. When I came to think about it, I supposed he was attracted to actresses.

There were still good things happening in life that kept my father amused. He came home from work one day saying to Sonia, "Your cousin Audrey came to see me today, saying: 'My chest hurts when I cough, Tommy'."

"She actually says 'corf' for cough, 'orf' for off and 'me' for my. So I asked her, "Has it been hurting long?"

"Well yes, it's nearly Easter now, and I think I did the damage on Boxing Day."

"What did you do?"

"I'm afraid I fell off my pony hunting my pack of Sealyhams. I didn't seem to have come to any harm. I got back on, and we had a lovely day. But after that, my chest hurt when I coughed. Otherwise I'm fine. I've been hunting the dogs two days a week as usual from Christmas to Easter, so there can't be much wrong. But now the season's over, I thought I ought to get it checked. My doctor says it's not my lungs: he thinks it might be my ribs I've hurt." Sealyhams, little white terriers like my father's 'Stephen', were fashionable in the 1920s and 1930s. They were extremely keen and good at catching rats.

"So I thought she might have broken a rib, and I sent her off to X-ray."

"Had she?" asked Sonia.

"*Had* she? She had. She's in her 60s, and she's been hunting a pack of Sealyhams two days a week for the last three months with *ten* broken ribs, no less. Either she's incredibly tough and brave, or she comes from the dark ages and cannot feel pain. I'm inclined to believe the latter."

When eventually Audrey died, two of her cousins, one of them Chaplain to the Queen, came to see her and arrange the funeral. They were sitting by her bed, heads down, eyes closed, praying when Cousin Angela heard a rustle. She opened her eyes a little and saw movement in the bed. The praying continued, but now Angela thought that Audrey was not dead, but might be waking up to hear it going on. She said to the Chaplain: "Stop, Alan. Look at that."

He stopped praying, and they both looked, and then saw not one but two black noses followed by the long bodies of Sealyhams come up from under the bedclothes beside their dead mistress. They stood on the pillows, defending her, barking vigorously.

Of course, all three of us, including Sonia, were delighted with this story.

Sonia used to give very full vent to her emotions, in a style I had never seen before. If the bath water was cold she shot out of the house, slamming the front door, leapt into her car and drove furiously down the front drive and up the back one spraying large amounts of gravel onto the lawns. She did this if she couldn't find her bra, or if she burnt the soup, or if nobody said how pretty her newly dyed red gold hair was. After two years, all the interior doors of the house hung loose on their hinges, the handles came off in your hand, Sonia's car needed constant repairs, and Brister the gardener was cross about the damage to the lawnmower caused by having so many stones sprayed up onto his lawns.

I resented Sonia having her new hairstyle done with a centre parting, just as my mother's hair in the photograph that once stood on my father's consulting room desk. Even though I had never seen my mother, I knew I did not want Sonia trying to be just like her.

When Aunt Ann next came to stay with us, I asked her if she could remember my mother.

"What was she like? Describe her to me, please."

"Your mother was really a very special person: quite outstanding. She was witty and such fun. She had a truly remarkable singing voice. Her hair was naturally the colour of ripe corn. She was so extraordinarily beautiful that when she came into any room, everything stopped. She was always the centre of attention."

About six months after my father and Sonia were married, I got a letter from Mary Wilson ('Willie'), my father's secretary, who had left I thought in a huff, just before he married Sonia. Willie had been a most wonderful secretary. Hugely intelligent, highly capable, she had been with us before the war, and came back afterwards. She lived in the house, I knew they slept together, she was the only girlfriend I did not call 'Aunt'. She was responsible for everything he wrote, in

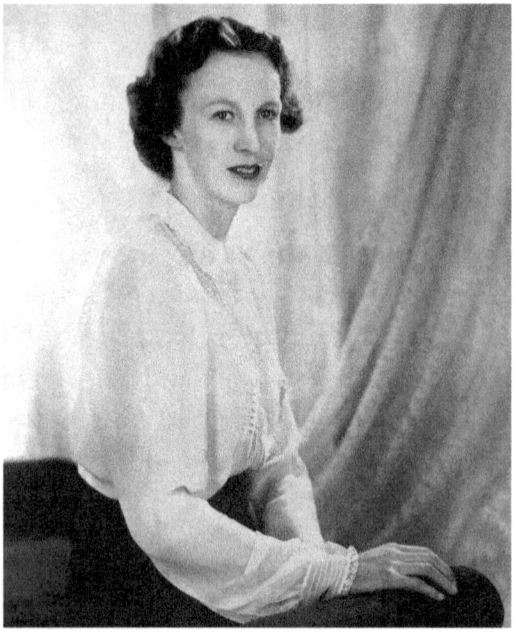

Sonia Barclay, Tommy's second wife, 20 years younger than him. She was Alison's step-mother, only 10 years older than her. This photograph (by Baron) appeared on the front cover of The Tatler and Bystander, (May 17, 1950). © Illustrated London News/Mary Evans Picture Library

particular for the much admired lectures he gave in America. It was her room I was playing in when I found the file with all the details about my mother.

Paper-clipped to the letter was a little photograph of Willie, showing her back and her long black hair, and over her shoulder she held a very small baby. The letter said she was extremely fond of her newborn daughter. I was so surprised I called my father and showed it to him. He read it, stared at me, and then tore it up into pieces smaller than a postage stamp. "Forget it," he said. "Forget it now, and forget it for ever".

I cannot forget it. Surely it must mean that somewhere in this world I have a half-sister, and I know nothing about her, not even her name. I greatly hope she has a long and happy life. When, two years later, Sonia had a daughter, I realised that now, like my mother, and like Sonia, I was one of three sisters (well, in our case, half-sisters) and we were to have very different upbringing and life prospects. I remembered Orwell's famous 'more equal' saying in Animal Farm (the book my father recommended to me after being enraged by my enthusiasm for communism) and thought, 'Some daughters are more equal than others'.

The Barclays endowed Sonia with an enormous sum of money, tied up in a trust that the newly-weds spent great efforts trying to break. They were able to get at it when after two years their baby daughter was born. They called her Léonie (long 'o' again: pronounced 'Leeonie'). The trust money was spent on making the six large Georgian rooms on the top floor into a great apartment for Léonie. She had a day nursery, a night nursery, a bathroom, a kitchen, and the Nanny had a bedroom and a sitting room. It was also spent on a ring with a very large ruby in it, a mink coat from Worth in Paris, and a month's holiday in the Caribbean (without the baby). I asked if they saw where the bookies go for Christmas, but apparently not. Sonia got almost everything she wanted, but she was not really satisfied: it never seemed enough. My father bought her a nice-looking horse called 'Roger' and all the expensive gear from Huntsman, Lock and Lobb to wear out hunting. She had to go up to London many times for fittings. It all looked splendid but it turned out she was frightened and did not want to hunt.

Sonia did have a generous clothes allowance from her parents. She appeared incapable of keeping any kind of account, and at Christmas there was always an explosive row because she had spent twice as much as she possessed. Her annual debts of well over a thousand pounds in those days (say, maybe £100,000 now) had to be paid by my father, who was of course himself seriously overspent. While these rows were going on loudly all over the house, Brister was fixing big cardboard letters covered in ugly variegated holly, to the beautiful banisters. They said, crudely, as they climbed the stairs, 'MERRY XMAS!'.

Sonia had difficulty reading; my father could not stop. He belonged to a postal library, which sent him about ten books a week, and he read one or two every night in bed. He read to distract himself: "I do not want to be alone with my thoughts," he said.

When Léonie (my official, acknowledged, younger half-sister) was born, Sonia's father Evelyn Barclay came out to Witton on his motorbike, walked up the lovely curved staircase in his brown leathers, goggles dangling round his neck, shouting "Where is it, where is it?" and burst into Sonia's room. He pushed past the monthly nurse, walked up to the cradle, peered in, and said "All bloody babies look alike to me", and repeated this mantra louder and louder as he went down the stairs again and out to his bike. If this was meant to be a kindly paternal visit on his part, it did not help. Sonia cried.

By the time the baby arrived, my father had had about enough of young love. He, who could make any woman fall at his feet, and could make his patients get up and walk if he told them to, was unable to handle Sonia's tempers.

Ever since he had fallen off O'Hara at that point-to-point, he had complained that his neck hurt. It was arthritic. He could not get to sleep. When I was four, and he read me Shadrach, Meshack and Abednego, long before the point-to-point, he had taken barbiturates to go to sleep. That is what those uncomfortable yellow capsules in his bed were: Nembutal. Now he did not just need 'Nembies' (about a dozen of them at a time, say, six times a normal dose), he needed a few 'Blue Bombers' as well. 'Blue Bombers' were sodium amytal, another barbiturate. After seeing his accountant he wanted to be unconscious, so he went to bed and took a handful of barbiturates. After Sonia went screaming down the drive he also wanted oblivion, and did the same thing.

He said barbiturates had a wonderful effect. There you were, your accountant had given a terrible warning, or Sonia was cutting up rough, you took a handful of those things and moments later a black curtain came down and you knew nothing, had no dreams, until you woke up. Sometimes, if he had taken a lot, he had difficulty waking up.

He needed uppers, as well as downers. So in the mornings he took 'Dexies': amphetamines. I have seen him handing out these little yellow pills, Dexedrine, to all the guests at a dinner party, saying: "Jockeys take these to keep their weight down, you know. Try some. They make you feel good, take away your appetite, and help you lose weight. They make you thin, and pep you up."

And because they admired and trusted him, everyone tried some.

One or two 'Dexies' every now and then seemed to do no harm. But Sonia hated the taste of alcohol. My father said: "You've got to be in good form, going out to dinner. Have a big gin and orange."

"Gin and orange makes me feel sick. I don't want any."

"Well you need something. Here, try a couple of 'Dexies'. They'll put you in very good form even before you get there."

So she took them, and became addicted to them, and they ruined her life.

At about this time, my father was Evelyn Barclay's favourite son-in-law. He used to drive over to Colney and together they raided Evelyn's excellent cellar for wine that had been laid down years before on the advice of a wise wine-merchant. They sat together on the broken sofa in Evelyn's smelly room drinking it, and gossiping and laughing and joking together. My father became Evelyn's confidant.

One day Evelyn, sounding very upset, asked my father on the telephone to come over as soon as he could. He confessed that he was having awful trouble with a former footman who had worked for him. The footman had lived in a cottage in the garden, and one summer his seven-year-old niece had come to stay for the holidays in the cottage. The footman was now accusing Evelyn of 'interfering' with his niece.

"He is demanding a huge sum of money to say nothing about it, not to tell the police, and go to court and so on. Appalling."

"That's bloody well blackmail: you can have him for that."

"It is blackmail all right."

"Well, that's a crime. You go to the police and tell them, and see how he likes it."

"I can't do that. I've thought of everything. I can't do it."

"You can't? Why not? Oh my God! Jesus Christ, Evelyn, it's true? You and this little girl, what was she called?"

"We had such a happy time. We went everywhere together. I took her out for drives, and to the theatre, and I think she and I got on very well. I believe she was fond of me." Evelyn was in tears.

"You're going to have to have to pay up then, aren't you? And if you do, how do you know the bugger will stop at that, and not keep asking for more? As far as I can see there's no other way out, but you really must make sure he's properly screwed down, and can't keep on demanding more."

So they arranged a meeting with Evelyn's financial adviser, who was a top man at the bank, and a solicitor, and I was never told what happened next. But it is interesting that long after Evelyn's death, to the considerable puzzlement of Norfolk society, we heard that Colney Hall 'had been bought by a former footman'. Was that the deal, I wonder? And perhaps it was Evelyn's final punishment for not keeping his dogs under control? I shall never know.

Sonia was at first enraptured with the baby, thank goodness, and for a while she seemed more confident and happy. Before they were married, however, my father and I had fun dancing sometimes. The Charleston, that heels-kicking-up, arms flying, toes-turned-in dance of the 1920s came back in fashion, and because we practised it for fun at school, I could do it. It is great fun, a bit daft, very silly really, but not what you would call a sexy dance. My father was a very good dancer, light on his feet and with perfect timing. He and I could give a bravura performance of the Charleston together at hunt balls, and he of course knew some rude words to it, about a butler who kept propositioning his mistress (and there followed a list of his improper suggestions): "But she said, I'd rather Charleston, Charleston, Charleston. I'd rather. . .". We had to stop dancing.

Sonia did not know it, and did not want us to do it. She did arrange, however, that I was to eat my dinner on a tray in my bedroom and not with them. Although I lived in the same house with him, I almost never saw my father, and was almost never alone with him. I found this disconcerting. So now where was my old friend and confidant? Where was my companion, my fellow horseman, my bookie, my playing-card and dance partner, my duet singer; where now were the rude jokes, all the naughty gossip? Not for me any more.

My father said, "I'm for an easy life. For *God's sake*, don't rile her." But it didn't take much to do it.

I wrote in my diary how horrible Sonia made life at home, and how awful were their rows, and she found the diary under my pillow and read it.

I heard the row, though I did not know what it was about. My father called me, told me what the trouble was, and with a glass of water in one hand, and a handful of barbiturates in the other, said: "I want you always to remember what I am going to tell you now. It is this: never, ever, put on paper what you do not want read out in front of the whole world."

And he swallowed the pills. I have not forgotten it.

I knew we were after the easy life, so, although I knew, and quite enjoyed knowing, I did not tell Sonia which of the women coming to their dinner parties had been his girlfriends. But Sonia had very clear sensitivities, and she often picked it up. Many times, correct in her guess, she asked me, "Was Aunt

Somebody one of his girlfriends?" I always replied, "I don't know" which failed to satisfy her, and when my father came home from the hospital, she flew at him, yelling accusations. The ensuing dinner party was a great frost, and my father got so drunk that his speech was slurred, and everyone was embarrassed.

When money was tight, we had to do without the butler-cum-chauffeur and the housemaid, and after the Oliver Cromwells left, Sonia employed a manservant with a lisp and a stutter, called Spooner. Spooner was not very bright. He was like Epaminondas, if he had been told to do something one way, that was the way he did everything. He had been told to use a serrated-edged knife for slicing tomatoes, so, that was the only knife to use. He used it to scrape the candle wax off the mahogany dining table which meant the table had to go away and be stripped down and French polished again. But he was sweet, and affectionate, and really pleased to be living with us, and always trying to help.

Somehow in his humility he managed not to rile Sonia, and she was good to him. One Thursday afternoon, his half-day off, he went out and did not return. The next day Sonia, upset and worried, went off to Norwich to report him missing to the police. She was told that he had been picked up on the quay at Lowestoft watching the boats come in, and trying to solicit sailors for sex. In those days, shockingly, homosexuality was a crime. He was now in Norwich prison, awaiting trial. She insisted on seeing the Chief of Police there and then, and ordered him to give back Spooner at once. She said he was very useful, she couldn't do without him, and (to my mind quite rightly) she couldn't care less what he did on his day off. Poor Spooner got three years in gaol. Sonia visited him every month throughout the time. She told him he could come straight back as soon as he was let out.

My father's reaction was completely different. He said Spooner certainly was not coming back. "Had I known Spooner was a poof I would have sacked him. I don't want queers living in the same house as me." His breakfast tray had to be put down on the floor outside his bedroom door, and he collected it himself. He announced that Spooner was to knock three times and go back downstairs at once. Playing it up for all it was worth and hoping to get a rise out of Sonia and me, he hissed "You keep that sod away from me". He certainly was not coming back.

But Spooner did come back, and stayed with us till the end. He was a small, anxious, balding, middle-aged man with thick-rimmed spectacles, a lisp and a stutter, and my six foot father seemed absolutely terrified of him.

Spooner's bedroom was in the old servants' hall near the kitchen on the ground floor. He asked if he could sleep with the dog, Sonia's slobbering black Labrador, Pluto, and Sonia said he could and I was absolutely never to mention it to my father. We had a real farce one Christmas when Spooner asked if his friend Nigel could come and stay. He said Nigel would be really helpful in the kitchen, and there was no need for another bed. I hated to think what would happen if my father discovered Spooner under his roof in the one bed with Pluto and Nigel. Nigel was most helpful, but we had to keep smuggling him into the larder or the boiler room to prevent him being found. I admired Sonia for her pluck and determination, and her unusual good sense. Not long after Spooner came out of prison, to Sonia's and my great relief, the law changed and same sex relationships between consenting adults became no longer crimes.

One Thursday evening, the usual night for dinner parties, Sonia called me to help her half an hour before the guests arrived. She and I worked together now, much more in the face of a common challenge. My father was lying splay-legged at the foot of the stairs, in the hall, through which the guests were to come. He was breathing very heavily, and had peed himself. We took him under his arms, his head hanging backwards, and dragged his almost unbearably heavy form to the library. I was terrified his damaged neck could not stand the strain. We left him on the floor. He looked grey and his husky breathing sounded like an old Pekinese asleep. Sonia locked the door.

I went and got the bowl, cloths and other items we used for clearing up incontinent old Gretchen's mess and cleaned the carpet. Sonia said he had been like this a few times before, but this was the first time I had seen it, because I had been away at school. I did at least get breaks from these horrors at Ashridge, my finishing school, while Sonia had to cope day in and day out. She turned out to be much tougher and more courageous and managed much better than I would have believed she could. That night, when the guests arrived, she told everyone he had been called out on an urgent case, which, when he came to at midnight, he found extremely funny because, as he said, orthopaedic surgeons never have urgent cases.

Sonia told me she was terrified he would make some mistake in theatre, setting off like a zombie for the Norfolk and Norwich to do a morning's list. One morning a week he operated on private patients at Grove House Nursing Home, and the matron there, who had known him for years and years, nowadays took him straight to her office as soon as he arrived, and sat him down and made him drink a mug of black coffee before he started operating, and she organised a delay of one hour before the first patient was anaesthetised. Even today, there are exhausted junior hospital doctors, on call at the weekend, awake and coping with everything for two nights and three days, who claim that though they have athletes' feet, tunnel vision and sharp tempers, the last thing that goes is their medical judgement. It is too important: they cannot afford to get that wrong. In this way my father said not to worry, he could do lecture tours in America, he could operate perfectly well, even if he sometimes seemed a bit woozy.

Chapter 30
The Gimlet

I walked into the drawing room one chill winter afternoon to practice the piano. The crimson leaves of the Virginia creeper were long fallen, but their stalks hung on, and a biting wind from the Arctic was rippling them up and down the house. This wind meant no one any kindnesses, and it blew the smoke from the big log fire back down the chimney and into the room.

My father was sitting in an acrid blue haze in his armchair in front of the blazing fire.

"What do you think this is?" he said. "Watch."

He had what looked like a whisky and soda in his hand. He poured a small bottle of little orange pills into it, and they started fizzing.

"See?" he said as he began drinking it. "A bottle of Junior Aspirin in a double whisky. The very thing. I shall go to sleep now. People think I take too many barbiturates, you know, that I'm addicted to them. But I'm not. Not at all.

They don't understand. I don't need 'Nembies' or 'Blue Bombers'. I just don't want to be here. I want to go to sleep."

I left him, undisturbed, to his sleep. But I felt hot between the ears, and very frightened, and could not settle to anything. I went out to the stables and shoved a pitchfork hard into the hay to get a strong hold of it, and took it out to the horses in the meadow, thinking all the time: ever since I can remember, he has made a fuss about going to sleep. The monstrous array of bedclothes he required, the necessary number of dogs in bed with him, wandering to the kitchen several times in the night to make himself sandwiches, and reading voraciously for hours. He never could bear to be alone with his thoughts.

And ever since I can remember he has taken Nembutal to go to sleep. Wanting to go to sleep is one thing; not wanting to be here quite a terrifying other. As the horses came over softly knuckering down their noses in greeting, wisps of hay flew in the wind and I thought, if you are a doctor and can write yourself a prescription for anything, and you don't want to be here, you can arrange for that to happen. The horses whisked the hay from me even before I had put it in the rack. I watched them happily eating, snatching skeins of it and crunching it up, and I desperately hoped he did not mean what he said.

I am sad to say that his addictions made him do many things he would rather never have done. He took Nembutal to speed up the long boring flights to America for lecture tours, and lying motionless asleep on the plane for six or seven hours at a time gave him deep vein thrombosis from which he nearly died.

A bossy and far too jolly Australian nurse who came to look after him got the sack for saying to him in his bath, "We'll soap ourselves all over, shall we?" A live-in day nurse and a night nurse arrived, but failed to discover that he hid Nembutal among the rocks of the water garden and kept himself topped up by visiting it daily for 'exercise'.

Sonia and I used to hear him searching round the house in his pyjamas at night, opening drawers in the butler's pantry, the door of the grandfather clock or the lid of the grand piano, loudly sniffing to see if he could find where we had hidden his new 'safe' medicine that could not kill him, and that stank horribly, called Paraldehyde.

When he went to be cured at Dundee he put a bottle of 300 sodium amytal on the table by his bed and challenged his doctor to count them. "I'm not addicted to them," he said. "You can leave them there all night and I won't touch them."

Sonia and I were surprised to hear that the doctor had done so. My father, even in this state, could obviously still talk the birds down from the trees. How would the doctor in charge have explained it if it had gone wrong? He had solemnly counted them all out in the morning, found 300, and said: "Well, now I'm afraid there is nothing I can do for you. You claim you are not addicted, and I suppose you have proved it. Before anyone can help you, you have to admit to being addicted. You refuse to, so I think you may as well go home."

He undid his barbiturate capsules and emptied the powder into a Macleans Stomach Powder jar belonging to Aunt Ann when she came to stay, and when she got home to Northern Ireland she took a whole tablespoonful of the powder and nearly died.

When my father had been very ill, in his Paraldehyde period, he had said to me: "I want you to listen to this, and promise me one thing. I have got life insurances, one for your mother and one for you, each for £10,000, but I have a huge overdraft at the bank. If I died, there would be very little cash around." Sonia would have great expenses at that time. "I want you to promise me that if I die, you will immediately give one thousand pounds of that money to her, in cash."

"Oh Daddy, don't die, please don't die", I begged.

"I won't if I can help it", he said.

I promised.

When I came home at half-term things were different. No nurses, all quiet. Sonia in the kitchen, cooking. We could not afford the cook and she had had to go. My father in the library, silent, reading. He had given up sleeping pills, alcohol, everything that nowadays would be called a substance, to misuse. He had done it all by himself, with no help from anyone. He must have had terrible trouble with insomnia, but he just made up his mind to stop it, and stopped. Nothing at all seemed amusing now: he was just withdrawn and quiet. He had nothing to say until one evening he asked me to come and look at the fish with him, his hundreds and thousands of goldfish in the water garden, offspring of the contents of the small jam-jar he had once been given by a surgeon in a Portuguese restaurant. Our water garden had three stone-edged ponds in it, each irregular but about the size of a tennis court, connected by a stream. The fish had multiplied magnificently, but they were a boring brown the first year, and the second year to his great pleasure they all together turned golden.

He turned to me with the saddest face.

"All my life I wanted to be rich and famous, and I was, and it was ashes and dust," he said.

"I've been to see my accountant. I am the last person in the world to be telling you this, but I do really believe, I know it sounds very dull, but I do believe that happiness is living within your income."

That was not the man I knew. Whatever had happened?

"I'm broke," he said. "I've got to sell Witton."

"Oh my God, Daddy. No!"

"I think it may kill me."

I thought so too. He seemed half dead already.

* * *

A few weeks later, I had to answer the telephone in the Hall in my finishing school.

"Hello?"

"This is Robbie. Is that Alison?"

"Who?"

"Robbie. Robbie, your father's secretary."

"Yes."

"I am sorry to tell you your father had a heart attack last night, and he is dead."

"Are you sure?"

"I am very sorry to have to say yes, I am sure."

"No, are you sure it was a heart attack: that he didn't die in a car crash?" I asked. That was what I feared.

"He died at home," Robbie said. "It was nothing to do with a car crash."

"Well thank you for telling me," I said, and put the receiver back on its rest.

What more was there to say? It was not a matter for discussion. It was utterly, utterly final. It was January 1954. He was only 50. I was 20.

The temporary head mistress said I was to stay with friends and not go home, and told me how to get to the funeral. On the way, on the train to Norwich, I saw Noons Barclay sitting in a first class carriage. On an impulse I went in, sat next to her, and told her what I had promised my father. I said, "If you see Sonia before I do, please tell her that". Noons was her always collected self, but she seemed to be in another world, silent, her face pale and drawn. After a bit she said: "Don't worry about that. There isn't any money. He cashed those life insurances just before he died." I said, "I wonder why?" and Noons did not answer. So I said, "Thank you for telling me that", and went back to my carriage. I was not first class. I supposed he must have needed the money very badly, and I felt for his anguish.

At the end of term, the last time I saw him, he seemed so silent and subdued, so unlike himself. He was sad about many things. Old Caravan, long past hunting and going blind now, had spent a last summer with other hunters in the freedom of the marshes before being put down. Gretchen too had lost the use of her hind legs and the vet had come and ended her life at home. Sonia told me they had had no sex for ages. Witton was sold, and they had moved back into a house in Newmarket Road, larger than the original one, but with nothing of the spirit and beauty of Witton. As in the old days, he had his consulting room in the house too. He called it, with disdain, "Living over the shop". I did think then, as he did, that it might kill him.

I do know that he went and visited Nobby Clarke, and Reg Watson-Jones, in the fortnight before he died, and they said they found him very quiet and subdued. He also visited John Charnley, of the 'Charnley hip'. John was the man who had hugely encouraged my father with his arthrodesis of the hip, but had since come to believe that artificial hip joints were possible, with the use of acrylic cement, and if so, a better solution. My father will have been told that, and will not have wanted to hear it. He would have found it very hard to bear that his operation was not the absolutely best, but quite appalling that McKee's might be better. Nobby, Reg and John all got knighthoods, long after my father died, about which he would of course have been delighted, and probably slightly envious.

Sonia told me she had found my father cold in the morning, he had been reading a book. She thought it a great coincidence that the book he had been reading was called 'The Long Goodbye'. He had had a heart attack. A post mortem was required to confirm this. The post mortem was necessary because he had neither complained about his health recently, nor consulted a doctor in the last fortnight. His old friend, Ken Latter, the chief physician at the Norfolk and Norwich Hospital, performed it and pronounced the cause of death: infarcts in his heart, a heart attack. I thought, there, it was a heart attack. At least he did not die in a car crash at the bottom of a hill, he just died: he did not do it.

But I worried. I remembered his insulin story. I knew, because my father had told me, that if you die of a heart attack, your life insurance is paid out. If you commit suicide, you get nothing. If you cash your life insurance before you commit suicide, at least you get the paid up value, at least some money, even if very little (in my mother's and my case, about £400). Even if he knew it was most likely that Ken Latter would do the post mortem, could he be certain Ken would cover for him? He cashed the life insurance four days before he died. He was, as I said, only 50.

At the crematorium, Sonia said: "Darling, I am going to have his ashes scattered over Norwich Staghounds country."

She told me that it seemed such a coincidence that the book he had been reading was called 'The Long Goodbye'. I knew the book. It was by Raymond Chandler, one of his favourite authors. It seemed odd to me, because I knew he had read it when it came out, the year before. I could remember him reading to me with delight, thinking of Grandpa's cruise to South Africa 20 years before, a bit where the hero describes a Gimlet: 'a real Gimlet is half gin and half Rose's Lime Juice, and nothing else'.

A real gimlet is of course something else, too. It is a wonderful little hand tool used for making small holes in things. 'A piece of steel of a semi-cylindrical form, hollow on one side, having a cross handle on one end and a worm or screw at the other'. It is extremely clever: in that once the hole is started, just by turning the gimlet it continues to make and enlarge the hole with no effort. No need to push and shove. The gimlet gets pulled further into the hole as it is turned; pressure is not required once the tip has been drawn in. Start using it to make a hole, and it finishes the job for you. Not a bad description of the way addiction to sleeping pills works.

My father's coffin was in his consulting room, which was full of flowers. On it was a huge pink bouquet from Sonia. I picked up a little round one, a ring of white roses surrounded by dark green leaves, with the message 'With love from Dorothy' and put it on the coffin too, saying to the undertaker "That's from my mother, his first wife, and it goes on the coffin too. Please leave it there". And he did. Aunt Ann said it was probably sent on behalf of my mother by her sister, Alice.

At the funeral party afterwards my father's brother Eric came up to me and said: "I'm going to teach you something Alison. There are times when there is only one thing to do and this is one of them. Drink this," and he offered me a large plain whisky.

"Whisky", I told him, sniffing it. "No, no, I hate the very smell of this stuff. I can't drink it."

Several members of my family on my father's side have overdone it on alcohol. My father's brother Eric normally only drank orange juice, but sometimes he broke free and drank so much whisky in one go that he could not remember anything. He told me once that he woke one morning in a strange bed. He looked out of the window, and saw the jagged outlines of Christmas trees sloping down a hill, blanketed in snow.

"Well now," he thought, "where the Hell am I?"

And he looked round a bit more, and found a strange woman in bed beside him.

"Where are we, and how did we get here?" he asked her.

"We flew here, Love," she said, with a strong Mancunian accent (Eric had taken over the Monarch Laundry in Manchester in order to establish English residency so that he could get divorced. In those days divorce was not allowed in Holy Ireland, but Uncle Eric managed it twice, courtesy of the Monarch). "You wanted us to come to Switzerland, don't you remember?"

It was a complete mystery to Eric: deeply shocking.

Now he was waving a tumbler that looked half full of neat whiskey at me: "Yes you can, go on, do," he said. "Force yourself. Come on, just like medicine, indeed just now it is medicine. Take it in sips, get it down."

Blazing heat roared down my throat, I coughed and spluttered. "More", he said. "And again." He bullied me, "All of it". Ah, now I knew he was my father's brother. But within less than a minute I could hold my head up, breathe out ferocious fumes, and look around me, smile at Eric, and realise that I could no longer feel my legs below the knee. The pain had gone. The tightness was loose.

"How like him," said Eric, "did you know he was horrendously in debt? Everything will have to be sold, and the Barclays will pick up the rest. He hadn't paid for the last four Bentleys. Typical."

"Four?" I asked.

"Yes, four. You know he ordered a new one every year? Well, he hadn't paid for the last four."

I giggled. Indeed, how like him. "Enjoy it while I'm here," he often said. "It won't be when I'm gone." And it was not. He was right.

"Now," said Eric, "Because everything is going to be sold, and I suppose you would like to have a memento of Tommy, I will steal you a couple of books. What do you want?"

I chose rather nice green leather-bound copies of 'The Oxford Book of Verse' and 'The Oxford Book of Modern Verse'. They have gold leaf on the edges of the pages. I could not resist 'The Oxford Book of Quotations', too, well thumbed and with the index pages falling out: a great favourite of his. We took them out of the shelves, went out into the hall and stuffed them into my bag. I am very pleased I have them. Apart from memories, they are just about all I have of the life we lived.

Chapter 31
A Frightful Mess

Cashing those life insurances will have gone nowhere in paying for the last four Bentleys, I thought. And those were nothing. He must have had huge debts; have known he was in grave trouble.

I always assumed that he died beside Sonia in bed. Fifty years after he died, when he would have been a 100 years old, an appreciation of him appeared in *The Journal of Bone and Joint Surgery*. It reported, 'One morning he was found dead in his library chair, without having made any complaint about his health in the preceding weeks. His death was put down to a heart attack'. It was written by his friend and colleague John Crawford Adams.

I went to see John Crawford Adams. Charming and hospitable, in his 90s, he cooked us an excellent lunch and was delighted to talk to me and my husband about my father. He gave a brilliant explanation of the Brittain arthrodesis and of his own improvements to it.

I asked him who had given him information about my father, before he wrote the appreciation. He said, "Nobby Clarke and Reg Watson-Jones". These were my father's two closest friends, the nearest thing to orthopaedic brothers that he had, who he visited in the fortnight before he died. I asked why he wrote, 'His death was put down to a heart attack'. That made it sound rather doubtful. Did he think it possible that my father committed suicide? He replied, "Nothing is certain, but I am afraid it does seem likely".

It was altogether different if he had been sitting in his library chair. And his death being 'put down to a heart attack' is, I am afraid, doctor-speak for 'but we don't really believe it'.

Not in that battered old chair that he had shared, in their time, with Stephen, Panda, Gretchen, Ferdie, and Anna, the armchair in which I had sat in his lap and heard war declared. Down the years, bright and clear as yesterday, I got the message. 'The Long Goodbye' was, of course, his last joke. Or the only way he could have had of letting us know, but no-one else, that his life like this was not worth living, and he preferred to be dead. I am afraid that what seems most likely to be true is that after he had let Sonia go up to bed, and was sitting there reading in the library, he took a massive handful of barbiturates. He would know that, because he had had none for six months, even his usual dose would be enough to kill him. He would have disposed of the bottle before he started. He probably washed them down with a whisky and soda and just had time to rinse out the glass and put it back in the kitchen. He went back to his chair, picked up his farewell book, and the curtain came down. Instant blackness, no dreams, all over.

When my daughter, Jess, became a GP in Norfolk, 45 years after my father's death, she had a delightful patient in Aylsham Hospital (that used to be the Workhouse in which wretched Abraham had been incarcerated). This patient was in a bed in the women's ward, and lots of very smart friends came to visit her, bringing enormous bunches of gladioli that did not fit on her little locker. "Darling", they said, "how awful to be in here with all these people: shouldn't you be in a private room?" "No of course not," she replied. "I love having everyone to talk to, and we all take great interest in and care for each other." Her husband, visiting, said to Jess, "I hear you are Tommy Brittain's granddaughter: is that right?" When Jess replied, "Yes" he went on, "I must tell you a story. After he died Sonia, his wife, said he wanted his ashes scattered over Norwich Staghounds country. Well when we got the ashes it was July. Norwich Staghounds country had wheat or sugar beet growing all over it everywhere. Not country for riding on. But I said 'Oh come on, nothing ever stopped Tommy doing whatever he wanted to do. He would want us to do it. We'll do it in memory of him'. And we did. Made a frightful mess but great fun."

Chapter 32
The Pantomime Cat

After my father's funeral, encouraged to distract herself, Sonia took up amateur acting again at the Maddermarket theatre in Norwich. She fell in love with the leading man, and had his baby less than a year after my father died. Her mother was furious, and arranged for Sonia to rent a cottage miles from anywhere. There she lived with Léonie, and there the baby was born and, as arranged by Noons, immediately taken away by nuns for adoption. When Sonia had to sign the adoption papers six weeks after the birth, she, distraught, refused, and guided by her sound human instinct, went in search of her Maddermarket hero. Together they went to see the nuns, and took back the baby. They married, and had three more girls, so Sonia had five daughters in all. I am sorry that as a result poor Léonie was made to do much of the childcare, and felt very left out of the family.

Unfortunately, Sonia's second marriage was not always happy. She had many different ways of getting hold of the amphetamines that my father had first introduced her to. She begged her doctor for them, she forged prescriptions, she changed her doctors constantly, and she went in and out of hospitals where they tried to wean her off them, but never succeeded.

Her husband, Donald, managed a smart shoe shop in Oxford Street, London. Léonie told me that her stepfather made sexual advances to her. She, wretched Léonie, was really pleased when he walked out one day, and never came back.

Sonia was constantly broke. Noons ended up sending 11 one-pound notes in registered brown envelopes to arrive on Mondays, and on this the family lived. In a Guildford nightclub Sonia met a plumber, who befriended her, and they used to go out on his plumbing jobs together. Then, one year just before Christmas, when she was 46, he left her.

She spent that Christmas with all her daughters, and having had quite a lot to drink, she wept bitterly that she was all alone, that she was losing her looks. Her children found her dead in bed on Boxing Day. She had taken a huge overdose of barbiturates. Léonie insists that it was not intentional suicide: she said Sonia was terrified of dying, and she would have taken those pills by mistake, probably forgetting that she had already had some. It was known that this could be a way that barbiturates killed you, and taking them with a great deal of alcohol could have been enough.

Sonia died without making a will, and the first thing the Barclays did was to find the man who was her legal widower. They sent two limousines full of pin-striped London solicitors down to a repertory theatre in the West Country and told Donald that they would fight and win if he tried to take her money, which he would now legally inherit. At the time he was being the pantomime cat in Dick Whittington, and apparently he simply said that they could keep the money: he hoped it would be of some use to his daughters.

Chapter 33
Out of the Bin

My GP told me, "Yes. This is positive. You are pregnant."

My heart hammered. "Am I really?" I was 28 years old.

"Yes, really. We had better book you into hospital to have it."

"For God's sake, no. Don't do that. I won't have it in hospital."

"Well where, then? There isn't really anywhere else. This is a first baby, and first babies are usually born in hospital."

"Not mine. I wish I hadn't told you I thought I was pregnant. I want to have it at home. Not in hospital. Can you force me to have it in hospital?"

So I explained to the doctor about my mother, and how I thought that just having a baby might send me mad, but having it in an unfamiliar place like a hospital might send me madder quicker. He was sympathetic, and said that if all went well with the pregnancy, and the midwife agreed, I could have it at home.

When I got home, and told my husband Anthony, he said he wanted to telephone his mother at once. She was very nice about it, but I could see that Anthony and I were both very shaken by this news. It was a relief that Anthony was quite sure he did want a baby. He thought it should be born in hospital, and if I was going to have it at home he definitely did not want to be there. He wanted to be out of the house. He said I mustn't scream. I was pleased when the midwife, later, said she had never heard one of her home-birth patients scream.

Anthony was there when I had her at home, and it was easy. I hugged my little warm baby to me in bed, a bit like cuddling Gretchen, though the baby had a quite different, sweet smell. They kept taking her away from me saying I might squash her. She seemed so serene, and plump, and slightly moist, and was to me, utterly beautiful, and I could not imagine squashing her. She had a dimple in the middle of her chin just like Anthony, and the midwife waved her about saying, "We can easily see who her father is, can't we?" But I spent the first night with her in a carry-cot beside me, and I kept waking and peering in to make sure she was real, and thinking 'I haven't gone mad yet. Could it really happen? Maybe I have less than a week with her? Oh God, please not'. I suppose she was about six months old before I believed I had got away with it, luck was with me and this time it was not going to happen.

Fifteen months after the first I had another daughter, also at home. This was a very different baby. This tiny morsel was born with clenched hands, and a furious red face, struggling and roaring with indignation. Very early on she learned a captivating smile. Looking at her, I had shivers down my spine, for here was the past come back to life. Everyone says that newborn babies look a bit like old men. This little girl had in miniature the exact same face as my father, and it seemed, his personality to go with it. As she eyed me up, I could almost hear her singing 'What shall we do with the drunken sailor?', or saying "Stop snivelling, will you?"

Much calmer now, I had time to reflect. I thought, if you had ever had a baby, you know, however mad you were, you surely would remember it. And sometimes wonder what happened to it? And where is it now? My poor mother must have lucid moments, I supposed, when she might like to know she had grandchildren. I wondered if I could find her, now, and if I should.

When my father died I had suggested to my Irish Aunts that I would like to see my mother. When she was committed to a mental hospital the breach between the two sides of the family had been almost complete. Her family's suggestion (not without reason, as they saw it), that he had driven her mad, had forced a wedge between the families: accusation versus pride. He could be totally unforgiving. The only communication had been the very rare formal letter such as I had read in the file from her sister Alice to my father, stating things like 'Dorothy needs a new pair of slippers, size 4'. In the days when my mother went mad, madness was regarded with horror, not pity. It was disgraceful, disgusting, a great social mistake to go mad.

At the time my mother was locked away, her sister, Alice, was already engaged to be married. Alice told me, in her old age, that friends had sympathised with her, saying how sad that now she would have to call the wedding off, and never get married, because of Dorothy's 'condition'. Fortunately, Alice and her fiancé had more sense, went ahead with the wedding, and had a long and happy marriage.

Ever since I found out what had happened to her, I was aware of my father's strong feeling that seeing my mother was definitely something he would rather I did not try to do, and I had never even asked him if I could. He was obviously afraid that both she and I would find the experience distressing, as indeed he would himself, if it meant in any way renewing acquaintance with her side of the family. When my father died, and I was 20 years old, I had suggested to my Irish Aunts that I would like to see my mother and they advised that trying to see her was a bad idea. They said, "No, Darling, don't, you will only upset her". They said they did not know where she was anyway, because when there was no more money to pay for the best mental hospital in the country, her sisters, my other aunts and namesakes, Alice and Betty, had asked to have her moved to a National Health mental hospital near where they lived, in Suffolk. Where, or what it was called, my Irish Aunts did not know.

I telephoned the Ministry of Health and asked for the names and addresses of all the mental hospitals in Suffolk, and sent them each a hand-written postcard, 'Have you got my mother, Mrs Dorothy Brittain?' One wrote back stating, 'Yes, we have her here. Her physical condition is sound, and her mental condition is better than it used to be'. I felt a peculiar hair-raising sensation at the back of my neck, and found myself drawing in long breaths. There suddenly she really was, in the flesh. What could I make of what they told me? She was physically fit, and still mad.

In some anxiety, but with strong support from my husband, I wrote back asking, 'Can I see her?'

When my letter arrived, Dr Cook, doctor in charge of the hospital, took it down the ward to my mother, and told her: "I have a letter from your daughter here, and she would like to come and see you".

She replied, "No thank you. It is too late now. Tell her I don't want to see her". And Dr Cook walked off down the ward with his head down, looking sad, and she could not bear to upset him because, as all the patients did, she loved him, so she ran after him and hugged him and said: "Don't look so sad, Dr Cook. I've changed my mind. Tell her I will see her."

But for that sudden change of heart, I would never have known my mother. Five weeks later, on a cold winter day, when the leaves were off the trees and the country looked dark and soggy, my family got in the car and drove to Suffolk. At the last minute, when we were nearly there, I panicked. "I can't do it," I said. "I think this is a great mistake. I don't want to see her. I don't know whatever made me think I did. Please stop the car."

"What are you afraid of?" Anthony asked. "Listen, she has been mad for so long that I bet she will be living in a small house with about five other dotty old ladies and one nurse in charge of them. We needn't be there very long. But having come this far, we must see her. She knows we are coming, and is expecting us. She will want to see the children."

"I need a drink", I wailed. "Whisky."

"No you don't," said Anthony. "And here we are."

We drove up a long drive and through a gate declaring 'No Unauthorised Persons Beyond This Point' to a Victorian former workhouse. It held 2000 inmates. A blackened red brick chimney shot up to the sky and belched smoke. I had visions of the hospital cremating dead, or old and unwanted patients, but Anthony said it was just a laundry chimney. We were taken to see Dr Cook.

He had grey hair and a kindly manner, like a nice uncle, and he enquired, "How long is it since you have seen your mother?"

What a question. I had no idea. "She must have seen me when I was a baby," I said, "I don't remember seeing her. I've never met her in my life."

I was obviously looking so terrified that he said: "So long ago? Don't worry. That doesn't matter a bit. You'll have no difficulty with her. She'd talk the hind leg off a donkey."

This was unbelievably worse than my worst imaginings, but there was no escape now. What could I possibly say to her? We left the children in the care of his friendly secretary. Dr Cook led us down dark corridors that smelled of cabbage, and up stairs that smelled of urine, repeatedly opening with his bunch of keys doors that had two brass locks on each of them. I do not know what I

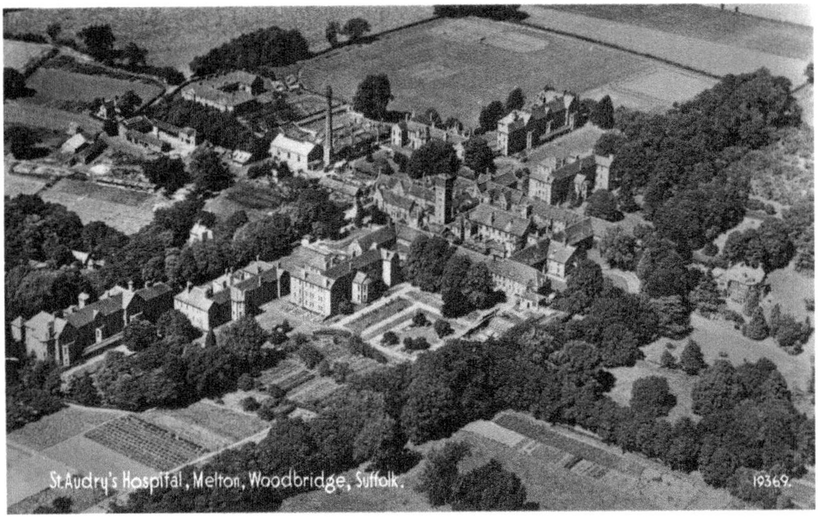

My mother's final hospital, St Audry's, Woodbridge, Suffolk, that held 2000 patients. Photograph circa 1950s. © Illustrated London News/Mary Evans Picture Library

was expecting. Someone slow and subdued and rambling on but not making sense, I supposed, after being locked up for half a lifetime. Finally he opened the door of a bright ward with big windows that must have had 60 iron beds in it, all neatly made up, each bed about one foot away from the next, and all the metal painted silver. No one was there. Then suddenly there was a click, click, clicking down the linoleum, and a tiny woman in high-heeled crocodile-skin shoes came walking fast towards us.

"You are terribly late," she said. "You must be Alison, goodness how tall you are, and you must be Anthony, Anthony Harris, tell me, are you a Jew?"

"Yes indeed," said Anthony. "Quite right. How did you know?"

"The name," she said. "The name. Now this is an absolutely terrible place to meet: we can't talk to each other here, so will you please take me out to lunch? A hotel anywhere?"

A self-confident, self assured, rapid little thing she was. Not at all afraid, like me. Driven by fear, I felt a furious urge to go to the lavatory, and fled. How could I have anything in common with her?

When I returned, we went to pick up the children. The older, Susannah, now nearly two, who loved everybody, gave my mother a beaming smile and said "Hello". The younger, Caroline, five weeks old with a shock of black hair, lay asleep, thickly blanketed against the cold, in her carry cot. My mother peered in and said: "Oh my God, just look at that. Tommy to the life."

I had not seen my father for eight years, and it must have been nearly 30 years since she had set eyes on her husband. I was amazed that she should have instantly voiced my very own thoughts. With enormous relief I realised we did have something in common.

The good Dr Cook suggested a hotel where we could have lunch. When we sat down, I dared to look at her. She was wearing a tweed coat and skirt that fitted her perfectly, terribly high-heeled tiny crocodile shoes, and a crocodile bag that matched. She was a miniature person, even in those shoes, about a foot shorter than me. Her hair was fair, probably dyed, I thought, and she had make-up, foundation, eye shadow, mascara, eye-brows pencilled in, and, horrors, dark purple lipstick painted on her mouth in an exaggerated cupid's bow (in the fashion of the 1930s) which made her look quite ridiculous. Oh no. How awful. She liked make-up, lots of it, and clothes. Perhaps she was just like my stepmother, Sonia, whose passion for make-up and clothes hugely irritated me. It dawned on me, to my horror, that my father was attracted to a particular sort of woman, and had married the same one twice. I definitely did not want a mother like Sonia.

Before our lunch arrived, she said "I say, is this butter or marge? Butter is it? Oh good. May I eat it?"

"Eat it all if you want to," replied Anthony.

And my mother put the butter dish, with its square lump of butter, in front of her, and ate it all with a fish knife and fork.

"Lovely," she said. "I don't know if you know, but we only get marge in the bin."

That's not madness, I thought, she had a perfectly good reason to eat that butter. Then she whistled loudly but quite tunefully while we waited for our food to appear. Other people in the restaurant looked up and stared at her. I wanted to bang their heads together: if only they knew. Thirty years of doing whatever seems to come naturally to you in a mental hospital is not all washed away in one visit to a hotel. Which of us would have perfect manners after that?

I wondered what she knew about the world outside, and she said it was not easy to find out. I asked why, and she said that although they did have television, it was almost impossible to see "because the loonies are always jumping up and down in front of it".

"The new bin, the bin I am in now," she said, "is much, much better than where I used to be. Here, you see, a doctor sees you once a week. Maybe Dr Cook only says, 'How's your knitting coming on, Mrs. Brittain?' but at least you meet him face to face and you can say anything you like to him" (Oh, shades of the donkey's hind leg? I thought). "In the other place, the staff were very cruel. They hit us. Not long after I got there they held me down and tore my wedding and engagement rings off my finger, and I never saw those again. You never saw a doctor, there really was no medical attention. I had to do a lot of doctoring myself: being the wife of a doctor, you see, I was the nearest to knowing what was wrong with other patients, and what to do about it. You know, things like colds and headaches, and tummy troubles."

I wondered if the medical staff of the highly regarded St Andrew's had any idea that the patients were happily making up for their lack of attention. I thought she had arranged a clever self-boosting persona for herself, and had managed to remain amazingly self confident in the face of terrible humiliation.

Here in the hotel she was bubbly and very happy, said the food was quite delicious and it was lovely to see the children and could she have photographs of them, so she could boast about being a grandmother? And she would like us to come and see her again, and take her out, and maybe, soon, they were going to let her out for weekends, and then could she come and stay with us? She wanted to see our house, to see if it was nice.

It seemed terrible to take her back to her prison, and leave her there. She leapt out of the car, kissing us both quickly and leaving purple cupid's bows on our cheeks, saying she had been afraid that we arrived so late that she might miss both lunch and tea, but was pleased to see that she would still be in time for tea.

"Go, and see Dr Cook" she said, "and tell him you have brought me back safely", and she scampered off.

Dr Cook asked how we had found her. I said accusingly "She doesn't seem very mad."

"No, no. Indeed not. That is why she is now allowed out a bit. But when she first came she had many 'episodes', when she became very upset, and needed calming down. Those are getting very rare now. She has not had one for many months."

"Is she better, then? What made her recover?" I asked.

"The wonder drug" he said. "Tranquillisers. Largactil. Once we had that and could give it to patients, they improved enormously. Largactil steadied them down, kept them on an even keel, and they were happier and much less trouble to themselves or to us. They, and we, both felt more confident, and we had greater trust in each other. I would not say that she has recovered, but she is a great deal better than she was, and I envisage her coming out for weekends to stay with her sisters soon."

"She wants to come and stay with us."

"Does she? Well that's good."

Well, maybe, I thought, but actually I would be terrified to have her to stay.

What if she went mad in our house?

On the way home I said to Anthony, "When I saw those clothes and all that makeup I was afraid she was just like Sonia; that that was the sort of woman Daddy liked to marry. But I have to say I am greatly relieved that she didn't do any heavy emotional thing, or make any kind of ghastly scene, as Sonia would surely have done. Do you think that's the tranquilliser?"

"No, of course not" said Anthony. "That's her real personality. She's like a little bird with a broken wing. Chirpy all the time. She seems to be unaware that there has been anything wrong with her. She's very sweet."

Sweet, I thought. Yes she is. Amazingly, for one locked away for so long, she seems to be a happy person. And she seems completely harmless: nothing to be frightened of. I scolded myself for being such a coward.

She did come and stay with us, several times. Each time, before she came, the hospital sent me a form to sign, saying that I had her out on licence, and I understood that she must go back after the weekend.

My mother taught her grandchildren to knit, the English way. She could not understand why we did not have servants: she believed we needed a Nanny, she would have done, of course, for me. She herself had had a cook general when she was first married, very useful. I had never heard of a cook general.

Once she asked me for sanitary towels. My father's sisters, those Irish Aunts, had said that lunacy was to do with the moon, and in women that meant that every 28 days there was danger. They said that Dorothy always got 'bad' when she was having her period. I gave her the tampons, shut my children safely in their playroom where I could keep an eye on them through the big serving hatch in the kitchen, and waited and watched her for any change in mood. There was of course, absolutely none. My blasted Aunts! I hated my fear, my suspicions of such an obviously sweet-natured, harmless woman.

Used to hospital ways, she was up and about up very early. One morning I came down with a hungry child on each hip and there she was, sitting at the kitchen table with a teapot, milk jug, sugar bowl and cup and saucer, not the old mug, milk bottle, and spoon from the bag of sugar that I would have used.

"My God, Mummy," I exclaimed. "Whatever time did you get up? You must be mad!"

"Oh no I'm not," she said. "That's where you're so wrong. I wouldn't be here, I wouldn't be out on licence, if I was mad," and she laughed happily at my discomfort.

Once the next-door neighbours had their mother-in-law staying, it was an uncomfortably warm July day, and, partly to amuse my mother, I invited them to tea on our lawn. The mother-in-law looked at my mother (thank goodness, by now, perhaps at her sister Alice's suggestion, she had given up the purple lipstick cupid's bow), and said: "I haven't met you before, Mrs Brittain. You don't live in Islington? Where do you come from?" The garden trees were that heavy July green. The lawn was burnt brown. The muggy hot air trapped within the garden walls did not move. I felt sweat trickling under my arms. Oh my goodness, I thought, whatever is she going to say? How shall I cover for her? In my mind's eye I saw the hospital with the big chimney, 2000 inmates, and double brass locks on every door. What should I say, quick? But my mad mother, perfectly in tune with the occasion, announced: "I live in the country, in Suffolk, in a tiny little village called Woodbridge. I don't know if you know it?"

Oh yes, I thought, you wonderful thing. Not much missing there. I winked at her, and she winked back.

She wanted to go to a musical, so we took her to 'The Boyfriend'. She kept exclaiming: "How ripping! How topping!" at every song. She was delighted, and said, rather loudly, in a quiet moment, "*We* used to wear crepe de chine knickers just like that."

Friends said what a lovely story it was, that after all those years in a mental hospital she was now sane. Was it not wonderful to have a mother at last?

Did I love her very much? And I had to tell them that I thought it was wonderful for her to be getting so much better, and to be allowed out, but I had to say with some shame, that unless you are brought up by someone as your mother, you simply never achieve that kind of love for them. You do not feel those strong ties of trust and affection for them that I imagine you can for someone who has mothered you. And there was no comparison with the emotion I still felt for Pinkie, whom at this stage I had not seen for 20 years.

My mother thought I was very clever to be able to put on nappies (I had a third baby daughter, Jessica, by now). She herself would not have a clue. She still could not see why I did not have a Nanny. She thought they were better at that sort of thing.

I said to Anthony: "We must take her out somewhere, to keep her interested, and stop her criticising me."

"Do calm down. She's just commenting, she's not criticising you. But I know, we could go and see Uncle Claude and Isa and have tea with them. He wouldn't mind, and he's probably grand enough to please her. Plenty of servants. I'll ring him."

Anthony's Uncle Claude was in the oil shipping business, and lived in a huge house in Godalming that was all Elizabethan one side, all Jacobean the other, designed by Lutyens and all built in 1910. It had a vast garden often open to the public, a model farm, and five or six real Breughels let into the panelling of the dining room walls. Claude's wife Isa said could I please get the dogs off the sofas, because the upholstery was petit point tapestry, all made by hand. All Isa's relations, at least seven Kaplanskys, were there for tea that day. We sat on the verandah, looking down the long perspective of the erupting herbaceous borders either side of a perfect lawn, and drank Lapsang Souchong out of lovely old china cups and saucers. We ate the thinnest possible cucumber sandwiches. My mother was obviously delighted, and dropped into a silence while everyone's mouths were full: "Anthony's so nice, you know, and d'you know, he's a Jew?"

The moment froze. In a state of rude shock, all the Kaplanskys, including Isa, stared at my mother, their cups rattling on their saucers, holding their cucumber sandwiches up in the air with C-shaped bites out of them, like little flags, in still and silent astonishment. I was mortified. How could she say such a thing? In the early 1930s, did ordinary decent people think thoughts like that about Jews? Maybe, I suddenly understood, that is how, although we knew about it, we took no steps to stop genocide, gas chambers, Belsen?

I put my hand on her arm to reassure her, but I think she was unaware of her faux pas. In inner turmoil, I would have done anything to undo what she had said. But I am happy to say that Uncle Claude, who knew my mother's history, and Anthony, looked at each other and grinned and broke into loud and confident laughter.

I asked her once, "Did they ever put you in a padded cell, Mummy?" I hoped she would say 'No,' or 'What is a padded cell?' Or even 'There was one, but it was never used'. I could not bear the thought of the terrible indignity of her being locked in a padded cell. She was so tiny that I imagined that even if she became violent the staff would easily be able to control her without that.

She replied, "Oh yes, Darling, often. It was very nice: a great relief".

"Very nice? A great relief? How?"

"Well you know, perhaps I had been helping to clear up tea, and I was in the pantry, mopping the floor, and along comes a lunatic and pees all over my nice clean tiles. I was so angry at the wasted effort I just cracked her on the head with the mop."

"Did you hurt her?"

"I don't know. I hope so. Teach her a lesson. So then they shout and blow whistles and come running down the corridor to get you. They push you to the floor and hold you down and give you an injection. And you come to in a padded cell."

"But why is that good?"

"Well, you're very, very angry, and you've got to work out your feelings, and let off steam, and you can. You can scream and yell, and throw yourself at the walls, and punch them, and lie on the floor drumming your feet up and down, and they can't stop you. From time to time they look through the little window, and ask 'Are you ready to come out yet, Mrs. Brittain?' and you can shout 'No I'm jolly well not' and carry on till you're bored. When you do finally come out you feel so much better. It really is a relief."

And I had thought that a padded cell would be the ultimate horror, the sure sign that you were not yourself, and nobody trusted you, and you had no future.

Yet what she said sounded absolutely believable, highly reasonable, and not at all mad. It had the ring of truth.

"And did you ever hear voices?" I asked.

"Oh yes, Darling, all the time. I couldn't think straight because of them."

"How horrible," I said. "What did they say?"

"I couldn't possibly tell you that," she said, grinning. "They were extremely rude."

I asked her what did she remember about becoming ill after she had had me.

"I don't know what happened," she said. "I think I tried to commit suicide by jumping in a river, because I was in love with a doctor, but they fished me out, and I ended up in a bin. I can't really remember any of it properly." Since she could not remember it, and I have never heard this from anyone else, neither of us will know if this was mad imagination or remembered reality. All it does tell is how miserable she was.

I did speak to my Aunts, her sisters Alice and Betty, in their early 90s, about those hideous events. The middle-sister Betty clearly recalled the fateful telephone call saying that Dorothy was ill. Betty was at home with her mother, who answered the call. Her mother held Betty's hand so tightly, digging her nails in, that Betty cried out, "Let go, let go, you're hurting me."

Betty, in her 90s, chose to tell me quite firmly, without my asking, that there was no mention of Thompson, the monthly nurse, or accusations of any untoward activities by my father. She said that if there was, of course she would have remembered it. Betty said Alice told the story, but Betty did not know where Alice got it from. Alice claims that my mother was terribly upset about the news of Thompson and she did tell me, and in this I believe her, that Dorothy never stopped loving Tommy, for the rest of her life. It seems extraordinary that two sisters, extremely close in age and affection, should hold such different memories. I simply tell their stories: I shall never know more than that.

I asked my mother about coming home: did she remember hitting Aunt Ann on the head with the mirror? She said she remembered it well.

"Tommy came to see me, and said he was going to take me away. He had to see the doctors to fix it. When they told him I could go, I rushed down to the front door and jumped into his car and asked 'Are we going home?' And he said 'Yes'. But when I got home, to my own home at last, I had to sleep in a different bedroom, not our own, not with Tommy. I asked 'Why not with you? I am going to, I must be. I am your wife. He said the doctors had said so. Well of course this made me wonder, 'Has he got a new girlfriend, then, and is he hiding her somewhere?' And the awful thing was he had, and I found her. I could not sleep, so I just went from room to room looking, and there, in that small room at the back, she was, lying asleep. That wasn't Ann, Darling. I would have known her. That was his girlfriend, and I decided to give her what for. That mirror was the only thing to hand, and it made a nice noise as it came down on her head. If she hadn't been wearing curlers, I might have killed her." And she laughed.

"That wasn't his girlfriend. I told you, that was Aunt Ann, remember?"

"Oh that's right. You told me that. I'd forgotten. I bashed it down on Ann. My God!"

Now she had come out of hospital, and was living with an old lady, being her housekeeper. She had telephoned me in floods of tears saying, "Dr Cook wants to get rid of me."

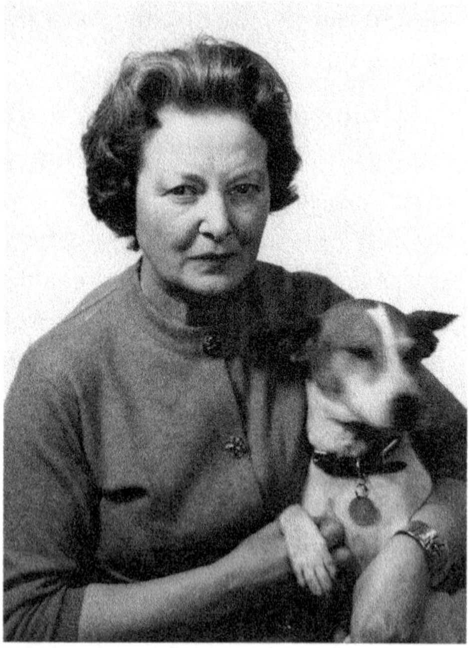

Dorothy having come out of her mental hospital, after 28 years inside. Now working as housekeeper to an old lady who kindly got her a dog called 'Laddie' to love. 1966.

"What did he say?"

"He said I could go and work for an old lady as a housekeeper. I am used to the hospital and I like it here. I don't want to go."

"Well look here. . . " I thought rapidly. "Why don't you make Dr Cook promise to have you back if you don't like it, and then you could give it a try knowing you were quite safe?"

I know now how lucky my mother was to have her sister Alice. It was Alice who kept in touch with her, and who worked with Dr Cook to find an old lady who needed a housekeeper to live with my mother and keep her company. It was Alice who led her out into the real world again and helped her to regain her freedom. It was wonderfully good of Alice. So Dorothy gave it a try and it was a great success. She wrote me a wonderful letter of joy, which began '*Darling Alison, I must tell you, I've got a room of my own, with a dressing table and mirror, and a bedside table with a bedside light. I have lovely curtains, and a carpet, and my bed is so comfortable*'.

'O God,' I thought, 'we all take those things for granted, don't we? And she didn't have any of them for 30 years. I never even gave it a thought before, that all hospitalised mental patients suffer such deprivations, and for an extremely feminine little soul like her, it really was painful'.

The old lady was kind and thoughtful. She made my mother learn First Aid, in weekly lessons, and take and pass her Red Cross Exam: an achievement she could be proud of. And she got her a dog: something for my mother to love. Her old lady was incontinent, and my mother telephoned me one evening and said "That's 17 pairs of knickers I have washed today!" But she did not seem to mind in the least, and she would have been perfectly amiable and good tempered about it. Once she rang for detailed instructions on how to make marmalade, which her employer wanted her to do. She said it turned out very well and they ate it all rather quickly.

The women she cared for were extremely old and frail. After a year or two, the first one died, and she went to a second, who did not last long, either. When her third employer died, she telephoned me and said: "That's three old ladies I've killed so far, do you think it's something I do?" And she giggled. She was joking, of course, but I thought how easy it would be for someone to accuse her of something like that. I was not worried, though, because as far as I could tell, her old ladies were very fond of her, and their children, her employers, would have supported her.

"You are naughty," I said.

"Yes I am," she answered.

On another occasion that she came to stay I asked her if she knew what had made her better, what had allowed her to come out.

"No, I don't know that."

"Was it drugs, do you think, Largactil, that stuff?"

"No, I don't think so, not that." Some time later she said: "I know what it was. It was money."

"What was money?"

"It was money that made me better."

"I thought you didn't have any money?"

"That's right, we didn't. So one day Dr Cook said to me 'Mrs Brittain, we're very short-staffed in this hospital'. And I said 'You're telling me'. He asked, 'I wondered if you would like to give us a hand sometimes, you know, help us out?' And I replied, 'What do you want me to do?' He said, 'Well, maybe give us some help in the canteen one or two afternoons a week, pouring tea, say.' And I said, 'No, certainly not, you're here to look after me'. Then he said 'We'd pay you, you know'. Well, that was it. I said, 'How much?' And he replied, 'Ten bob a week'. 'Cash?' I asked. 'Yes, cash.' 'Can I spend it myself? Can I go into the village and buy what I want with it?' 'If you go in with a member of staff, yes you can'. So I started work, and I got paid, and I could buy my own knitting wool, and make-up, and hold my head up high. That's what started my recovery, and made me better. There you are. It was money, Darling."

I wonder if regaining self respect is a useful part of recovery for some mental patients? If the National Health Service gave a little sum of money every week to each of its mentally ill patients, in return for some small task they had to do, might that be a useful aid to recovery? It would be cheap at the price. When I telephoned the hospital where my father had paid for her all those years, and asked what treatment she had been given, they said that whether I was her only child or not, the recent Data Protection Act prevented them telling me anything. But they did kindly tell me that they had encouraged patients to do occupational therapy, which was thought to be the best thing for the mind. They encouraged knitting. Certainly, my mother knitted non-stop. But I cannot forget that she said with such emphasis that what cured her, was neither Largactil nor knitting. "That's right. It was money, Darling."

Chapter 34
The Rain in Spain

Eight years after she came out of the hospital, my mother has a brain tumour. The children and I have come to the Maida Vale branch of the National Hospital for Nervous Diseases to visit her. She is sitting up in bed, knitting.

"Oh my God," she says, "Look at that. Caroline is still the very image of Tommy. How she reminds me of him." Caroline is six or seven years old now.

She does not seem very ill. She seems exactly her old self.

"What are you knitting, Granny Dorothy?" Caroline asks.

"A bed-jacket, Darling, do you like it?" and she holds it up for Caroline to see.

"Yes I like it. What is it for? And who is it for? We haven't got bed-jackets."

"It's for me. You wear it sitting up in bed, and I am going to spend some time in bed, now."

She says they do not know what is wrong with her, nor does she. She feels perfectly all right, only she keeps falling down. They are going to operate on her to find out. She seems completely unworried: and chatters away about brushing Miss Pretty's hair and suddenly falling down, and being out shopping and finding herself lying on the pavement. The bed-jacket is pink, and has an extremely complicated pattern. The girls lean over her as she shows them how to knit one, slip one, and pull some stitches over the others, making a pretty bobble. Absorbed, they repeat the instructions after her. Has she not had enough bad luck in her life? Why should this happen to her? She has only had eight years of freedom, and is this the end? My head is screaming with rage as I arrange the flowers we have brought.

On the way home in the car, the girls are singing in the back. They have clear, pretty voices, and are singing verse after verse of 'I ain't a-going to grieve my Lord no more'. They are in tune, and in harmony: Susannah is singing it in thirds below the others.

You can't get to heaven, if you don't wash up,

'Cos the Lord won't have, no dirty plate and cup.

We are just home when they reach the penultimate verse:

If you get to heaven, before I do,

Just dig a hole, and pull me through.

I saw my mother one more time. She had had her operation. Her head was thick with bandages. She introduced me to her 'very useful assistant'. I recognised the royal blue uniform, and held out my hand, saying "How d'you do, Sister. I'm Mrs Brittain's daughter".

"Not Sister." My mother contradicted. "I said, she's my assistant." Sister, who was large and West Indian, did not look best pleased.

"You're lucky to be in here all nice and dry and warm", I said. "It is streaming rain outside."

My mother holds up the bag of urine connected to her, and swinging it carefully, sings loudly, in tune and in time with its swings, "The rain in Spain falls mainly on the plain".

Then they put some screens around her, and, waiting on a chair outside, I can hear them asking her questions, and I can hear her answers. "Do you know what day of the week it is?" She says, firmly, "Friday", but it is Sunday. Does she know who the Prime Minister is? "Winston Churchill" she answers, but it is Harold MacMillan. Can she count backwards from a hundred in sevens? "Here goes", she says, and gives out a set of random numbers, none of them right. What have they done to her? She was all right before they operated. I hate them.

Then the consultant comes to speak to me. I ask him if this tumour has anything to do with her schizophrenia?

"No. We think not. The operation went very well. We have taken out much of the tumour, and we are very pleased that so little damage has been done. She is talking very well" (as if she ever was not talking). "But after those little tests, we have decided there is nothing more we can do for her. We are sending her back to Ipswich."

When I get home I telephone a friend who is a psychiatrist, and ask him why the hell they have done that to her. She was all right before her operation, and now look.

"Everyone goes mad in their own special way", he says. "She has gone back to her schizophrenia, by the sound of things."

"But why, why? What did they do to her? She was fine, and now she's nuts again."

"Tumours keep on growing. A brain tumour grows all the time, but it is encased in a rigid box, your bony skull. As it grows and presses on the brain, it causes the most intolerable pain. The best thing to do is to operate and take out as much of it as you dare. That leaves space for it to go on growing without giving terrible pain, and hopefully some remaining bit of it will kill you before it gets too big. They are proud of themselves because they have taken a big piece of it away, and yet they have left her a walking talking woman. The fact that she talks nonsense matters not to them."

I only hope it did prevent and relieve the suffering she might have had. She died nine months later, at the age of 60, and I went to her funeral. I sent a wreath of white roses, as she had done for my father, and a woman sang "Oh for the wings, for the wings of a dove. . ."

On the way home after that last visit I remembered the final verse of 'I ain't a-going to grieve. . .'

And that is all, St. Peter said,
He shut the gates, and went to bed.

Chapter 35
A Happy Release

I had seen my father with so many women. I often wondered, if my mother had not gone mad, would he have been faithful to her, would they have had a long and happy marriage? I never knew my mother as she was when they met. She was by all accounts the leader of three lively sisters, with a happy disposition. They say she looked astoundingly beautiful, was full of fun, interested in everything. She was a talented violinist with a hugely promising soprano voice. She dressed with a great sense of fashion. She loved him till the day he died.

My father paid for her hospital stay till the end of his life, all the time he knew Pinkie, and through his divorce and then his marriage to Sonia, by which time Dorothy was no longer in any way his responsibility. At one point I believe he acted recklessly to save her (and he never knew the result because by then it was long after he was dead) but by that action he succeeded in giving her those eight years of freedom she had at the end. It does seem likely that they could have been very happy together.

The wedding sounds as though it was delightful, and everyone seemed very pleased with it, but wait a minute, maybe her mother, Bella, did not want Dorothy to marry Tommy? Her wearing black velvet for the wedding may have been a sign of her distress. Certainly the two younger sisters thought it was done on purpose to give a message of disapproval. And Alice's description of them all coming back into the house from the church, and Dorothy's mother telling Alice, "This will end in suicide or murder" does sound as if Bella, at least, was extremely worried about the marriage. Did that cause enough stress to drive Dorothy mad a year later?

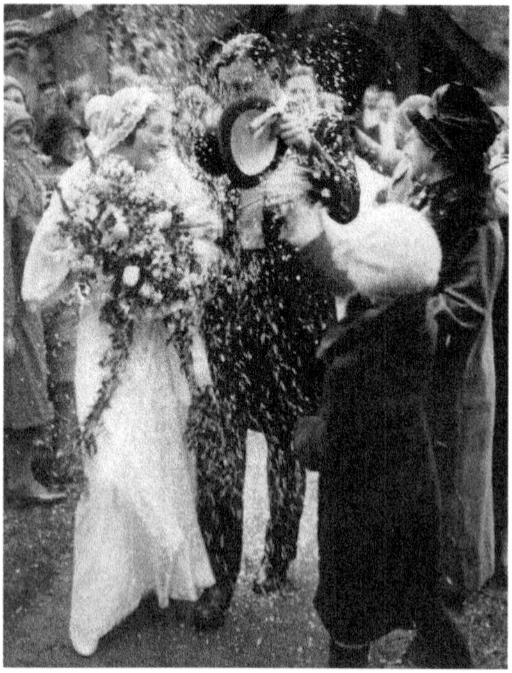

Happily Married: Dorothy and Tommy, Alison's mother and father, coming out of the church in clouds of confetti, 1933.

What is it like when you go mad? You are witty and talented, the brightest and best of three lovely and well-loved sisters, life is exciting, the best part is just beginning, and snap, in a few days everything goes wrong, and the chances are it will never go right again. Was the stress that caused this due to the mutual disapproval between your family and your new husband, or the extreme hormone changes caused by the arrival of your new baby? Was it both? Can it be undone? No. Is there a cure? No. What happens now? How will you adjust to a new life where you are locked away forever, where no one listens to you, no one believes you, people talk behind your back and make arrangements for you without telling you, there is no one to love you, you do not have a husband, a baby, a house, a bedroom, a dressing table, a bedside light, a carpet or even curtains?

What happened after my mother went into a mental hospital, less than a week after I was born? Certainly I was not told. A conspiracy of silence began from the start, to hide the truth from me. When I was about four my nursery governess agreed with me, when I asked her, that she thought 'maybe', my mother was 'in Feather' that I mistook for the word 'Heaven', not that I had any idea what that was. Pinkie told me that my mother had been 'very ill' when I was born, which was why I was only christened when I was nine, in Heydon. In Dublin, when I was 11 my cousin Happy told me that her mother (Aunt Doris) had told her a secret about my mother and said she must never tell me, "Ha, Ha"! So my nursery governess knew, Pinkie knew, so did Happy, all my father's friends knew, even Mrs Robley-Browne knew: everyone except me knew this secret. All my Irish Aunts knew, but they chose not to tell me. Of course, all my mother's side of the family knew, but I was not allowed to meet my mother's sisters. I could not ask, and had to find out for myself, when I was 13. When I did find out, I was told I was wicked. My poor father was so devastated by the loss of his wife that although he knew he must one day do it, he could not bring himself to tell me. Being mad was so shaming that it was kept secret.

I asked my father if he had visited my mother once she was installed in St Andrew's Hospital, after there was, presumably, no further hope for her recovery. He said yes, he did at first, but then he was asked not to, and told it would be better for her if he did not because it upset her terribly, and they found her then very hard to handle.

Not long ago I was tidying my jewel case and looking at the silver baby's bracelet and the small garnet brooch that my mother's sister Alice had given me after my mother died, saying they had belonged to Dorothy. I then remembered that my father had given a magnificent emerald engagement ring to Pinkie (the one he finally threw into the Bay of Naples), and an equally spectacular ruby ring to Sonia. He might not have been so well off in those early days, but he would have been likely to have given my mother a ring he could probably not really afford as an engagement ring. What happened to that?

Thinking about it I remembered a conversation with my mother, one of the first we had when she came to stay with me and my young family when she was first let out of hospital for weekends on licence. She said the hospital she was in now (a National Health hospital in Suffolk) was much better than the one she had been in. She remembered with horror a few days after she went into St Andrew's a group of nurses jumping on her. Nurses there were called 'Companions'. These companions held her down on the floor and she screamed as they pulled her wedding and engagement rings off her finger, and she never saw the rings again. It sounded awfully true, but she was mad, was she not, she was out on licence, so I could not be sure she had not made it up. When you are mad people do not always believe what you say.

When my mother was admitted, St Andrew's was considered the best mental hospital in the country. Those rings have never turned up, there is no record of them. Now I know I grossly misjudged my mother: I never heard her tell a lie. I am shocked to have to admit that that ring story has almost certainly got to be true.

Your husband, the one outside person who you can beg for help to come and take you away, no longer comes to see you and disappears. The only possessions you have, the promise of love in the rings he gave you, are stolen. You are still alive: that's all. And maybe not even that.

I did ask a friend, another psychiatrist, how different the woman I knew as my mother, whom I only met after she had been incarcerated for 30 years, would be from the woman my father had married?

She replied, "You already know that insulin coma therapy and electroconvulsive therapy cause brain damage. I am sorry to say that long-term schizophrenia produces its own brain damage, too." And then she described to me exactly the woman I knew, almost as if she had met her. She quoted my mother's lack of anxiety at attacking Aunt Ann with the mirror, at hitting the peeing patient with the mop, at odd remarks about Jews, and at laughing about 'killing' three old ladies, and said that such things are what you see in a 'burned-out schizophrenic'.

"To recover as much as she did, she obviously did extremely well. Most patients who have spent 30 years in mental hospitals have no one on the outside who still loves and cares for them. She would probably never have come out if it had not been for the support her loving sister, your Aunt Alice, gave her. But she will no longer have been able to show or feel profound emotion."

All I can say is I am incredibly glad my mother recovered as much as she did, and that she was able to leave her mental hospital and have those years of freedom. And perhaps I understand why, although I felt extremely protective of her, I was never able to feel any profound or overwhelming emotion for her as my mother.

In care in a mental hospital, you lose status. You are physically hemmed in. If your 'Companions' attack you and steal your rings and you complain, you have no redress. No one believes your story. Time goes by and those who once so loved you no longer come and see you or let you know they remember you. No birthday or Christmas cards. Your status can go down so low that you are actually quite forgotten, until you no longer really exist.

Five girls from two families descended from Charles Trefusis, 21st Baron Clinton, born between 1912 and 1926, were described as 'imbeciles' and placed in

Earlswood Hospital (built in 1855 as an 'Asylum for Idiots') in Redwood, Surrey. Two of these sisters, Nerissa and Katherine Bowes-Lyon, neither of whom learned to speak, were the children of our Queen Elizabeth the Queen Mother's brother, John Henry Bowes-Lyon, and therefore her nieces and our present Queen's first cousins. Burke's Peerage recorded Nerissa's death in 1940 and Katherine's in 1961. In fact Nerissa died in 1986 and Katherine in 2014. This was the Royal Family's secret, never told. There were 46 years in which the dates of death might have been corrected, but only silence remains. You can be killed off by Burke's Peerage but go on living for another generation.

John Crawford Adams MD, FRCS, Consultant Orthopaedic Surgeon of St Mary's Hospital, London, wrote a centenary memoir of my father – 'A Notable Centenary: H A Brittain and Ischio-Femoral Arthrodesis' – in an orthopaedic journal. He writes with affection and enthusiasm, but the part towards the end is untrue:

> 'Here was a man who seemed to have everything: wealth, a fine home with a devoted wife, work and recreations that he enjoyed to the full, and a happy relationship with his patients and staff. Yet, as often happens in life, there was a dark shadow that clouded a great part of his life – a grief that he had to bear alone. He had married quite early in his career and had a daughter. But sadly his wife developed postnatal depression of such severity and persistence that she had to be cared for in an institution. This went on for many years, until eventually she died. In a way this was a happy release for her and a late opportunity for Tommy to pick up the threads of his domestic life.'

By the time John Crawford Adams wrote that, all my father's friends were dead as was my father, so John had no one to ask. He must have simply made up the untrue fact that my mother had died when he said, because actually she outlived my father by 16 years.

With postpartum schizophrenia, not only can everything worth living for be taken from you, but even the fact that you are still alive. A word or two from someone who does not know what they are talking about can rub you out. First you become a secret never to be told, then you can be erased. They just say you are dead, it is recorded that you no longer exist. In this simple way you can be finished off, and here is the evidence that sometimes this happens.

What had I said when my school friend Pixie asked about my mother?

"She's dead, I think."

Chapter 36

A Broken Spout

I did see Pinkie one more time. We stayed a weekend with my daughter Jessica and her family in Norwich. Jessica's sweet children were tiny, so I guess I must have been about 65.

That Saturday we see in the *Eastern Daily Press* that magnificent Melton Constable Hall is up for sale. Once Elizabethan, it was remodelled in the second half of the 17th century and is said to be 'the finest example of a Christopher Wren country house'. No one has lived in it for a long time, and a film crew is feared to have misused it while it was empty. This is the day of the View. The whole of Norfolk society has not been inside it for years, and this is their, and our, opportunity. Everyone who loves, or owns large country houses is there, and I meet several friends of my youth. They are all in their 60s too, and even as we recognise each other, we are a bit embarrassed to see evidence of the passing years.

Then, round one of the huge pillars on the portico, comes someone I am sure I know. He has blonde hair going grey, and a furrowed brow that reminds me of Mary Anne and William's father, Preek. He comes straight toward me, holding out his hand, and says: "Hello, Alison. It is Alison isn't it? I'm William Bulwer Long, Mary Anne's brother. You remember me?"

Well yes, now that he says it, of course I remember him. William, at six years old, my bridegroom-to-be. I am so relieved he has told me who he is, "William! William Hanslip Bulwer Long! Good Heavens! How nice to see you. How are you? What are you doing now? Where are you living? In Heydon?"

"Living at Heydon, as always, and doing a bit of farming, you know."

"Oh, living at Heydon. You are lucky. William, this is my husband, Steve", and I introduce him and they shake hands. "Tell me, is Heydon still the same?

I haven't seen it in years. I often dream about it. And Mary Anne, is she there? How is she?"

"I don't think it has changed very much, you must come and see it. I live in the Hall now, and farm. And Mary Ann is there, with a husband and children, and well I think."

"And Pinkie. . . Pinkie. What happened to Pinkie? Is she still alive? If she is I would love to see her. . ."

William's brow furrows more, and he says "Pinkie is very sad. She lives in the village, but she has Alzheimer's disease, quite badly, now."

Then he looks at me harder. "Pinkie doesn't know anything about anything any more. Her short-term memory is gone, absolutely gone. But I do wonder about you and her? She can still remember some of her past. She has gone back so far that she can no longer remember her husband, who is dead now, or her three children, which is just as well, because two are in Australia, and her son is not around. But you are from her long since past, so far back that she just might remember you."

"Shall I go and see her?"

"Would you?" he said, "Would you really? You will have to expect anything.

She may not remember you, and sometimes nothing at all can make her quite angry. But if she *does* remember you it will make her so happy. Would you just try, and not mind if it goes wrong?"

"Of course I will", I said.

"She's living in the cottage next to the shop. She doesn't answer the doorbell. You'll have to go round to the back and knock."

"All right, I will."

"Well thank you. And good luck."

The small 18th century soft-coloured red brick cottage is on the public house side of the shop, near the track to Church Farm, where we used to ride the Nelsons' heavy horses at harvest. The same shop with the old bowed window where we bought humbugs with our sweet ration. It looks a bit smarter than I remember it during the war. The side gate of the cottage is open and we walk around to the back. I can hear the rattling sound of raking gravel, and Pinkie is there, wielding the rake, doing a pretty efficient job with it.

"Hello, Pinkie. Do you remember me?" I say, nearly choking.

"Oh *Alison*! How lovely to see you. It's been ages, hasn't it? Come in, and I'll give you some tea."

"This is my husband, Steve," I say, and try to introduce him. But Pinkie just says "Come in".

Pinkie still has the lovely heart-shaped face, and the hazel green eyes that I remember. She is wearing an old dark green jersey, a colour that always looked good on her, and a tweed skirt. Her hair is grey now, and a bit untidy, but then for whom is she to tidy it up? The window in the little kitchen sheds light on the earthenware sink with its wooden draining board, her tiny kitchen table and chair, and the electric cooker. In the darker parts at the back of the kitchen are many cardboard boxes. She makes us tea in a pot with a broken spout, and lid only about half of which is still there.

We go next door to the tiny back room with the tray, and some mugs and biscuits. She pours two mugs of tea, looks round, looks at my husband with some doubt, and pours a third. In this little room there are also piles of big cardboard boxes, the sort that removers use, at the back. As we sit down I can see that her nice old brown moccasin shoes have got big holes in the soles, and I can see her bare feet through them.

"You'll have to forgive me", she says. "I've only just moved in you see, and I haven't unpacked yet. I ought really to be living at the Hall, you know, and I can't think why they put me here. I was born in the Hall."

"No, don't worry. What a nice cottage to be living in. Please don't apologise. It is lovely to see you."

"So, how lovely to see you too, Alison. You've come back to Heydon," she says. "Do you remember it?"

"Of course I do. I remember it all the time. The church, the green, widow's row, the well, the blacksmith, our ponies."

"Mickey Mouse" she says. "And William's naughty little grey Shetland that used to run away with him and get him shoved off under the low branches of the chestnut trees in the Park. Threepenny Bit, we called him. And Aunt Bee's bath chair. Can you remember ruining that? Goodness, you were naughty."

"I'm sorry," I said. "But I did enjoy it."

"I thought as much." She smiled her beautiful smile. "And do you remember hanging William up over the well? Fur was furious."

"He did it for me," I said, "to show how much he loved me. He wanted to marry me."

"You might have killed him," said Pinkie. "And he didn't marry you, did he?"

"No, of course not," I said. "I was far too old for him."

Pinkie smiled. "Two years older," she said.

"And the dogs," I said. "I remember inky black Jonathan with his furiously wagging tail stump."

"Yes, my Jonathan," said Pinkie, "And Gretchen. Do you remember when she had Jonathan's puppies? He went two miles to find her."

We chattered away about what we remembered for nearly an hour, until it began to get dark. I never mentioned my father, because what would have been the point? We were completely happy in each other's company, as we had always been. This was my Pinkie, as I always remembered her, and we were terribly lucky to catch the moment, so lucky that it was not a few months later, when she might no longer remember me.

We hugged goodbye, the old familiar hug. It could have been 50 or more years ago. As we left, she said "Do please come again." And I said "Yes, of course we will". But I realised, sadly, that by the time we are next staying in Norwich, and able to go to Heydon, Pinkie will not know who I am.

I was glad my husband put his arm round me as we walked back to the car. I needed that.

We met William in his battered Honda pick-up driving out of the Park gates, and he stopped and asked: "How did it go? Did she know you?"

"Oh she did, she did," I said, "And it was lovely. She remembered everything about us and the war, and we talked for ages. She said she had only just moved into the cottage."

"Oh dear," said William. "She's been there two years, and she refuses to unpack. She just lives in a bit of her kitchen and downstairs bathroom and a bit of her back room. She hasn't been upstairs yet. But if she knew you and you were able to chatter about old times, that will have made her very happy."

"And me too," I said. "Thank you so much for telling us to try it."

When we got back to Norwich my daughter Jessica asked me, "How was it?"

"Lovely," I said. "I am so glad we went. For me there was still the very essence of the Pinkie I remember, and we were able to talk about so many things that had happened during the war while I lived with her. She gave us tea. And something strikes me. She gave us tea out of a very old brown teapot, with a broken spout and only half a lid. And her shoes had holes in the soles and I could see her bare feet through the holes. That family is not poor, you know. William is living in considerable comfort in the Hall. Why don't they treat her a bit better? A pair of shoes and a teapot wouldn't cost much."

"Oh no, they are treating her absolutely perfectly," replied Jessica (Jess is a general practitioner, and has patients with Alzheimer's). "That, sadly, is what the disease does to you. I'm afraid that she would never use a new teapot: she wouldn't know what it was. If you took away the old one, she would never have tea again. And she wouldn't recognise a new pair of shoes. They have probably bought her some but she won't wear them. She is going to wear the old ones till they fall off, and then she will go barefoot."

"Oh is she really that ill? I didn't think she was. Because her memories of the wartime with me are so clear, I couldn't believe she had so very much wrong with her."

"I'm afraid the old shoes and broken teapot are typical of the way her brain is closing down: she cannot manage new things. But it is good that she is coping, and that her family looks after her with such understanding. Don't worry about it, no one could do any more for her. You were very lucky to visit her while she still remembered you so well."

I am so glad we saw her. And that I was reminded again that she was still the woman I had loved and learned from, and who I would have liked to have been my mother.

So many memories were stirred, and came flooding back. What about my father? Could he and Pinkie have been happy together? I have never seen him happier with anyone than with her. In her company, he had been absolutely shining with delight. Pinkie appeared to glow with him around too, and she dearly loved both him, and me. She knew we were both a bit naughty, but she was quite capable of coping, and actually she rather enjoyed it. Had there been no senseless nonsense about his divorce, and if the bloody war had not dragged on for so long, I believe they might have had a very happy life together.

But it did not happen and, disastrously, my father married someone else.

Chapter 37
The Monster

There is something else I was not told. Not being told does not mean I do not know. Not knowing does not make it go away. I nearly know. I wish I absolutely did. I suppose it is true. It is something I have to deal with whether I know it or not: did he kill himself? Well, he must have done. Nothing else makes as much sense. If he did, could I have stopped him?

There were sleeping pills in my father's bed when I was four and five. I guess they helped him cope when my mother went mad. When Pinkie had jilted him, with anguishing thoughts of her disloyalty rattling round in his head, I bet he turned to barbiturates then, if not in the intervening years. He would have found the humiliation and loss unbearable, it would be much harder this time to pick himself up, dust himself down, and start all over again.

By the time he came home from the war he probably needed sleeping pills every night to sleep. He may not have known, or wished to recognise, and the medical profession may not then have been fully aware, of their addictive properties. They were fashionable drugs in his day, but today his two medical grandchildren have only theoretical knowledge of them. They have never prescribed them. Nowadays they are no longer used. Surely after many years of taking them, and knowing he needed such extraordinarily large doses, he might have worked it out for himself? But it is the nature of addiction, that one will not look it in the eye. And when he finally did, and gave up, he did not realise that the monster was still treading silently behind him, breathing down his neck.

He thought sleeping pills dealt with long boring flights to the States on his successful lecture tours. But they gave him deep vein thrombosis. His illness caused him to stop earning, his ingenious operation was performed less and less, he had to sell his lovely house, his debts were so large that he would never be able to pay them, and, aged only 50, loved, adored and worshipped by huge numbers of people, he was found dead in his armchair, holding a book called 'The Long Goodbye'.

On 20th March 1954, Richard Howard, his well-loved colleague wrote:

> I would like to pay tribute to my late chief, Mr H. A. Brittain, with whom I was closely associated as a registrar and later as a junior colleague. I owe my present position to him, and seldom has a young surgeon had a more stimulating and happy discipleship. Wherever he went he left his mark – here was a man who could not be ignored. Loved and almost worshipped by countless patients, he must have become used to adulation, and yet, strangely enough, humility was one of his virtues. But it was the right sort of humility – private not public. He was a gifted conversationalist and writer of the English language, with an incisive mind; and he loathed pedantry and plagiarism. Loving life with a youthful zest, he always made it exciting for others: dullness and boredom were alien to him. The orthopaedic department here in Norwich has lost its first and probably its greatest orthopaedic surgeon, but his memory will live on in the basic principles of orthopaedic surgery that he taught so thoroughly, and in the enthusiasm for the truth which he has bestowed on all those who came under his influence. (*British Medical Journal*)

In that same year his old friend Nobby Clarke (later Sir Henry Osmond Clarke) wrote an obituary assessing his contribution to orthopaedic surgery as being of the very highest quality and extremely influential:

> Only the best in life was good enough for Tommy. . . his sense of proportion and his very well developed sense of humour eventually overcame all his defects to show to all who had the patience to look at the real generosity and depth of his character.
>
> Everything he did he did well, and to the very utmost of his capacity, whether at work or play. He had been a hard-working rugger forward, a good golfer and squash player, an able swimmer and an accomplished

> dancer. Late in life he took up riding and pursued this pastime with tremendous zeal. . . he was hunting a few days before he died.
>
> At his lovely home at Witton in Norwich he entertained on a most hospitable scale. He was a wonderful host with a cultured knowledge of food and wine, witty, generous to a fault, well read and a raconteur of the very first order. (*Journal of Bone and Joint Surgery*)

Yes, I was lucky to have such an exceptional father. He loved life. He was such fun to be with. He was always exciting. He made it so for everyone who spent time with him. Everyone wanted to have some of him. Ebullient, witty, whacky, he was always saying. 'Now let's have some fun. Let's see what makes it go'.

And though no one knew it at the time, I was exceptionally lucky in that I had all the best of him, and the longest time with him. Of course, it should have been my mother who had that, and it is a tragedy that she did not.

What a huge excitement those first summer weekends at handsome old Hyntle Place must have been for my father. My mother was the oldest of the three little sisters looking for fun. They were lively, lovely and exciting, petite and neat, and their mother was an excellent hostess. They threw themselves into everything and soon my father did too. They were all laughing, exploring the garden, playing tennis, telling jokes, playing the piano and dancing, and passing the wine around. The girls teased the young men, told naughty stories and squealed with joy. The men were surely dazzled. These girls were astoundingly pretty. After supper they got out the dressing-up box and played charades. They reminded my father of his own younger sisters in Ireland, but seemed fuller of sparkle, far more amusing.

It was a hard choice, but the one he really thought quite striking was the oldest one, Dorothy, with the lovely smile and astounding singing voice. She seemed to like him, which was nice. He hoped he would be asked again. He was, more than once, and he fell in love.

When I finally met my mother, after my father was dead, one of the first things she told me was how exciting it was when he arrived one weekend with a new sports car, and took her for a drive. He stopped the car, and asked "Will

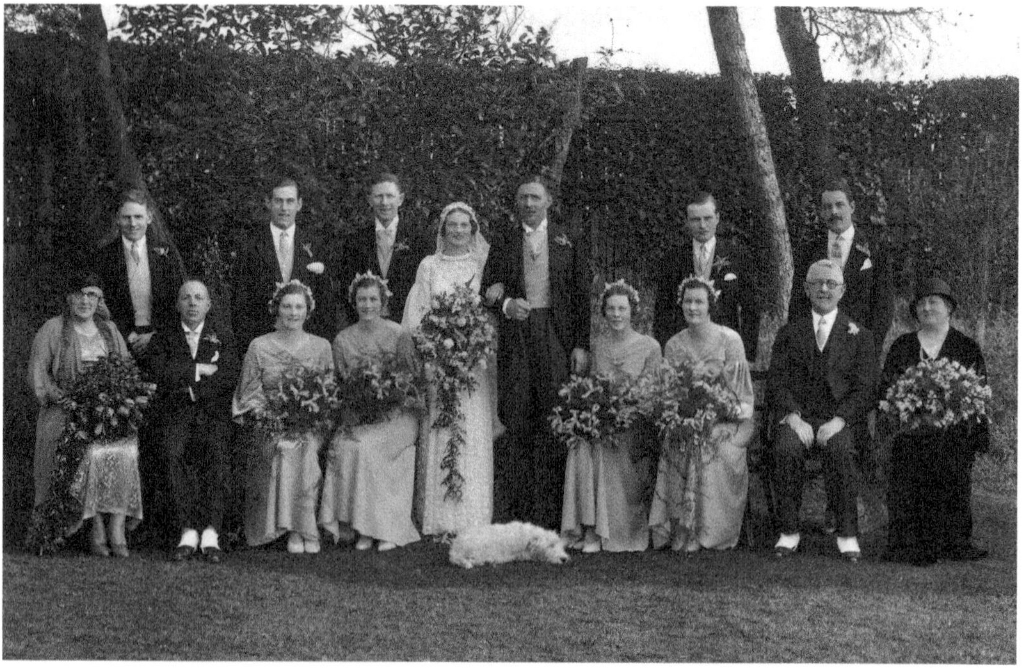

Wedding photograph of Dorothy and Tommy, January 1933. Within a year of this being taken, everyone in the picture has conspired never to tell Alison what happened to her mother. They were, top row (left-to-right) - Ian Payne-James (Alison's uncle, medical student), unknown, Eric Brittain (Alison's uncle, her father's brother), Dorothy Brittain (Alison's mother), Tommy Brittain (Alison's father), Hugh Maingay (doctor, close friend of Alison's father), unknown. Bottom row (left-to-right) - Elizabeth Brittain (Alison's grandmother), Jackie Brittain (dentist, 'The Little Bugger', Alison's grandfather), Betty Payne-James (Alison's aunt, her mother's sister), Ann Brittain (Alison's aunt, her father's sister), Alice Payne-James (Alison's aunt, her mother's sister), Phyllis Brittain (Alison's aunt, her father's sister), John Wesley Brittain (Alison's grandfather), Bella Payne-James (Alison's grandmother, wearing black velvet) and (at front, middle) Stephen the Sealyham. Dorothy and the dog are forgiven.

you marry me?" and she said "Yes". She described it 30 years after it happened, including the tea-coloured silk dress she was wearing, as if it was yesterday.

I was told by Alice and Betty in their 90s that, "Dorothy threw herself at Tommy". She never forgot him. She was writing to him in Italy with love in 1943 (from St Andrew's Hospital) during the war. She exclaimed with delight every time she saw her granddaughter Caroline that she was "Tommy to the life".

She should not have gone mad. There was no warning. She should not have failed to recover under treatment. She should not have spent 30 years locked in a mental hospital.

My mother had a psychiatric disorder suffered by only one or two mothers in a thousand. Today called postpartum psychosis, it is one of the least understood and most serious complications of childbirth. It is different from the commoner depression after birth felt by one in a hundred mothers, and it is not the schizophrenia for which it is sometimes mistaken and that it may resemble. But it does hold a very high chance that the mother will kill herself or her baby.

First described by Hippocrates in 400 BC, it may have no exactly known cause. Research mainly concentrates on the role of the immune response and the endocrine system, both believed to contribute to this mental illness. It does run in families, but who will get it is hard to know. Of sudden onset, triggered within a few days of birth, it is a medical emergency for which a mother needs to be kept in hospital. If she will not go in willingly for treatment, she may have to be sectioned, kept in and not allowed out. It has been said that the frightening problem for a practicing psychiatrist is deciding whether the mother is a danger to herself or her child, and to err on the side of extreme caution. With today's treatment swiftly put in place, there should be recovery.

About three-quarters of the patients with this disorder show delusions, for example believing they are being persecuted. My mother did have these, and she heard 'voices'. She also telephoned her sister Alice from her nursing home bewailing her distress that her husband was making love to the monthly nurse, Thompson, who was caring for their baby in the nursery in her new home. My father, when I asked him about this in my late teens, said no, they had been married only ten months and he loved her, and I think I knew him well enough to be sure I believed him. He said if what Alice said was true then that must be the first sign of Dorothy's psychosis coming on.

If a mother has this psychosis today, what happens?

The ideal treatment is to keep the mother safe, under 24-hour observation, with her baby if possible and with her partner at least able to visit her daily. Given the severity of the symptoms, pharmacological treatment is necessary. There was none available when my mother became ill. Nowadays a mother will be given mood stabilisers, tranquillisers and antipsychotic drugs, encouraged to talk with a psychiatrist trained in her treatment, and be helped to look after her baby herself as much as she can.

There are 17 mother-and-baby units that can take urgent referrals of this kind in the UK: more are needed and empty beds are rare. Under the best treatment today, the obvious signs and symptoms of the disorder gradually die down. Usually the mother will only stay in hospital for a few weeks before she is deemed to be no longer at risk of suicide or infanticide. She can then go home, behaving normally again. She will typically be followed up for two years, but recovery is usual after a year. Relapses are possible. A mother is considered to need watching and contact if she is having another baby, though many go on to have further children with no problem.

Since treatment today can control the behaviour and distress so that the psychiatrist can safely believe that the mother is no longer a danger to herself or her child, and it is safe to allow her home, it is mercifully no longer considered necessary that a mother with this disorder should be locked in a mental hospital for the rest of her life. Indeed a mental health nurse has recently told a mother with postpartum psychosis, "You have the best mental illness, because although the symptoms are the worst we see, you are likely to recover".

My mother should have remained a much loved and wanted wife, the mother of more children, and it is plain that she loved her husband to the end of her days. Through losing Pinkie, final divorce and unhappy remarriage he continued to pay till his dying day for his first wife's care.

If she had not gone mad I might have had brothers and sisters by the time the war came and I was five. I am pretty sure my father would have volunteered to serve his country because he thought he should. He was like that. When he was sent abroad I suppose my mother and we children would have moved to be near her family in Dedham, to live in lovely Constable country, in close supportive touch with her family, safely away from the Norwich suburbs where German bombs threatened, until the war ended. Never mind horses, ponies, dogs, cats and hens: I might have had them or I might not. Far more important: I would have had my mother. Instead, she spent nearly half of her life secured in mental hospitals.

Her madness destroyed my father. Had she stayed sane, he would not have needed to try sleeping pills. He would not have struggled to get her treatment. If he had, and that treatment failed, he would not have felt he must recklessly snatch her away from Moorcroft House without securing his legal position, and then pay for her to stay at St Andrew's Hospital for the rest of his life. Had she remained incurably insane in spite of every effort, he would have been able to divorce her in five years and thus had a chance of happiness with another wife. By the time that all went wrong he had made a huge success of his medical life, of his life with innumerable friends, of my upbringing, of his beautiful house and fast cars, of his horses and hunting, of everything that he could enhance and improve, but alas, little chance of making emotional sense of the rest of his life.

At the time they had married, he was tough and adventurous; she was beautiful, talented and determined. They seemed a couple very likely to make a success of a long and happy marriage. It was absolutely nobody's fault that she went mad, but it produced terrible wreckage.

If I force myself to think about it, I do know what the trouble was. My father was a betting man, an optimist. We all know that marriage is a gamble. You dare to bet it will all go well, you bet you can make each other happy. I do not think my father was blinded by love. He knew he was taking chances. He leaned over the rails in the paddock, drinking in the excitement, choosing the winner as wisely as he could from the most beautiful fillies in the ring. They were glossy, lithe and fit, they looked like potential winners. Reassured that they seemed to have respectable ancestry, that other people liked them and spoke well of them, and he could see no obvious disadvantages, he laid what seemed like sensible bets. There was no indication that his horses were not sound. No sign that my mother would go mad. No feeling that any of these fillies could not stay the course. No knowing that the divorce courts, and the war, would take longer than Pinkie could wait. Nothing to warn that his horses would not come in. There was no telling, during the thrill of his engagement to my stepmother and renewed hopes for happy marriage at last, that she suffered a crippling lack of self-confidence reflected in an uncontrollable temper. Like nearly all addicts he refused to believe he was addicted and he was in no suitable state to be married. Sadly, for both of them, neither was able to cope with the other.

When he placed the three most important bets of his life (on Dorothy, Pinkie and Sonia) he had no way of knowing he did not stand a chance.

Chapter 38
Bread and Milk

After my father's funeral my kind Aunt Ann and Uncle Douglas had me to stay in Cheltenham: Douglas was now headmaster of Dean Close School there. For days and days I walked miles round Cheltenham and the hills above it. I had to keep walking to keep my uncontrollable rage at bay. As I walked, I kept thinking about what had happened. Did he kill himself? If he did, could I have, should I have, stopped him?

So what then became of me? I was devastated by my father dying. I was crucified by his funeral, and I absolutely refused to go to his memorial service. "It will be full of his old girlfriends saying 'Your father was so *wonderful*!' What the hell do they know? I hate them all. No, I will not go." When letters came to me I opened them and if they were letters of condolence I tore them up without reading them. I got good at it after a bit and was able to guess what they were and tear them up without opening them. I got some satisfaction by carefully burning the torn-up bits in the fireplace. I found I could not stay calm, and veered without warning between rage and tears.

One letter was from Dorothy Neville-Rolfe, the headmistress of Ashridge, the finishing school I had now left. I tore it up, but then she telephoned, and I answered. She had come back from a sabbatical year, heard that my father had died and asked me to come and see her.

I had first met Dorothy-Neville Rolfe when no other school would have me, because I kept getting expelled, and I had found she was the only one who had trusted me. She had said to my father that she would like to talk to me alone. She had asked me then to think for three days whether I wanted to come to her House of Citizenship, and then to telephone her and say yes or no. Depending on my answer, she would tell my father if she would offer me a place there, or not. I said, "Daddy will be listening. He can hear every telephone in this house going, and will know I am ringing". She gave me the cash in coins and said, "Walk to the telephone box in the village when he is not around, and ring me up and tell me. Understand that I cannot have highly disruptive girls in my school. I would need you to try to keep time, and to try to learn with everyone else what we are trying to teach you. In return you will have as much freedom as I can possibly give you."

I had telephoned and said I wanted to come, and she had been as good as her word. Her school was wonderful. For the first time I loved a place of learning, was fascinated by what we were taught and enjoyed being there.

This time Dorothy said, "You got a double distinction, did you know that?" I replied no, it did not matter anyway, now that my father was dead.

"Yes," she said. "And did you know that he died leaving no money?" Of course I knew that. He always declared, "Enjoy it while it's here. I won't be when I'm gone."

"You will need to earn a living now", Dorothy told me. I could not imagine how I could do that and thought it would be easier, quieter and simpler to die. I could arrange that. I said nothing.

"If you could learn typing and shorthand you could get a job." I could not see how I was going to learn that. "You did well here", she said. "The staff and I like you." I thought yes, but it is all over now: you may as well shut up.

"If you are prepared to put in the effort, we are prepared to have you here one more term, free, during which you will learn shorthand and typing. You will do a year's work in one term. It will be tough. Will you do that?'

I looked up at her. She was smiling at me. She meant it. What a chance. I leapt at it. And suddenly I was crying.

We had all had to learn Citizenship, and then could choose, History of Art or Shorthand and Typing. I had no problem with that choice. I absolutely loved History of Art, and Susi Swoboda from the Courtauld Institute, who taught it. We had been to Italy for a fortnight in summer, and a whole new world opened up for me. What fool wanted to learn something so dull as shorthand and typing?

Er, me it seemed. That extra term was horrible. I had spent time in the Ashridge library learning to write like Michaelangelo. Beautiful straight downstrokes, lightly curved tops and bottoms of letters, and that nice line running through a double 'ee'. I was a perfectionist.

Shorthand is anything but. It is scribble, scribble, scribble. . . fast and infuriating. You must write it fast and, if you do, you write nonsense and cannot read it back. I was sadly aware how bad I was. Not any good. Useless. I hated myself but swallowed hard and got on with it. Not until shorthand outlines run through your brain at the same time as you hear spoken words or read anything will you get near the speed and accuracy you need. I am afraid that the shorthand short forms for '*administratrix*' and '*plant and machinery*' are engraved on my heart, and will be found there after I am dead. I dreamed shorthand outlines: they were my nightmares.

Typing was terrible. You had to plonk away to the tune of a well-known march on the gramophone. If you made a mistake you could try rubbing it out and typing it again, and the teacher would examine it with a magnifying glass and if she could see where the mistake had been (and she was very skilled at that) you had to type the whole page again. You could not leave the room until all mistakes had been properly corrected. You might have to type the same page five times and miss coffee or tea, but first and foremost you were going to get it perfect. You cleaned your huge heavy typewriter perfectly every morning. A perfect typeface. No bloggy ees with black insides. And all this and producing all the proper kinds of layout had to be learned before you tried getting up to any speed. Your third and little fingers, that had to be used in touch typing, ached painfully all the time, even in bed at night.

Ashridge standards were stupendously high. It produced the best secretaries in the world. If you were good enough you could get a job in the Foreign Office that eventually might lead to being the First Secretary (a diplomat, I mean, not a typist) in an interesting embassy in a fascinating place. I knew girls who had done that.

We had to learn to answer the telephone (in front of all the rest of us, who were encouraged to heckle) and produce off-the-cuff excuses for our (imaginary) boss who should have been heading an important meeting in 10 Downing Street but had gone to get his hair cut. "A secretary," we were told "is a wife in everything but the sex". If your boss decides to take you with him because you will be useful at a conference, you are to choose the hotel and book it, and make sure that you book the rooms on two different floors.

Oh for God's sake, horrible humble stuff, did I want to do that?

Dorothy called me in. This term she no longer wanted me climbing the roofs of Ashridge (quarter of a mile long, fascinating) at night. She had been shocked to see, out of her bedroom window, someone in a long white nightdress climbing about on the tiles by moonlight at one o'clock in the morning. She knew it was me, thought it was dangerous and wanted me to stop. I explained that there were ladders on most roofs, and it was quite easy. But she asked me not to. She had been good to me. She deserved that I do as I was told, and I stopped. It had been a relief to climb. Now life felt gritty. I just hated everyone and everything.

At the end of term I was only just good enough. Accuracy fine, telephone chatter fine, spelling bearable, Snob's Bible good enough (we had to know how to address Dorothy Sayers' Lord Peter Wimsey, his Harriet and their entire family on every occasion) but speeds at shorthand and typing terribly slow.

Ashridge kindly got me a job with the British Red Cross in Wilton Crescent, just off Hyde Park Corner. I went for an interview. They said "We are a charity so we pay very little. We expect our girls to have a private income, so we hope you have one." Well no, not me. But I did not dare tell them I did not. I was told I had a job in the Foreign Department and I should find somewhere to live.

I was no good at London. The hem of your petticoat was black with grime after only one day's wear. London was grey with dirt, busy, noisy and I had no idea how to get from one place in it to another. I was in the front seat on the top deck of a bus hoping to see where it was going when it went past the place where friends lived where I had meant to get off. Now I simply did not know what to do. I burst into tears. A woman got up from a seat on the other side and sat next to me.

"Hello" she said. "Can I help you?"

"No you can't," I replied. "Go away. Please go away."

I was utterly humiliated. The bus stopped and started several times, and she put her arm around me and said, "I can see you are crying, so tell me why." "I am looking for somewhere to live," I said, and hating myself I cried even more.

"You are a lucky young lady," she said. "Because I run the London Society for the Protection of Young Women and Girls. And I can help you to find a room."

And she did. She did. She found me a very cheap tiny room in the attic of a house in Earl's Court, talked to the landlady, helped me to book it, and showed me how to get by bus from it to Wilton Crescent. I bless her.

So there you are. I had a job and somewhere to live. I could earn my own living. Only I could not. I was paid six pounds a week. Three pounds and ten shillings went on my room and all but the last ten or fifteen shillings on the bus journeys. I got no money till the end of the first week. I ordered half a pint of milk delivered every morning and ate with it half a small loaf of white bread and the same again every evening. I did without lunch. We got free tea and coffee at work. I lived on free sugar lumps. Most of the time I was quite hungry. I had a group of friends from home who lived nearby in a flat. They worked in and around Sloane Square and went home to Norfolk at weekends, where their mothers loaded them up with fruit and vegetables from their walled gardens. Some of that they kindly gave to me and I was very grateful.

My job was to type letters for my boss, head of the Foreign Department. She was a woman: no men worked in Wilton Crescent. I had to type five copies of every letter. That meant using four pieces of carbon paper, and absolutely no mistakes. The top copy was signed by my boss and sent off. The next copy I punched two holes in and put it in the Foreign Department's files. Then numbers three and four had to be taken by me downstairs to the Library, for cross-referencing. The last very faint copy had to wait in a tray on my desk. Once a day a very well-bred girl, presumably with a private income, who had bad cerebral palsy, would climb the stairs, take the copy from my tray and carry it down to Lady Limerick. The oval stone staircase was beautiful, with lovely decorated iron bannisters. That silent girl used them to haul herself up with two fingers twined round them. Lady Limerick, the ultimate boss, sat at a most enormous desk in a room that took up the whole first floor of the elegant Georgian house. It had three huge sash windows and was full of light. She possessed a red ball point pen, a 'Biro', very rare in those days, I had never seen one. She studied the copy she had been given, and if it had not been typed to within one inch of all four margins (we had five sizes of writing paper to choose from) she marked the extra space and wrote on it, in red, 'Waste of paper in Foreign Department' and sent it with the struggling young lady, back up to me. I then threw it away. I wept that the Red Cross should treat that disabled girl in that way. She found that stair climbing so hard, and it was so completely unnecessary. I wanted to throttle Lady Limerick.

I was very hungry at first, until I got more used to it. If someone at work had a birthday they often had a cake and sometimes I was given a slice, which was lovely. The bus would pass shops with food in, and I remember longing for a lamb chop that I saw with a label saying 'three shillings and six pence'. I did not know that you paid for meat by the pound. That sign 3s 6d meant the price for a pound of chops. Actually I might have been able to buy just one. I thought, 'too expensive, no'. Cabbage was cheap, and I often ate quite a lot, raw. I saved any odd pennies and about once every three weeks I had 2s 6d. If I had the money and I saw in the window a very small cardboard box of potted shrimps for half a crown, I went in and bought them and bolted them. Eventually I bought a tiny aluminium saucepan with a rack for poaching an egg. I found I could afford eggs, and I ate two poached eggs a week with my bread. The trouble was you needed a shilling to put in the gas meter to make the gas ring work to cook an egg.

We had had a cook at home who would not allow me in her kitchen. The only thing I knew how to cook was an omelette to eat after hunting. But you needed butter for an omelette. I could not afford butter. I could buy a big potato and boil first one half on one side, turn it over and cook the other side. It was good with salt, and my landlady gave me some.

If there was a disaster somewhere in the world the British Red Cross would send 100 blankets to wherever it was. Nice women everywhere knitted woollen squares with wool they had left over from knitting some other garment. These were sewn into blankets, and good and warm and quite jolly they were. It was my job to order them, or the hard grey army blankets that we sometimes gave, from the warehouse and get them sent off. We arranged for someone to count them when they arrived. By far the largest amount of my correspondence was sent to one disaster area or another enquiring about missing blankets. How many exactly had not arrived? Where were they? Would somebody kindly find out and let us know. I was sorry to have to write again but I had had no reply to my first letter. I knew we had sent the right number, so what had happened to those missing one or two? It was important for the British Red Cross to know. I thought it was bloody not important. Whoever took them surely wanted them. They would keep them warm. Let us have pity on them. I thought we should bloody shut up. What a waste of time, and bloody effort, and indeed paper. Paper: note this Lady Limerick, haven't you bloody well got anything better to do?

One day my landlady came upstairs to see me, very flustered. There was a gentleman outside in a bowler hat who wanted to come upstairs and see me. I asked why. She said he wanted to give me a letter and would not give it to her. Bowler hats reminded me of hunting, but it was early August and hunting seemed unlikely. I said "Let him come up, and you come too please, to keep me safe." The landlady was shocked. She said "He comes from a solicitor," and I could see that she thought he was coming to arrest me for some crime and she did not want criminals in her house. They came up together. He wore the hat because he was, he said, a solicitor's agent, and he handed me an envelope. "What is it?" I asked. He replied, "You can look if you like. It's yours now." I opened it and it was a cheque for £400, the paid-up money from the insurance company where my father had taken out, and then needed to cash, the life insurance for £10,000 for me. That £400 would be nearly £3,000 today.

"Oh God, poor Daddy!" I let myself down and cried in front of them, and could hear my father's voice saying "Stop snivelling".

I took out a Post Office Savings Account and put £100 in it, in case I should ever need an abortion. I knew girls who had had an abortion and I knew the name of a doctor in Harley Street who would do one and in my time I gave that name to several friends. Girl friends said you must always keep aside £100 in case. No indeed, I did not want a baby. It might drive me mad. And even if not, how would I raise it? I could not afford to feed a baby, could I?

I sent the other £300 to Dorothy Neville-Rolfe, saying I hoped she could put it towards a scholarship so that another girl in my situation could learn to earn her living. I absolutely needed the self respect of not being in debt. I could hear my father saying, "I'm the last person to tell you this, but happiness is living within your income." In this way, I could sort of make it up to him. I could hold my head up high, and smile. Dorothy understood me, accepted the money, and we remained very good friends for the next 20 years until she died in 1976.

My Aunt Pat (my father's cousin, and one of his lovers (an Aunt in both senses) who had helped furnish Witton) found out where I was living and came to see me. She brought such a huge armful of gladioli that she could scarcely get into my small room. We had to ask my landlady to lend us a pisspot to put them in: they would not have fitted into anything smaller. She said she had come to take me out to dinner. We went to Claridges and she ordered a large rump steak and chips and salad.

In my head I said: "Oh Daddy, Daddy, you loved Pat, and Claridges, and rare rump steak. Why aren't you here now?"

My mouth watered crazily but I was so unused to eating meals that I could not get it all down, and we pretended we had a dog and ordered the extra to be put in 'a doggy bag' (rare in those days) for me to take back to my room for another day. She asked what was I doing in London in August. In August everyone should be in Scotland. She thought I should be too. She would be, tomorrow.

Then she said she knew I was terribly sad about my father dying. She was too. She had found a wonderful fortune teller, someone in touch with the other world, with where my father was now, and this wonderful woman was able to get through to him and give Aunt Pat news of him. She was extremely expensive, but Aunt Pat was so relieved after interviews with her, it was so good to hear from him. She, Aunt Pat, would love to pay for me to go and see her and hear all about him too. I said I did not believe in fortune tellers, what 'other world' was she on about, what could she possibly know? I would rather leave things as they were. But I could tell that it mattered enormously to Aunt Pat, that I should go. She had brought me a great armful of flowers, a dinner that would last me a week, and she knew this meeting would make me happy. What would it cost me to go and listen, to cheer Aunt Pat up, by hearing out some stupid lying woman pretending she knew my father now. Now that he was dead. Surely I could take that on the nose? Better say yes than no.

It was gruesome and hurt me far more than I had believed it might. The wonderful fortune teller wore many sparkly shawls. We sat at a table opposite one another. She produced a large glass ball that she said was a crystal that would let her get through. I was to keep quiet and breathe deeply while she reached the other side and found my father. Eyes tightly shut she snuffled and grunted, drew in deep breaths and announced that she was over there and calling out for him. "I want to speak to Tommy, to Tommy!" She knew that everybody loved him but I loved him most of all and he loved me most of all. She could not promise that he would speak to me. But she could give me a message from him and tell me what he was doing these days. Did I know that he had given up being a surgeon? He was now looking after mentally ill people. He was a psychologist. He was curing huge numbers of patients, dealing with them one by one, and they all loved him and had great respect for him. His love for me was extra special, and next time I came she believed that he would be able to say something to me.

I looked at her glass ball and with a tremendous effort stopped myself from picking it up and banging it down as hard as I could on the top of her head. I went out to join Aunt Pat who was crying. So I cried too. I thought the fortune teller had no idea how lucky she was, and how narrow was her escape. Thank heaven Aunt Pat went to Scotland straight away.

I got a cold. It turned into a cough. It would not stop. I could not shake it off. One of the friends in the nearby flat said why not go to a doctor? Under the National Health Service (so greatly hated by my father) a doctor was free. She found the name and telephone number of one who lived near us.

He listened to my chest and weighed me. He asked what I did for a living. I was not to go to work until I was better and he would write a letter telling the British Red Cross that. He said that I weighed under seven stone and was five foot eight inches tall and in his opinion I might have tuberculosis, be undernourished or both. He would send me for an X-ray. What was I paid? I told him I could not afford to pay him and he said I did not have to. I went back some days later for the X-ray result and was told I did not have tuberculosis.

Then he got tough. He said that I plainly could not afford to live in London. I should get another job that paid better: a lot better. What did I eat? That was ridiculous. I should be eating meat and fish and cheese, and vegetables and fruit. Very interesting that in the big city you could find people who were starving.

I was starving. I ought to go and get a job in the country, where money went further.

I found him terribly humiliating. I really did not like being told that, I felt sorry for myself and I left in floods of tears.

Of course I heard my father saying, "Self pity is the worst vice".

But the doctor who saw me was right, and he probably saved my life. I resigned from my job and kind Aunt Ann had me to stay in Cheltenham while I recovered. My old school friend, Carol Barnsley, got in touch with me and suggested we live together in Oxford, and I could get a job in the country. She was now working for a Diploma in Education after getting a good degree from Oxford in Chemistry, and we found somewhere to live together. A job advertised in the *Oxford Mail* said 'Girl, young, wanted for Reader's Department, apply Production Manager', and I applied. I said I had ten School Certificates and three diplomas from the House of Citizenship, I could do shorthand and typing and had worked for the British Red Cross. The Production Manager looked at my letter of application and Curriculum Vitae in amazement and I could tell it was all wrong. So I said "I can read," and that was obviously better. I told him, when he asked, that I was 21 and he said "Oh dear, we want a girl of about 16. Probably can't read." I told him I'd be better than her, and I wanted any job on the *Oxford Mail* so that I could work my way up and become a journalist. I was given a job taking Births, Deaths and Marriages on the front desk, and it paid much better than the British Red Cross. Carol and I had a lot of fun learning to cook together and eventually I did end up being a journalist.

Chapter 39
Saving Grace

Bless her kindness and thoughtfulness, Aunt Mabel invited me to stay in the West of Ireland with her family and friends for the summer holiday in a house on an island in the Kenmare River estuary. I did not want to go, but the Aunts left me no choice. It was a horrible journey, and I kept asking myself why I had not had the sense and courage to kill myself instead of being squashed in this hot smelly car beside my two sweaty male cousins, and driven all the long day from one side of Ireland to the other. Now I had no control of anything and I had had enough. I was being carried off to unknown territory with frightful Fitz. I would jump off a rock as soon as we got there.

Exhausted, wrung out, we arrived after dark and had to lug enormous amounts of equipment into rowing boats with water in the bottom of them. Oyster Bed Pier was dark and slippery, the boys rowed us over, then we had to drag our soggy luggage up rough uneven rocks to the house. We had a bowl of soup and went to bed. I will get up early and find a good rock, I thought.

My room was the size of a cupboard, up under the pitch of the roof of the lean-to house extension, with just a single bed and a chair and hardly any standing room. I fell into bed, and was amazed at the strong and lovely smell of the honeysuckle that climbed the wall outside my window.

The house was the only one on the little island, but although it was very small, and lit by gas and candles, a lot of people could stay there. The tiny rooms were furnished with fine mahogany bunk beds with inset brass handles to the drawers, made to the same design as those of the first class cabins of the Lusitania, a luxury liner that had been sunk by torpedoes off the nearby coast of Cork. There were going to be at least six cousins and six grown-ups there with us most of the time. I must find that jumping rock.

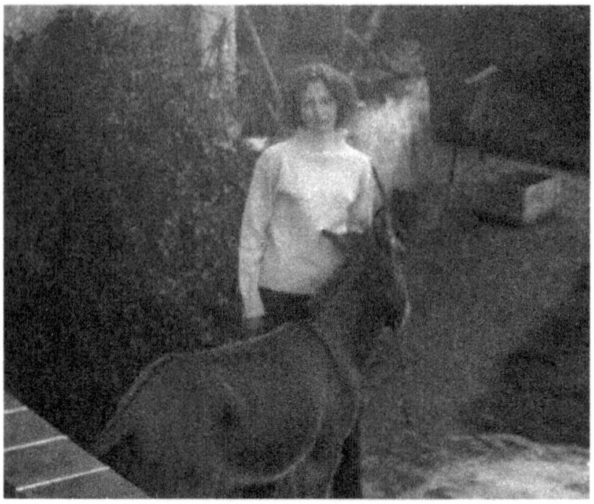

A lonely donkey left on the island to clear the furze (gorse) wants to be loved.

I got up very early, when no one else was about, and went outside to see the honeysuckle. A vision of the estuary was laid before me. Green wooded hills sloped down to the glassy sea, there was gorse (it is called furze in Ireland) and heather and little paths around the island, and I found a donkey, who was very pleased to see me, and have his neck rubbed and scratched. I would look for the rock later.

I was relieved to find that no one paid any attention to me. They were all having such a busy time arranging how to have their holiday, that no one badgered me. A real pleasure was finding that Uncle Fitz had mercifully grown out of me, or rather, I of him. No longer ten years old (I was 20 at the time), I was safe from his heavy good nights. I could do what I liked. I spent hours looking into rock pools. And hours watching gleaming gannets diving like arrows into the sea for fish. Sometimes I talked with Dinny, who milked the cow that he had swum over from the mainland with her calf for the summer.

Several times a day I stroked his donkey, who was lonely: no donkey likes to be on its own, and this one was plainly pleased to have me as his companion. I picked blackberries with everyone else. We messed about in rowing boats when the sun shone. We pulled up lobster pots and cooked the lobsters for dinner.

Fitz fished in mountain lakes in mainland Kerry for trout. The wife of the farmer who had let him do the fishing gave us all tea with homemade butter from her small black Kerry cows, and homemade soda bread cooked in a bastable on her open turf fire. We sat on a one foot high bench to eat it, with our feet on her earthen floor.

Uncle Eric tried to poach salmon at night in the Sneem River with a net stretched across its mouth. I was told that only men and boys could poach, and I could not go. One despairing day in the last week I had borrowed a boat, although Uncle Fitz told me not to because girls could not row. I just wanted something hard to do that needed concentration, to distract myself and stop brooding. I had rowed out to Inishkeragh, an island a long way out into the estuary, landed, wandered round it, and rowed home. Uncle Fitz was livid when I returned, and claimed there was a mad bull on the island, and I was lucky it had not killed me. I never saw it. Fitz probably made it up. But his son John said that I had rowed further than any of them had ever done. So I pointed that out to the poaching party, and they let me come. We put socks on the rowlocks to muffle our oars, and with every sweep of them watched the beautiful curved waves of phosphorescence given off by the disturbed plankton in the bright water. We drank three bottles of cherry brandy in the coastguard's house. One of the coastguard's jobs was to prevent poaching, but on this occasion, in Irish style, he was on our side. When we came out to pick up our prey in the early hours of the morning, the net glowed alive with phosphorescence. The salmon saw it as clearly as we did, and we were just as pleased at seeing the huge salmon leaping almost lazily over the golden net than if we had caught any. The cherry brandy warmed our way home.

Most nights we rowed over to the Great Southern Railway Hotel at Parknasilla (which had been built in anticipation of the arrival of a railway that never reached it). After several days a cousin insisted on dancing, and I danced with the others, till the small hours. Coming home, the moon lit the rocky path up from the shore, and above my head I had never seen such huge and brilliant stars. The scent of honeysuckle filled the house, and the sound of the waves rocked me to sleep. I gradually forgot my misery and began to like life again.

We all spent hours in Winnie's bar on the mainland in the little town of Sneem. While there we bought everything we were going to eat, and brandy and gin. Winnie told us about her brother, a priest in New York, who had sent her a postcard inviting her to come and see it, and hadn't she sent him one back writing, 'I've something here you'll never have there. I have time to live'.

I began to understand that there were things in the far west of Ireland found nowhere else in the world. There was its luminous beauty, the people were incomparably friendly and kind, there were no impossibly high standards that must be matched, all the natural things worked together. There was fish for gannets, furze for donkeys, gin for Mabel, brandy for Fitz, dancing for all of us, the bright stars in the night sky seemed to close around us. We all knew, and

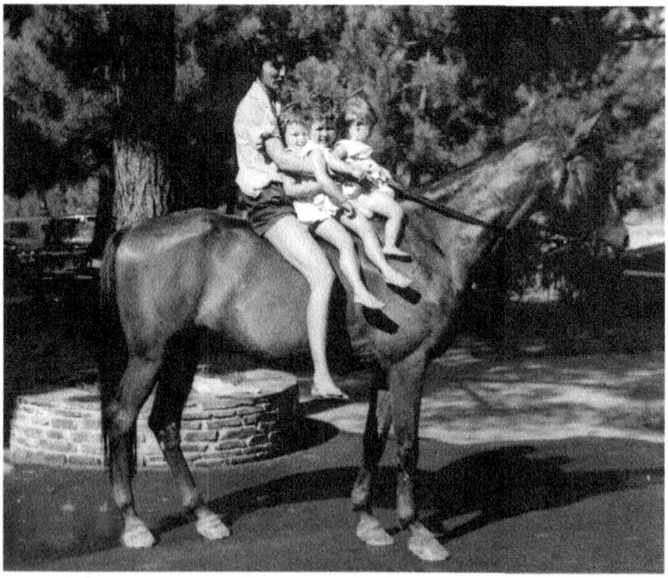

Alison grateful to be the happy mother of Susi, Caroline and Jessica.

there was no need to discuss it, that we were surrounded by generosity of spirit and affection. We all found, with wonderful relief, that we had time to live. I knew and accepted that I could be no help to my father now. I decided that if ever in my life I had the chance to live, with a donkey or two, in a little house in the West of Ireland, I would do so. And so, a dozen years later, I did: and it has soothed the souls of three generations of my family for over 50 years since.

If only my father or my mother had ever known such peace.

* * *

That first morning on the island in the Kenmare River estuary, I remember seeing seven magpies all together, a very obvious and cheerful family. They are fun to watch, they always seem up to some mischief. Seeing one single magpie is bad luck of course, unless you acknowledge its presence. You may flap your arms up and down, or say "Good afternoon, elegant bird". Better still, say "Good morning, Mr Magpie, how is your lady wife?". That shows you think there are two of them and it is not just one bird denoting sorrow. They mate for life, so seeing two for joy is very common, especially in spring.

In Ireland, they say you should salute a magpie, tell it the time and always treat it with respect, to avoid the sadness that it may otherwise bring you. There, they are generally called 'Francagh', a Frenchman, which implies that people thought they came from France, rather as the name Brittain implies that our family came from Brittany and were called Bretons. Young magpies, on hatching, often stay near the nest or hang around for the rest of the summer, still being fed by their parents. This may account for the fact that they are quite often seen in numbers. A clutch of six eggs is quite usual, so that seeing seven at once, two parents and five young, is not an impossible sight

Counting them, I wondered what secret they were guarding. That led me at once to think, one day they might make a good title for a book.

Acknowledgements

I discovered for myself the bare bones of why I had no mother, and seized the opportunity to read my father's private papers at the age of 13. I am hugely grateful to a lifetime of family and friends for helping me finish the job. The first person to be thanked is Pixie Marlowe (now Wathen) my 12-year-old school friend, who insisted that I should discover about my mother – "What did she die of? Where is she buried?" and who started my search.

I thank Anthony Harris, my first husband, who was absolutely sure, as I was not, that he wanted children. I am grateful to him for calming my fears, and for his support in helping me to meet my mother for the first time.

I am of course enormously thankful to my lovely daughters Susannah, Caroline and Jessica for all their help, over many years and in so many ways.

I knew nothing about book publishing, and am immensely grateful to knowledgeable friends who helped: in particular my publisher (and diligent researcher into my families' histories) Gavin Jamieson, and also to Richard Dawkins, David Kewley, Mark Le Fanu, Jan Maulden, Jason Payne-James and Marion Stevenson. And also to Jana Lenzova, whose beautiful cover design was a present to me in honour of my mother, whose silhouette is behind the seven magpies on the front.

Friends and the families of my youth told me stories I did not know that fitted together to make a picture of what had happened: David Barratt, Judy Don, Robin Don, Mary Anne Shippam, Lord Somerleyton (nephew of Nick Crossley), Mark Wathen.

Many thanks are due to David Goldberg, a psychiatrist friend since his medical student days, when I had my first child, and who later, now Sir David, explained my mother's illness and updated me on how different it was for her then and would be now. Two more psychiatrist friends did a great deal to show me where to find out facts, and to describe my mother's illness although they had never seen her: Simon and Susan Britten.

I am very grateful to my friend Christopher Bulstrode, an orthopaedic surgeon who drew my attention to an article celebrating the centenary of my father's birth, in *The Journal of Bone and Joint Surgery*. This led me to get to know the author of the piece, John Crawford Adams, another orthopaedic surgeon who proved extremely helpful in understanding my father and his contribution.

It was a great help to talk for the first time to someone other than my family who had direct experience of this illness: Ellie Ware of the charity Action on Postpartum Psychosis.

I must thank members of my family on my father's side who knew so much more than I: my aunt Ann Graham, and my cousins Judy Brittain, John Fitz-Simon, and particularly John Graham.

And also members of my mother's family who told me at last all their side of the story when I talked to them at length in my 70s: my aunts Betty Baynes, Alice Mason, Angela Payne-James; my cousins Sally Gotelee and her husband Michael and, this time wearing a family hat, Jason Payne-James.

I have spent 40 wonderfully happy years with my husband Stephen Cobb and my gratitude to him is utterly beyond measure. He has been a brilliant help with this book.

No book would have been written without the energy and help of all these people, and many more unmentioned, and I have limitless thanks for them all. Sadly, many of those named above are no longer alive to receive my thanks, but my gratitude is no less for that.

Action on Postpartum Psychosis

A donation from each sale of this book will be made by the author to Action on Postpartum Psychosis, a charitable network that helps women and families affected by postpartum psychosis feel understood, supported and less isolated.

Action on Postpartum Psychosis is the national charity for women and families affected by postpartum psychosis (PP). PP is a severe mental illness which begins suddenly following childbirth. It should always be considered a medical emergency. Symptoms include hallucinations and delusions, often with mania, depression, sleeplessness or confusion. Over 1,400 women experience PP each year in the UK but most women go on to make a full recovery with the right support.

Action on Postpartum Psychosis exists to raise awareness, campaign for improved services and provide information and support to women and families.

To find out more about what we do, visit www.app-network.org